~~Crystal~~,

May the gift of peace
and hope be yours forever.

Truly,

Karen Wells

BLESSED TRAGEDY

BLESSED TRAGEDY

Restoring New Life with Hope and Faith After a Head Injury

KAREN WELLS

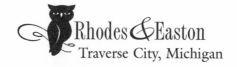
Rhodes & Easton
Traverse City, Michigan

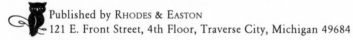Published by RHODES & EASTON
121 E. Front Street, 4th Floor, Traverse City, Michigan 49684

Publisher's Cataloging-in-Publication Data
Wells, Karen.
   Blessed tragedy: restoring new life with hope and faith after a head
   injury / Karen Wells. – Traverse City, Mich.:
   Rhodes & Easton, 1997
        p.   ill.   cm.
   Includes bibliographical references and index.
   ISBN 0-9649401-7-5
   1. Wells, Karen. 2. Christian biography—United States. 3. Head—wounds
   and injuries—Patients—Biography. I. Title.
BR1725.W45 A3   1997   97-67343
362.1' 9751 [B] dc—21   CIP

PROJECT COORDINATION BY JENKINS GROUP, INC.

00 99 98 ❖ 5 4 3 2 1

Printed in the United States of America

To my parents, Bill and Dorothy Wells,
for showering me with endless patience,
unconditional love, understanding, prayers,
and encouragement; and most of all,
for planting the seed of the knowledge of God's love.

Contents

PART FOUR — THE REFRESHING RAIN

PART FIVE — THE RAINBOW

Acknowledgments

THOSE WHO HAVE MADE it possible for me to share my story are those who have walked beside me on my journey of recovery. I have seen God's work of carrying me on this journey through their presence—both physical and spiritual.

I truly feel blessed to have had a highly-skilled and tenderhearted team of physicians caring for me. I have appreciated their personal touch, patience, comfort, and willingness to give me their valuable time. I thank James MacKenzie M.D., for being most instrumental in orchestrating my recovery, and for being my physician and friend; Diane Cornellier M.D., for guiding me through my seizure disorder; Julian Hoff M.D. of the University of Michigan; Michael Holliday M.D., for helping in the repair process; and Don Long M.D., for his unlimited perseverance and ability to finally put the pieces back together again.

Many health care professionals cared for me throughout my recovery, each in a unique and valuable way. For their sensitivity and genuine concern, while leading me through a major self-discovery process, I'd like to especially thank: Cindy Monroe, Speech Pathologist, for her constant encouragement, patience, and the ability to begin to open my eyes to reality; to Margo Million M.S.W.; Sherri Helman M.S.W., C.S.W.; Glen Johnson Ph.D.; and Vince Cornellier Ph.D. They taught me how to let go.

To the staff on Meyer 8 at Johns Hopkins Hospital, who became my Hopkins family during my extended stays, I say thank you. You shared more than your expertise in health care—you shared yourselves. A special thank you to Jennifer Accinelli R. N., who took the time to talk and share her faith, helping me to remain at peace while in the midst of the storm. I thank Mary Kay Conover-Walker R.N. and Susan Schnupp R.N. for all of the help they extended in a warm and genuine way.

I thank all of the patients and family members of patients I met, who bonded with me while in the midst of their own storms. My connection with each of them was very special, as we were drawn together by sharing the same determination to survive. Thanks to all, especially Beth, Barbara, Rose, Anna, Jim, Judy, Andy, Mel, Mary Jo, and Fran.

Members of churches from all over the country were praying for me and I give them thanks for being there in spirit. I was overwhelmed by the care, support, and prayers of Emanual Lutheran of Flint, Michigan; Messiah Lutheran of Alpharetta, Georgia; Prince of Peace Lutheran of Traverse City, Michigan; and Atonement Lutheran of Baltimore, Maryland. A special thanks to Ellen Commarato, Kathy Potter, Carla Melendy, and Susan Haar, who spent countless hours visiting and entertaining me while I was at Johns Hopkins Hospital. Thank you for reaching out to me as you did. Pastor Paul Koelpin also spent many hours talking and praying with me, sharing God's word and reminding me of God's hope, and I thank him.

I thank the contributors of this book, for their time, energy, and patience. Thank you Jerry Jenkins for encouraging me to bring it to completion, to Alex Moore for the coordination of this book, to Mary Jo Zazueta for her great work in editing, to Eric Norton for his creativity in cover design and bringing together my ideas, and to Barb Mosher for her feedback in the initial stages of editing. A special thanks to Emily Helman for using her talents to help me share the feeling of my thoughts visually.

I credit my basketball coaches for helping to build a foundation beneath me, beginning at a young age, while seeking to fulfill my athletic dreams. Thanks to Mary Prange, who was not only my teacher and coach, but a spiritual mentor. I thank Sharron Sheridan, for instilling desire and determination to succeed; and Karen Langeland, for helping me mature and prepare for the real world. I have the utmost admiration for these individuals and I can only pray that I have positively affected their lives half as much as they have affected mine.

I don't know where to begin to thank my friends, everyone who stood beside me, walked through the storm with me, held me, cried, talked, laughed, and sat quietly with me. God has surely been working through you—my angels—to guide me along my path of recovery. You have wrapped me in love and held me with patience, touching my life in a very special way.

I especially want to thank Karen and Kerry Ferguson, Joy Schmuckal, Carrie Mayes, Dosie Kermode, Paula Helminiak, and Ron and Gloria Hodgins. I'm so very thankful for my church family at Feast of Victory Lutheran, who graced me with countless prayers, cards, support, and love. My "Traverse City Family," my Small Group Ministry group, helped me grow spiritually, feel needed, and acquire the strength to persevere. A special thanks to Karen and Mark Klug, for being my angels in such a great time of need. Diane Palm (Fetter) and Paul Fetter, their combined friendship will compare to no other. Pastor Jim Helman has been another spiritual mentor and shepherd. He is the most gifted pastor I've known and has helped me walk through the storm and look to my Heavenly Father, with faith, hope, and trust.

Once strangers, sharing common prayers, fears, and challenges, the Kampens became a part of my family of close friends within a very short period of time. I am forever indebted to them for all they did for me. Ken and Carol welcomed me into their home, loved me, and took care of me as if I were their daughter. Kathleen, in the midst of struggling with an inoperable brain tumor, connected with me as a friend and as a sister, sharing her support, laughter, and positive outlook. I am confident all of the Kampens were placed in my life for a very special reason—my angels, my soul-mates.

To Aunt Jean and Uncle Howard, I extend a warm-hearted thank you, for all you have shared and done for me throughout my recovery, especially being with me at Hopkins. Your love and devotion is anchored deep within my heart.

So dear to my heart are my brother and sister. I thank Lamar and Kay for loving me, protecting me, and helping me to keep my focus on my Savior. Their endless praise, encouragement, and patience was so critical to my feelings of acceptance, at a time when my heart felt broken. They have walked with me along this journey, cried many tears, and shared many joys. Their tender hearts have filled me with peace and happiness; we are of one blood, one soul, one heart, united with God's love.

The seed for my restored life was planted many years ago when my parents first introduced me to my Savior. Had they not taught me about God's promise, had it not been for their continuous prayers and praise, I would probably be wilting somewhere along my road of recovery. Instead, I have blossomed through faith and hope of our Lord. Thank you Mom and Dad for not only giving me life, but for providing me with the understanding and knowledge to walk with God on my journey. Thank you for your unconditional love, patience, and devotion.

Thank you God, for a second chance. Thank you for new life. Thank you for your love and healing hands.

Introduction

I have promises to keep,
and miles to go before I sleep.

Robert Frost

IT WAS A SOUND I had never heard before, but one I will never forget: crashing bike frames interrupting the silent hum of cyclists spinning down a quiet, tree-lined road along the shoreline of West Grand Traverse Bay. It was July 9, 1989. I was a twenty-seven year old competitor in the Cherry Festival Bike Race in Traverse City, Michigan. We were only five miles into the race, on our way towards the tip of the peninsula; thirty-five miles of challenging terrain and beautiful scenery.

I heard the crash behind me as I stayed with the leaders of the main pack. The sound brought fear closer to reality, but I still couldn't look back and chance losing control of my bike. I could only picture in my mind a dozen bikes, within one second, made into carbon fiber and aluminum pretzels. It was not enough, however, to replace my relentless competitive drive. Despite fearing that my husband, friends, and teammates were involved in the crash, I did not hesitate to keep going. I had to keep going.

Athletes often carry a sense of immunity from career-ending injuries, believing we bear a muscular coat of armor which will protect us from all harm. On this day, the thought of injury to myself and others was far from my mind. I was concentrating more intensely on my strategy, my desire to achieve my goal, and my pursuit of success.

The athlete's game is generally played with a great deal of emphasis on the physical element of life. The body often feels like a machine, and the athlete's ultimate goal is to make it run as smoothly and efficiently as possible. We are willing to pay a very high price to do this. There is frequently an air of confidence among athletes and a great sense of pride. Our ultimate motivation is to win.

However, there is always a need for a balance of physical and mental preparation. Moments prior to the race I prepared myself mentally by reviewing the layout of the course, visualizing my increased needs for physical exertion at various points. This helped me pace myself, conserving energy for more difficult parts of the course. This is an essential ingredient to racing success. Knowing what lies ahead gives a racer a significant advantage.

I was very confident of my mental and physical training as I strategically maneuvered my bike within the pack. I knew what it took to be successful, the physical preparation, giving 110 percent effort, fighting through pain, focusing on a goal, and having fun. I was in top physical condition, coming off victories from seven of the nine events I had entered already that summer. I was confident this was going to be a good summer, and the beginning of reaching higher levels of competitive success.

Following my pre-race strategy, I maintained my position within the lead pack of male cyclists, ignoring the crash behind me. If I was able to maintain this position, I knew I could win the women's division of the race. There were no other females who could endure this speed.

This was an unusual race in that both males and females competed together. It was to my advantage. My training had primarily been with men, which helped me develop greater strength, making me stronger than most women, who were not able to stay with the men during training. With this thought I planned my race strategy.

If I stayed to the outside of the pack, towards the front, and stayed close to the wheel of one of the top ten riders, I'd be able to break free from the large pack. Most women would never know I was ahead. With my bike helmet on I had occasionally been mistaken as a male. In this race it, too, would give me the edge.

The pace would speed up, then it slowed down. Riders stretched apart from one another, then snapped back closer together, much like a giant rubber band. We flirted with imminent danger, while feeling invincible, riding shoulder to shoulder and within inches of one another's tires. This took great concentration, as we worked to steady our line while trying to keep the pace as consistent as possible. Each time a rider would speed up I dug deeper for strength to stay with them, knowing the only way I could maintain this speed was to stay within their draft.

When riding behind another cyclist, or in this case a large group of cyclists, a draft or vacuum of air is formed behind the lead riders. This allows other riders to ride just as fast, while using approximately 30-35 percent less energy than the leaders. This was what enabled me to stay with the stronger and faster pack.

This race was a local event, and thus there were many cyclists within the pack who were my friends and teammates. I knew from training with them that I was capable of staying with them throughout the race. I appreciated hearing the guys' encouragement, as they recognized I was keeping up with them. At one point, while riding beside Mike Ray, one of our club's top racers, he said to me, "Way to go, Karen." He acknowledged the strength and endurance it was taking for me to remain with the pack.

Along with the reassurance from my teammates, my own confidence prevailed. I knew I was strong and ready to withstand anything; or so I thought. Like any other race, I was nervous and a bit fearful of the unknown: my opponents. Athletes, however, try never to show emotion, especially fear, lest we may appear weak and give our competitors the edge. Thus my race preparation involved thinking and planning, not knowing I would need to be prepared in a very different way—emotionally and spiritually.

At this stage of my existence, this was also the manner in which I played the game of life. I rarely shed a tear or expressed fear, feeling a need to remain strong, as if these emotions were displays of weakness. I thanked God for blessings received, and prayed for help when feeling desperate, but I did not weave Christ into my life, as much as one should. I failed to give my fears to God and use Him as the source of my strength. I was too focused on my own attempts to control.

As our lead pack of twenty riders broke free from the main pack, we began working together to pick up the speed. Upon reaching the first hill, the majority of the pack took off, trying to drop the less-experienced and weaker riders who had managed to stay with the pack. I made it to the crest of the hill with the leaders and powered down the hill at forty-two miles per hour, staying with them as others fell behind.

With anticipation of a cash prize to the first cyclist who reached the top of Smokey Hollow hill, each cyclist was jockeying for a break away position. We were on relatively flat terrain and moving at a speed of twenty-eight to thirty miles per hour, a relatively fast speed for this level of competition... then... the next thing I remember, I was being lifted into an ambulance.

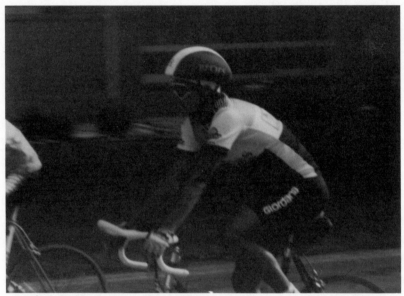

July 9, 1989...Traverse City, Michigan...twenty miles before the accident.

Time was snatched from me when a cyclist in front of me lost control of his bike, taking down several riders around him— including me. I was right behind him and had no time to respond. My body was catapulted head first over the handlebars. My head hit the pavement at a speed of thirty miles per hour. I remained lying unconscious as others who had fallen got up, gathered their bikes, and continued the race. Meanwhile, the leaders, riding in front of the crash, sustained their pace toward Smokey

Hollow hill, with the sound of crashing bike frames once again being engraved in their memories.

Those who saw me lying lifeless on the pavement, rushed to my side, while others called for help. Vojen Baic, the area's greatest supporter of young athletes, was following the lead pack of riders in his car. He saw it happen in front of him, as a slow motion replay might show cyclists falling like dominos.

Vojen later told me what happened after my last memory of the race, which was at the point of the first hill, several miles *before* my crash. He tells the details of the crash like this:

> I was right behind the group when a cyclist lost control of his bike. He was trying to drink from his water bottle, in anticipation of the big hill climb, I suppose. His front wheel became locked with the bike in front of his. When he tried to regain control, his front wheel turned ninety degrees, causing him to be thrown over his handlebars. He had time to react and put his arm out to break his fall, breaking his collarbone. Karen, you were right behind him and obviously never saw it coming. You went over your handlebars, too.
>
> But you had no time to put your hands out to protect yourself. Your head hit the pavement first, and then your body instantly went limp.
>
> It happened so suddenly, within one second.

My husband was in the pack behind me. As he rode past, he saw me lying on the ground. He quickly turned around, not knowing what had happened. Many other friends later told me they too came to help me, and how devastating it was to see me lifeless on the ground.

I have no memory of any of this. It feels more like a story than reality, even though I'm the main character. This increased the difficulty I experienced in my recovery, understanding and believing the reality of the crash and the incredible impact it would have on my life.

At the starting line of this bike race, the only sign over the road was the START/FINISH sign. There were no signs telling me that in less than one hour, while traveling at a speed of 30 miles per hour, my head would hit the pavement, leaving me unconscious by the side of the road. It did not tell me that within this time, my road to fulfilling my athletic dream would end; my entire life would change. Nor did it tell me this tragedy would be the greatest blessing in my life.

I was on my way to higher levels of competitive success. Little did I know, the higher levels of success were not going to stem from athletic endeavors. They would be higher levels of consciousness and spiritual well-being, with an overall greater value for life.

Never in my wildest nightmares did I ever believe it would happen to me. It had been such an ordinary day, surrounded by familiar sights, sounds, and feelings. Yet something happened that was totally out of my control and will remain with me the rest of my life. I will live with a closed head, traumatic brain injury, forever. Nonetheless, I can finally (and honestly) say, I would not want my life to be any other way.

When the gun went off at the start of the race, it was actually signaling the start of a new and very fulfilling life, one that would manifest more emotional and physical pain than I had ever experienced, while bringing a wealth of happiness and peace. A *Blessed Tragedy*, a consequence of one second of my life.

Part I

THE CALM

Sailing To Success?

*Never take life for granted, because just
as quick as lightning can strike, life can
change or be taken from you.*

KAREN WELLS

I LEARNED COMPETITIVENESS AT a very young age. It is a cultivated behavior that currently consumes our society. Competitiveness can lead to success—and often despair. It's something which can spark desire and motivate you to work hard and to learn, but when taken to an extreme, competitiveness can dominate your life.

With each passing year, competition became deeply intertwined in my life. I only knew its positive effects. It helped me strive for greater heights, motivated me to work harder than I thought possible, and built my self-esteem. It became instinctive, eventually ruling my life, encasing my true personality, often distancing my relationship with God.

The athletic arena is often an optimal competitive experience, where one can learn to rise above challenge. I know it well, it became my second home at the age of eight. This was the first time I can recall playing basketball in my driveway, dreaming of the day when I could play on a team like my brother, Lamar and sister, Kay. I fulfilled that dream, along with many others, in subsequent years.

I was a humble player and a quiet kid, never wanting special attention or recognition. I was just one member of the team, and teamwork was a critical factor in basketball. I was also motivated by the incredible feeling of God's love, despite being very young, an attribute learned from my parents. I desired to give back a portion of His countless blessings, by using them to the best of my ability.

I enjoyed the challenge of playing and working hard to improve. I loved to learn and see my progress, and I welcomed coaches who took a special interest in teaching me. I was fortunate to have two coaches in elementary and high school, Mary Prange and Sharron Sheridan, who not only taught me the game of basketball, but who were also interested in building a foundation for life beneath my quest for success; the quest which often stands in the way of athletes seeing what truly is important and valuable in life.

I began distance running when I was in the fifth grade, before running became popular. I ran around the block in my high-top canvas Converse basketball shoes, hoping it would help me increase my endurance for playing basketball. Running became a natural part of my life at a very young age, and greatly lessened my fatigue both on and off the court. I learned early in life that I could always go further and faster than expected. This attribute of running carried over into other aspects of my life as well.

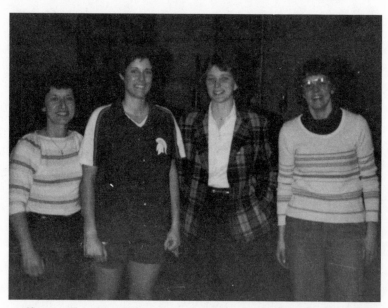

Sharron Sheridan, author, Karen Langeland, and Mary Prange. (1982)

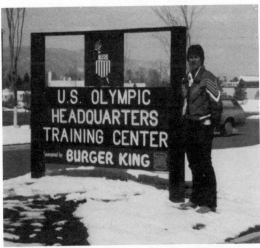

Women's Basketball Olympic Trials in Colorado Springs. (March 1980)

From high school I became a highly recruited basketball player. I chose Michigan State University (MSU), where I played four years on a full scholarship. My decision was based on my recognition that Karen Langeland, MSU's women's basketball coach, would continue to teach and guide me both on and off the court. I looked forward to the opportunity to play with higher caliber athletes who would challenge me. I knew that without challenges, without competition, I could not learn and improve.

MSU was precisely what I needed to satisfy my longing to be challenged, to learn, and to fulfill another dream. I valued the learning process more than the prestige of playing for a Division I school. Along with this level of play came more intense training. I was never afraid to feel physical or emotional pain. I knew fatigue was a sign of building strength, while the emotional pain of overcoming fatigue built character. It would have been easier to give up at times, but I promised myself, and God, never to give up, unless I had a good reason.

IN MARCH OF 1980, FOLLOWING MY first year at MSU, I was invited to the trials for the USA Olympic Women's Basketball Team at the USA Olympic Training Center in Colorado Springs. My invitation was a result of

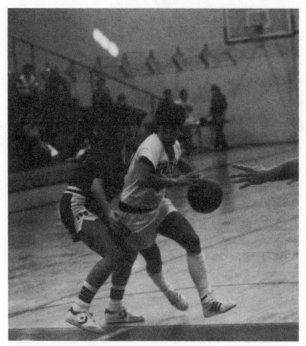

My 26-point performance. Michigan State University versus Illinois State. (1982)

reaching the top twenty-five list of players during the Junior Olympic Team trials the previous summer.

The thrill of receiving an invitation was breathtaking, for my ultimate dream in life was to play in the Olympics. However, upon receiving my invitation I was very pessimistic about my chances of succeeding. If it weren't for my parents, I would have turned down the invitation, due to a lack of confidence in my playing abilities. My parents refused to allow this opportunity to pass me by. Their encouragement and willingness to fly to Colorado with me to the USA Olympic Training Center was a treasure I shall cherish forever.

When faced with such a prestigious honor, I lost sight of my standard of success and why I was there. Suddenly making the team, the ultimate goal, became more important then participating. Competition was casting its dark shadow over my motto for success and the importance of my work ethic.

Fortunately my parents were there to guide me, saying words I will never forget, words which changed my entire attitude for the tryouts and for the rest of my life. They said, "Karen, you are here because someone noticed you are a great player. It doesn't matter how much time they give you to play, just do your best. That's all anyone can ever ask of you. This is your dream, so have fun and treasure every moment."

My success has always ridden on the value of participating and giving my best, yet in the midst of being an arms reach away from my highest goal, I kept losing sight of who I was. The fierce competition would have smothered me, had it not been for my parents. Excessive competitiveness was seeping into my life already and would only flow deeper and deeper within me before I recognized its effects.

Although frustrated with the limited time we were given to play before the coaches began making cuts, I tried my best to relax and have fun. By refocusing, I played well enough to make it into the final thirty players, before the next cut would select the Olympic team. Therefore, just as my father said, "You're the thirty-first best player in the country." I'm just as proud of this accomplishment as I am for not giving up.

THE FOLLOWING THREE years of playing for MSU were extremely memorable and rewarding. During the off-season I worked hard at my conditioning program. I added cycling to my routine, hoping to increase my endurance without adding to the risk of injury. Riding the thirty-six miles around Houghton Lake, where I spent most of my summers, once seemed like a long car ride. Yet I gradually built my endurance to the level of being able to ride my bike around Houghton Lake. I was learning how perceptions were relative to accomplishments, and accomplishments were relative to work output.

In the summer of 1980, I welcomed the opportunity to enter my first cycling race around Houghton Lake. Even though cycling was only a means of training for basketball, it was fun to accept the challenge. Cycling was a thrilling sport for me, but in all my years of riding a bicycle, both as a kid and adult, I had no knowledge of my need for wearing a helmet. I road without one, on the brink of serious injury, with only one mission in mind, physical growth.

I loved to put my body through conditioning programs, feeling the emptiness of a muscle's fatigue. It was fulfilling to experience muscles screaming for rest and then pushing them to go further, drawing on reserves, pushing the limits of their capacity. Seeing how far I could push my body physically was actually the easiest part of the challenge. The mind is always most resistant of pushing limits, but can be taught to survive pain, fatigue, emptiness of strength, and the burning desire to quit. Pushing harder took me to new frontiers, where I learned what my inner physical and mental capacity held. This is an authentic potential for life being demonstrated through athletics.

I use the game of basketball as my analogy to the game of life. My coaches are my parents and teachers, while my teammates are my siblings and friends. We play together, striving to achieve common goals. The score is not as important as how we play. How we play the game, our way of participating in life is what governs success.

I walked away from MSU and my basketball career with more than I ever dreamed possible, much of which I had yet to recognize as the major fabrication of my life. Despite not setting any records or winning the Big Ten Championship, my contribution to the team was immeasurable and hardly unnoticed. My work ethic, determination, and unwillingness to give up paved my road to fulfilling my success in basketball, and became the ground work to fulfilling much of my success in life.

I was awarded the Big Ten Conference Medal of Honor for athletic and scholastic achievements in my senior year. For me this award represented the reputation and respect I gained from my dedication and perseverance. Some might say my athletic abilities came naturally, but most who really saw the whole picture knew it was my work ethic that took me beyond mediocrity.

God had given me the potential, but in order to capitalize on it I really had to work hard.

Before graduating from MSU, with a Bachelor of Science degree, I was offered a Graduate Assistantship with the Women's Basketball program and Physical Education Department at the University of New Hampshire (UNH). This allowed me the opportunity to study for my Master of Science degree in Exercise Physiology, while at the same time keep a hand in basketball and competition.

It was very difficult for me to make such an abrupt transition—from being an athlete to being a coach. I craved competition. It became very stressful to be in a position where I didn't have control over how hard my players worked or how dedicated they were.

I chose to release my stress by running again. I still craved hard workouts. I then participated in a local running race, which sparked my interest in racing and individual competition. I had to put that on the back burner, however, because of an intense work load with coaching and studying.

My time at UNH was critical to my growth and to the decisions I made for my future. I enjoyed coaching, while also being very intrigued by my study of exercise physiology. My outlook on coaching might have been different had I worked with a more honest head coach. Instead, I imagined a career as a coach as being too political. I was scared of falling into a competitive trap, one which would control my life.

Not only did I become very intrigued with exercise physiology, but also with new insights to valuable aspects of life outside of basketball. I started looking at things more philosophically, trying to understand the way of the world, subconsciously searching for my relationship with God.

An example of this occurred one fall day as I was walking into the Field House at UNH. The sun was shining. The colored leaves on the trees were beautiful. I had no sooner stepped through the door, when a bolt of lightning pierced through the heavens, striking a tree nearby. Within one second the tree split into pieces. Leaves that once reached to the sky, now extended from broken branches on the ground. Their future had been instantly altered, yet for this moment their beauty prevailed, despite being severed from the trunk. Others, once hidden deep within the tree's web of branches, were now more visible, radiating even more brilliance. One lightning bolt, one second of time, one penetrating change of life.

For several days I couldn't stop thinking about the bolt of lightning and how quickly something can happen when one least expects it. And furthermore, how devastating one second, one bolt of lightning, can be. I was reminded of its impact each day when I walked past the tree on my way to the Field House. It was a reminder, "Never take life for granted, because just as quick as lightning can strike, it can change or be taken from you."

When I left UNH I wanted to carry this reminder with me for my life journey. So I cut a lightning bolt out of felt and hung it in my car. Several years later, my parents found a gold necklace with a lightning bolt on it. I wear it everyday as my reminder. It became my motto, a reminder of how life can change so quickly, yet remain beautiful.

F OUR MONTHS PRIOR to completing my master's degree I began my search for employment. I didn't have to look very hard, in fact a job fell into my hands as if it were destiny. It seemed as though everything throughout my life had fallen into place quite easily. Before one phase was completed, the next phase was already in place, without much planning or effort. Life just seemed easy. I frequently asked myself, "Why am I so fortunate? What did I do to deserve this?" Even though I knew the answer was nothing, absolutely nothing. God's blessings are richly bestowed upon us, without any merit or worthiness.

I was offered the position of Exercise Physiologist at Munson Medical Center, a major regional referral center in Traverse City, Michigan. I accepted. There was no question in my mind this was where I wanted to begin my career. I was excited at the prospect of a new challenge. All of my instinctual competitive drives were about to carry over to my new career.

In fact this was the arena where competition began controlling my life, taking on a negative overtone. Athletically it was healthy, within my career it became an affliction eventually carried over into my personal life. And where was God during all this? Walking beside me the entire way, as my eyes focused on other things, primarily how much "I" could do. I maintained only a distant relationship with Him.

I remained very goal-oriented, striving for excellence in all that I did. A healthy balance of physical, emotional, spiritual, and vocational wholeness had disappeared. I was feeling a very strong need for control, control of self and sometimes other situations. I began following my own set of blueprints, not God's, despite having recognized how God's plan was laid out so nicely.

A FTER MOVING TO Traverse City I began competing in more running races, with my sights set on someday competing in the Ironman Triathlon in Hawaii. When I found out my boss, Garry Demarest, had competed in this event, I was even more motivated. Garry encouraged me to participate in my first triathlon and to purchase my first cycling helmet. I really didn't see the critical need for a helmet, but it was required to race, so I began wearing one. It's like buying an insurance policy. One feels invincible, and thus the purchase seems worthless. Little did I know this helmet was the most valuable insurance I would ever own.

Moving to Traverse City opened a whole new dimension to my already competitive life-style. My desire to reach greater levels of athletic success, which seemed hopeless after the 1980 Olympic trials, was revived. I was back in training, having no idea of my full potential.

The first three years I competed were transition years, changing my body type from that of a basketball player to a long distance endurance athlete. By my fourth year of competing I had become very well known in racing networks as the top female cyclist and triathlete in northern Michigan. I ranked in the top three in running events. By the spring of 1989, my body was in the best condition of my life. I was even stronger and had more endurance than when I played basketball at Michigan State.

By this time, I had experience in a variety of events, including marathons, half marathons, 10K and 5 mile races, triathlons, cycling criterions, road races, and time trials. I enjoyed testing my abilities in these events and was thrilled with my success in all of them. This motivated me to keep increasing the intensity, quality, and quantity of my training. I pushed the limits, wondering how far I could go with these newly-discovered forms of competition.

My competitive success was still not driven by popularity but by an internal desire to achieve, to go faster, and to be stronger. Unlike a plant which grows both above and below ground, my competitive roots were growing deeper and deeper, while everything about me above ground remained the same.

As my physical training and subsequent athletic success established a major role in my life, I failed to recognize that some very important segments of my life lacked appropriate attention. I was working so hard at

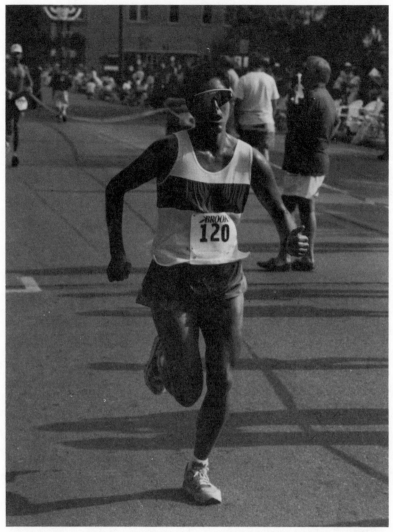

First Place finish in Traverse City, Michigan Triathlon. (June 1989)

building my physical and occupational self, I failed to work on my emotional and spiritual self.

I needed to spend more time nurturing my faith and getting in touch with my feelings, but success began to stand in the way of seeing such a need. Life seemed very comfortable. I had success without hardship, stress, or tragedy. Thus, I felt I was on the right path. There didn't seem to be a

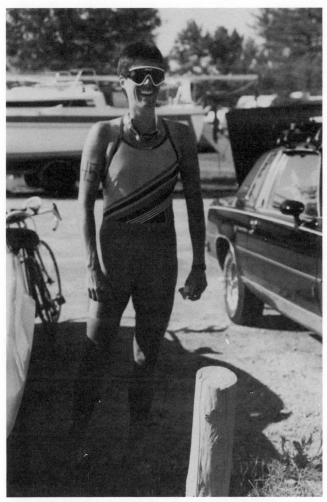

First Place finish in East Jordan, Michigan Triathlon.
(July 1989)

need for spiritual growth in my life, since everything was going so smoothly. Why try to fix something if it doesn't appear broken? After all, nothing would ever happen to me.

Part II

THE BOLT

Two

It Could Happen, It Did

*Faith is delighting in the fact that though I am
a vessel marred, unsightly, broken, I am
filled by God's own hand with Christ, His treasure.*
UNKNOWN

I FELT A JERK beneath me. I was lying flat, firmly secured to a board. I couldn't see what was happening—but I sensed something was wrong. Before attempting to move, I struggled to open my eyes. Feeling the absence of time, I thought to myself, "I must have fallen asleep, but why in the world am I tied down?" I was struck by fear.

The first thing I saw were lights on the ceiling. Seeing the life-support machinery and paramedics surrounding me helped me conclude it was the ceiling of an ambulance. I was very scared and confused. The report from the paramedics indicated that after I regained consciousness I kept asking, "What happened to me? Am I okay?" Damage to the short-term memory center in my brain, which no one knew at the time, was not allowing me to remember anything they were telling me. Thus, I kept repeating the same questions over and over again. It was obviously my biggest concern.

My memory loss of the crash is difficult to understand, but truly a blessing. I'd rather not have a haunting vision of this traumatic event. The story itself is enough. Even the fact that the paramedics were telling me

17

what happened, and I couldn't remember, was a protection from the emotional trauma that could have overwhelmed me. The brain does some pretty amazing things to help us cope with life's difficulties. In this case, it completely shut down in order to preserve life and cushion emotions.

I felt confused, spaced out, and had no idea why. Why were they not telling me what happened and what was wrong with me? I remembered being in a bike race, but could not tell anyone what day or month it was. It was as if I had been placed in a time capsule and sent somewhere out into the future. Memory loss can really play games with the mind. No matter how many times I asked what happened, I was not able to remember hearing the answers.

We frequently think or say, "It'll never happen to me," when considering the chances of an accident and/or a disabling injury. On the way to the hospital, on a back board and in a cervical collar, those thoughts haunted me. How could this be real? I felt out of control. I managed to wriggle my toes and fingers, to make sure I was not paralyzed. My biggest fear was a broken neck, paralysis, or a fractured skull, and just the thought and fear of this began to overwhelm me.

Had I known I was suffering from a traumatic brain injury my anxiety would have lessened. Of course I had no knowledge of what this label meant, nor the dramatic effect it was about to place on my life. No one knew the extent of my injury.

The pain began in the ambulance. My head felt like it had been crushed. I envisioned blood all over me. The pressure in my head was incredibly painful. One eye felt as though it were going to pop out, as if a knife were being stabbed through it. I continued to move my toes and fingers, self-evaluating the extent of my injury. As long as I could still move them, I figured I was okay.

The back of the ambulance seemed to be rotating and I couldn't focus my eyes. Yet, I didn't want to close them. I wanted to keep in touch with what was taking place around me. I thought this must be a nightmare, and if I could just focus on opening my eyes, maybe I'd wake up. It didn't seem to work. Darkness soon filled the ambulance and the words of the paramedics faded.

I cannot remember being wheeled into the emergency room, but I do remember lying on a stretcher in a room with curtains hanging from the ceiling. A stranger was standing next to me apologizing. He was wearing cycling shorts and holding his arm as if it hurt. I found out later he was the cyclist in front of me who caused the crash.

While I was in the emergency room, several friends who had followed the ambulance, began to comfort me. The worried look in their eyes was surely greater than my own, especially once I heard the x-ray and CT scan results:

Munson Medical Center
CT OF THE HEAD

FINDINGS: Normal sized ventricles, without evidence for hydrocephalus. No abnormal shift of midline structures. No acute intracranial hemorrhage or extracerebral fluid collections. No areas of pathologic radiolucency. No abnormal intracranial calcifications.

IMPRESSION: 1. Normal.

Since the results came back normal, I believed I was home free. The only thing I thought I'd have to deal with was my headache, but this seemed like a minor detail.

Before the accident I never experienced headaches. My empathy for individuals who frequently suffer from headaches began to significantly increase the longer mine persisted. I needed the nurses to turn the lights off because the brightness intensified my pain. To escape the piercing pain that penetrated my head with the tiniest movement, I remained as still as possible.

I became nauseated, a probable combination of the pain and fear. They admitted me once a room was prepared. I faded in and out, not remembering when they moved me from the emergency room to my hospital room. The only piece that sticks in my mind is when I asked the nurse to pull the shades on the windows. The sunlight pierced through my head like daggers.

I didn't get much sleep that night. The nurses had to wake me frequently, to check on me. One might think I'd worry all night about my future, but because I was in complete denial of my injury, I had very little to worry about. I was just anxious to resume my training and get back on my bike.

Through the night I kept trying to remember the race and the accident. It was all such a mystery to me, as if I had never raced that day and didn't have an injury. It seems more real when one can see the injury, a bruise, swelling, or blood. This injury took a long time to be seen, to be accepted, to be real. For the moment, it was just a story someone was telling me.

As I look back, I'm amazed how quickly my focus turned to how the accident affected my plans for next week's race. The thought never occurred to me that I should be worried about how it would disrupt the rest of my life. It certainly did not fit into my planned schedule for the summer or unbeknownst to me, for my life. The only plans it fit were God's, and at this point, I wasn't even capable of not liking it.

U PON AWAKING THE morning after my accident, my thoughts were immediately directed toward how soon I could get back on my bike. I knew I had to first convince my doctor I was well enough to be discharged from the hospital, even though I was not feeling very well. The headache I was enduring was like nothing I had felt before.

When the nurse walked in and started to open the curtains I quickly asked for them to remain shut. The pain was intense. Often times I found myself holding my left eye closed, putting pressure against it with my fingers. It felt as though it would pop out of my skull. I remained as still as possible, avoiding all unnecessary movement which might increase the pain.

I attempted to get out of bed, but was met with immense pain and dizziness. I couldn't stand without holding onto something, as if I were standing on a merry-go-round. I was determined to make it to the bathroom without assistance, an opportunity to rehearse what I needed to do when my doctor came to see me. Sweat covered my brow from the anxiety my condition was creating within me, yet I refused to let go of my determination.

I had been admitted to the hospital where I worked. Once word got out about what had happened and where I was, coworkers began coming to my room. It was early Monday morning. This was another test for me.

Could I converse with others without them knowing how I was feeling? I didn't want them to suspect I was in pain.

First Sue Peters, the Vice President of Human Resources, the division of the hospital I reported to, stopped in. She was the first to ask the most common question, "What happened?" I answered by telling the story that had been told to me. It still seemed like a story to me, as I was no where near being ready to take ownership of it. As I spoke, I found myself struggling for words, not realizing this was also a result of my head injury. I spoke very deliberately, again attempting to hide anything abnormal.

Ronna Hoffmann, my boss, also came to see me. I could tell by the type of questions she asked she had a very different concern than most of the others visiting me. She seemed very concerned with how I was doing emotionally, in addition to physically. I was touched by her way of showing she cared. The boss/employee relationship seemed to be set aside, and her concern was more out of friendship.

How was I doing emotionally? I was in the first stage of my grieving process, denial. I was already struggling with the reality of my injury. Having no memory of it and not being able to see it made it difficult to understand how it could be real. I began denying there was anything wrong as soon as I heard the first results of my CT scan. At the time, it seemed quite odd to me that others were expressing such deep concerns for me, when I truly believed there was nothing wrong. I wanted desperately to believe the negative CT scan was the answer to everything, denying there was a chance my injury might be severe, despite those results.

M Y DOCTOR, JAMES Mudgett M.D., entered my room just before noon. He was my family practitioner at the time, and also a very active individual and friend. We shared the competitive instinct and drive to push our bodies physically. He knew without asking that I was anxious to be discharged and return to my schedule. After a brief conversation, he asked me to stand up and walk to the door, wanting to check my equilibrium. I knew if I moved slow enough I could pass the test. I did.

He stated there was no reason for me to stay in the hospital, adding it was only a place which might cause me to get sick, given all the bugs floating around. He said I'd be better off recovering at home. He discharged me with orders to call him if I had any problems at home. He prescribed Motrin and Tylenol for my headache.

I was thrilled with his decision to send me home. I couldn't wait to not only return home but also to get back on my bike. I was confident I could resume my training and racing schedule, including a race planned for the coming weekend, and not miss a beat. After all, I believed there was nothing wrong with me.

I WAS DISCHARGED the day after my accident and immediately began planning my strategy for returning to competitive action. I thought it was just a matter of getting my balance back, finding a way to get rid of my headache, and then I'd be back to normal. I never had headaches before, not to mention one that felt like a knife stabbing through my head.

After coming home from the hospital, I immediately tried to get back into my normal life. I went to the basement to do laundry and noticed my helmet next to my dirty cycling jersey and shorts, the ones I had worn in the race. It was the first time I had seen my helmet since the accident. It was shattered. "This could have been my head. This is real. It is not just a story," I thought. My hands quivering, I picked up my helmet, drew it close to my chest, sank to the floor, and cried. I knew something was wrong with me, something was wrong with my head, and I was scared to death to admit it.

I found myself bumping into walls and needing to lay still, otherwise I would become extremely nauseated. I could not walk through a doorway without colliding with the door jamb. I had several collisions with floor lamps, end tables, and anything that stood close to the daily traffic pattern in my house. Even lying still was difficult. It felt as though I needed to hang onto the bed, so as not to fall off. As soon as I closed my eyes, everything would spin.

After returning home, I had several conversations with family and friends on the phone. I became very frustrated with my inability to speak as I used to. There was a noticeable delay in my word finding, causing my speech to be extremely slow. I couldn't put words together to make a sentence. My speech was broken. It was getting harder and harder to hide my injury. The need to hide stemmed from not wanting to be "broken," resisting change, and my competitive desire to keep training. I tried desperately to remain active, not wanting to stop training. I wanted to forget this ever happened to me.

I tried to go for a run, making it less than the length of a city block before I fell to the ground, vomiting as the earth spun around me. I managed to get home, and while it seemed like the longest run of my life, I had traveled only a short distance.

This was only the beginning of what always seemed like the longest journey of my life, recovery. I thought I was traveling down a road that would lead me to my old self again, but this journey was actually pointing in a different direction. I needed to travel a long way before I would realize I'd never return to the self I knew before the accident.

I had lost many pieces of my old self, but had yet to recognize I was left with something even better. Buried beneath many frivolous pieces of my life was the most valuable part of myself, me. I had been living under a suffocating blanket of trivial needs...competition, training, playing, working, riding, and running faster. This was through no fault but my own. One of our greatest threats to our personal well-being is our own arrogant pride. We are not victims of society or Satan. We have the ability to make choices. We are victims of ourselves.

My injury rescued me from this needless cover. Some might think an injury of this nature would cause one to change and lose their identity. I, on the other hand, found mine. Underneath the insignificant aspects of my old life was an individual longing for deeper emotional connections with others, one who found pleasure in touching the hearts of others. Yet all this was concealed by needless aspects of life I had thought were important.

Through my injury, I came to discover more joy in crossing, not finish lines, but barrier lines separating individuals from one another. Thankfully, throughout the period of my life when I was focused on competition, I did not abandon those who were important in my life, my family and friends. I must say, however, I was far from relating in the most desirable way.

At this stage of my recovery, I did not know what direction to turn. I still wanted to believe nothing in my life had changed, while at the same time I pleaded to God, "Help!" I prayed for the strength to accept anything that He was allowing to happen. I kept reminding myself He was not going to give me any more than I could handle. I could handle change as long as I had directions. I knew I wanted to continue participating in my game of life. I could never be content being a spectator.

As symptoms of my head injury persisted, I became a bit more nervous about my condition. This prompted a call to my physician, Dr. Mudgett. He encouraged me to come into his office, so he could evaluate me. After looking in my ears, nose and throat he said, "All is okay. I don't see any bleeding. Don't sit around and get depressed. Go back to work." While this surprised me, it was exactly what I wanted to hear. I welcomed the chance to return to work and attempted to do so the next day.

My first day back I found it very difficult to accomplish anything. It seemed as though I was five steps behind in everything I tried to do. I could not process words from a conversation. No one seemed to be speaking my language. Words seemed foreign to me.

When I tried to talk to people my speech was very slow. I had to concentrate on every word I said. Often times I could not find the next word, thus creating a huge void in my speech. I knew there was a word for what I was trying to say, but could not for the life of me think of it. Sometimes I'd say a word which made no sense at all, something totally out of context. It was as if there was a short circuit in my brain.

Nothing felt natural. I could feel the strain on my brain as I worked hard to be *normal*. I was still afraid others would notice something was wrong. As I walked down the hallway I had to keep one hand on the wall, to steady myself. When I stopped to talk with someone, I held onto the wall, to prevent my body from swaying.

In the latter part of the morning, I had a meeting with my boss, which was extremely difficult to pull off. I felt a need to be *normal* and to prove there was nothing wrong. I spoke very deliberately, so she wouldn't notice that I was stumbling for words. She breezed through her agenda with me. I comprehended one to two percent at the most. I was not about to acknowledge this to her. She never questioned my behavior. She did, however, question my quick return to work. I reassured her my doctor had recommended it.

I struggled through the day, confused, frustrated, and exhausted. Everything I did seemed to take three times the amount of energy. Near the end of the day, one of my other supervisors found me in my office, I had blacked out. I had been trying to read some reports at my desk. I remember straining to keep the words in focus, but then all of a sudden Marianne was talking to me. I could not understand what she was saying at first. All of her words were muffled and blending together. I just nodded and said, "I'm okay," hoping she'd go away. Finally, what she was saying began to make some sense. She began encouraging me to seek an opinion from a different doctor, or talk to Annelle Kasper, one of the nurses I knew who worked for a neurosurgeon.

I took her advice and called Annelle, nurse practitioner for Dr. Zimmerman. She advised me to come into their office the next morning so she could check me over.

I was nervous about seeing Annelle, fearing she'd clearly recognize the problems I was experiencing. I was also too scared not to do anything about the uncertainties of my injury. Annelle had already heard some of the details of my injury from others at the hospital, intending to see me before I was discharged.

I tried to explain to her everything that had happened to me over the past week, but had a very difficult time communicating everything to her. It seemed as though my speech was getting worse. I stuttered and felt slow, but kept remembering how I was told by Dr. Mudgett that everything was okay. Thus, I figured it was just my imagination that I was not doing well.

Annelle relayed her evaluation to Dr. Zimmerman, who then ordered repeat CT scans and Magnetic Resonance Imaging (MRI) of my brain. Like x-rays, these tests allowed him to see my injury. Annelle explained to me that head injuries often times do not show internal bleeding on the initial scan, thus Dr. Zimmerman ordered the CT scan to be repeated. She said most bleeds show up 48 hours later. The MRI was ordered because it gave him a better three dimensional picture of my brain.

The MRI was a new experience. I had heard of some people having difficulty with this test due to claustrophobia. The tube which your body is moved into for the test is extremely tight fitting. I was not sure how I was going to respond, but remained calm and confident. I had no problem once I realized it helped to keep your eyes closed and visualize being somewhere else.

Within a few days I had to return to Dr. Zimmerman's office to discuss the results of my tests.

Munson Medical Center
CT OF THE HEAD:
IMPRESSION: No evidence of intracranial trauma. Persistent mucosal thickening in the sphenoid sinus.

Munson Medical Center
MRI OF THE HEAD WITHOUT CONTRAST:
FINDINGS: The brain is normal in appearance with no subdural hematoma, mass effect, or abnormal signal demonstrated. However, there is fluid within the maxillary sinuses bilaterally with near complete opacification of the left maxillary sinus. The sphenoid sinuses are also involved.
IMPRESSION: Normal brain. Bilateral maxillary and sphenoid sinusitis.

On the day of my appointment I bent over to put on my shoes. Suddenly, clear liquid came pouring out of my nose and onto the floor. My husband, who was standing there waiting for me, said, "Wow, what is that?" I didn't have an answer for him, although my first instinct was that it was spinal fluid. The liquid was clear, like water, and ran from my nose like a faucet. I quickly discounted it, still denying there was anything wrong.

Dr. Zimmerman spoke with me at great length about my head injury and reported that the MRI showed fluid in my left maxillary sinus. He suggested this was due to a sinus infection, and I should return to my general practitioner to be treated. I told him about the fluid that flowed out of my nose when I bent over. He indicated this was logically the same fluid and could be cleared up with antibiotics. He suggested I begin with Sudafed 60mg. four times a day and aspirin for my headache.

He discussed the types of head injury that require professional assistance and rehabilitation. Still not believing my injury was severe enough to require rehab, I just listened and said I'd follow his recommendations.

He referred me to Munson's NeuroRecovery Program for cognitive testing. This measured whether there was any damage and deficits to my brain. He also recommended a minimum of two weeks off work. I was a bit confused by this, due to the opposing recommendation of Dr. Mudgett. He had sent me back to work, while Dr. Zimmerman wanted more tests and told me not to work.

I became even more alarmed when I returned to Dr. Mudgett and he refused to give me the necessary HMO referral to a neurosurgeon. Dr. Zimmerman had agreed to see me initially before all the paperwork had been processed, but needed to receive a referral for further treatment.

My faith in Dr. Mudgett was diminishing at an increasing rate. It now seemed as though this injury might be more severe than he believed. Even I could figure out I should not have been sent back to work.

Within a few days, I selected and had my first appointment with a new primary care physician, an Internist, Dr. Joseph Stafford. He reviewed my medical records and talked with Dr. Zimmerman prior to my first appointment, which made me feel cared for. During my initial appointment, I was very comfortable with him, as he listened sensitively to my entire story, including why I was changing physicians. Being aware of the fluid in my sinuses, he started to treat me with antibiotics to clear it up.

Three

Hang On, It's A Medical Roller Coaster

The key to everything is patience.
You get the chicken by hatching the egg...
not by smashing it.

ARNOLD GLASOW

AT THE SAME TIME Dr. Stafford was treating me with antibiotics for the sinus fluid, I was also following Dr. Zimmerman's referral for cognitive testing at NeuroRecovery. While I really wanted to go back to work, I was becoming more worried there might be something wrong. Deep down I think I knew there was, but I was still afraid to admit it. I continued to follow the advice of my current physicians, realizing I was not a specialist in this type of rehabilitation.

It took two days to go through the cognitive assessment with Cindy Monroe, the Speech Pathologist. In the afternoon following the first morning of testing I saw Annelle and said to her, "Since I know I passed the first part of the test with flying colors, can't I return to work?" Little did I know, she had already received some of the results from Cindy.

She was very quick to inform me, "Karen, you have not done well. You flunked. You won't be going back to work, not even in two weeks."

This was a tough one to swallow. My perception was that I had completed it perfectly. This ignited more fear of continuing the testing process. I really did not know what this meant. I had a hunch there was more to my head injury than I was aware of. What else might be wrong with me that I was totally oblivious to?

She proceeded to write a list of Do's and Don'ts for me, recognizing that what she told me verbally was not registering. I needed everything written down in order to be able to recall it.

Once the assessment was completed, I was informed I had some deficits of short-term memory, concentration, abstract reasoning, and reaction time with decision making, among others. This was very hard to reason out. I had an injury I could not see, nor did I remember how I got it. Now they were telling me I had deficits, including problems with abstract reasoning. How can I ever expect to abstract reason through this one?

I tried to make sense of it by reading and learning more about head injuries, and what kinds of things survivors go through. This seemed to help a little, but it still did not make my injury seem real to me. It seemed so much like a nightmare. I was expecting to wake up and realize it was just a dream. This never happened.

As time went on, I sometimes felt like ending the nightmare myself. I didn't want to accept not being whole. I did not want to grieve the loss of parts of me I would never recover. I did not want to admit to anyone, especially myself, that I had lost some skills my brain once performed very easily, skills it no longer had the capacity to do.

The writings of Bernie Siegal, a physician and author of three books, helped me tremendously. I first read *Love, Medicine and Miracles.* Even though it was written for cancer patients, it helped enrich my positive attitude. If these people could survive, I could too. It helped to read about someone who, in my opinion, was struggling with more than I was. It helped me remember, there is always someone worse off than yourself if you look around, and you don't have to look very far.

The book also gave me some very effective tools to enhance my perspective. I began to realize that life is built around perceptions. If I perceived this injury to be disabling, it would be. But if I perceived it to enhance my life, it would. How we react to stress appears to be more important than the stress itself. I strongly believe how I reacted to my head injury has been the link to my survival. Most importantly, it has linked me closer to God.

Had I thought of this injury as a form of punishment from God, or being victimized, or even blaming myself for my inability to avoid the accident, I would still be struggling today. I would be wading through the streams of self-pity, anger, or guilt. On the other hand, since I have chosen to react in a positive way, I am able to see the beauty of my injury. It took me a long time to sort out my feelings about it, but beneath all the broken pieces lies a very beautiful portrait of feelings.

I played the song by Wilson Philips, "Hold On," over and over again. The lyrics repeat "Hold on for one more day," and "I know there's pain." The song helped encourage me to take one day at a time. Holding on for one day at a time was about all I could handle. Anything more than that would have overwhelmed me.

I felt so often like I was pretending. Pretending I knew what was going on. I pretended I heard what was said and that I understood. I slowed my speech down so it would come out correctly. It felt like my brain was only running on two of its six cylinders. Each time I would listen to a conversation and suddenly recognize I was lost, anxiety would sky rocket inside me. I did not know what to do. With some people, I became comfortable asking them to repeat things or to slow down. With others, I let it pass, hoping I could wing it.

I often times felt as though others were making more out of my head injury than what was really there. The words, brain injury, alone were very frightening. I sometimes felt I was making more out of it than I should have. On days when I did not have the strength to get out of bed, the effects of my injury seemed ridiculous. How could I possibly not have enough strength, determination, or desire to get myself out of bed? But it was true. This was extremely discouraging, coming from one who had been so active and eager to jump out of bed early every morning.

I received written results of my cognitive assessment from Cindy, also sent to my physicians. Upon reading them I was floored. How could this possibly be true? It says I'm operating at a sixth grade level when I have a Master's degree. My auditory short-term memory was at the 9th percentile, while my visual recall was at the 98th percentile. Abstract reasoning and vocabulary skills were at the 25th percentile, and this was just the tip of the iceberg.

Seeing the results on paper moved me closer to realizing this was real. It also scared the daylights out of me, wondering how I would ever be able to keep my position at the hospital. What would I do?

My boss, Ronna Hoffmann, had showed interest in helping me through my recovery, and seemed to genuinely care about my well-being. I recognized at this point that I would not be able to hide my deficits from her, and thought it was probably best if I was up front with her and told her the results of my assessment. My intuition told me to share it. I knew deep down she could help me. I knew she had the ability to help me overcome obstacles by the support she had already displayed in the organization as my Director. She is a very intelligent woman, who I thought might think of ways I could modify methods of performing my job, without jeopardizing my performance. There was also an overwhelming fear of her ability to fire me from my job because of my brain damage. But the fear of trying to conceal them was greater.

It was a major step for me to give my results to Ronna. I didn't have the ability to tell her in person. She did not need an explanation. I simply walked into her office and told her how I was tested and asked if she was interested in reading the results. She seemed quite shocked I was offering her this information, but she took it and said she would read through it as soon as time permitted.

Within a few days, after having read the results, she called me and asked if I would like to talk about them. I agreed and said I would appreciate any help she could offer. We met and talked about ways in which my work environment could be altered to assist me in my productivity. She recognized there was a need for her to alter her method of communication with me and made several suggestions.

She began slowing her speech and offering to repeat or rephrase anything she would say. She wrote everything down for me that was important to remember, as well as waited long enough for me to take notes on our discussions.

My intuition had been right. She did not place any blame or shame on me at all. It really helped being honest and open with Ronna. She was very willing to help me. This began to open my mind a bit and motivated me to work harder at freeing my inner thoughts and emotions. It was part of paving the road to recovery.

Ronna also encouraged me to work hard in cognitive rehabilitation. She showed interest in what I was doing and how I was feeling about it. I had reservations about whether I really needed rehab, even after seeing the results. I still was in denial. Having Cindy Monroe as my therapist helped. She was very sensitive to my feelings and knew I thought I didn't need to be there.

I met with Cindy three days each week to work on very specific tasks, ones that were found deficient. Each session drained my energy more than I ever thought possible. I never realized how much energy the brain required. Now that mine was using 3-4 times the normal amount, it was very apparent to me. I left every rehab session completely exhausted, as if I had just run a marathon.

The more work I did with Cindy, the more I realized the extent of my cognitive damage. When she gave me directions on how to do something, my initial thoughts were always, "This will be easy." Then when I attempted to perform the task, I couldn't do it.

I was never quite sure whether I was improving or not. Cindy always praised me for my efforts. My confidence in being able to perform the "easy things" reversed itself as I became more and more aware of my shortcomings. By nature, I'm a very hard worker, and despite being skeptical of my abilities, I worked very hard to see improvement and regain my confidence.

One of the skills I worked on in therapy was reaction time with decision making. Cindy was very perceptive when I told her of my recent incidents with the police. Within two weeks of my accident I was stopped twice by the police for driving through yellow/red lights. As a result, Cindy tested my reaction time. She found I was above average in reaction time, as long as my brain did not have to go through the thinking process. When I had to use my decision making pathway, I was three times slower than I should have been.

I also was stopped one night for suspected drunk driving. I was not drunk, nor had I had anything to drink. It was dark and the headlights of vehicles driving towards me were blinding, intensifying my headache. I was driving extremely slow and hovering towards the side of the road to avoid the lights. I did not explain to the police officer my dilemma. I simply passed the breathalyzer test, walked as straight of a line as I could, and went on my way. I think he was quite surprised I passed the tests. I was humiliated.

When driving at night I frequently had to stop by the side of the road to vomit, because my headache would be so painful. I tried wearing sunglasses while driving after dark, but I realized this was not safe. Eventually, I began to avoid driving at night.

I COULDN'T REMEMBER anything people said to me, unless I wrote it down. I was very thankful I had been an organized person prior to my injury, because this made it easier for Cindy to train me to take good notes of everything I heard. Everything anyone said to me had to be translated into pictures in my brain, since my visual skills remained intact. I quickly realized how much people depend on memory for everyday living, and how much extra energy it requires to change the pathways in the brain.

Talking on the telephone was very difficult, because it was not a visual form of communication. I could only hear the words, and unless I associated pictures to them, it was impossible to remember anything. When someone gave me a number to remember, even writing it down was difficult. I was slow to hear, process, and record. I would record the numbers in reverse order, like a dyslexic, even though I was certain I had recorded them accurately. In fact, I would have bet money on my accuracy. But when I repeated the numbers to verify what I had written, they would be in reverse order. Sometimes it was very embarrassing, especially when I needed to write a phone number down. If I got it wrong and the individual had an unlisted number, I could not contact them.

Now, I repeat numbers several times. It took me a long time before I felt comfortable asking people to slow down. I would just try to get it right, although most times I was not so lucky. This can easily be detected each time I get my phone bill. When I look at the long distance phone numbers I have called, there are always a few unfamiliar numbers, ones I have transposed.

During this time, I came to know a man quite well. He happened to have a phone number that was the reverse of my parents. Eventually it became amusing, but I felt bad for wasting his time.

I would completely forget conversations ,and spent twice as much energy trying to figure things out, because I was too embarrassed to ask for things to be repeated. Sometimes I felt so confused I simply wanted to escape the situation completely. It was difficult to focus. I did not have the energy to concentrate.

There are simple situations where memory is vital. One day I forgot I had put my right contact lens in and began putting the left one into the right eye on top of the one which was already in place. The discomfort I immediately felt helped me figure out what I had done. On another occasion, I cleaned my contact case very thoroughly, before remembering I had not taken my contacts out of the case to put them in my eyes. One was salvaged, laying by the sink. The other had been washed away.

One out of every two days, when putting my contacts in, my first motion was to reach for my eye and attempt to pop the lens out. The message from my brain to my hands did not quite connect. Since both movements were so natural to me, my hands moved freely before my brain had a chance to catch up.

Anytime there are multiple sensory inputs to my brain, I cannot process even one of them. I lose everything. This never seems fair. It was so easy before. I could talk on the phone and have the radio on. I could be in a room of several conversations, and still be able to carry on a conversation with the individual in front of me. Now, it is as if everyone's voice is amplified. Although I can hear the noise of their voices, I cannot comprehend a word they are saying.

The speed at which I can process information is noticeably delayed. When I am too embarrassed to ask for something to be repeated, I will just nod and hope it is appropriate. Often times it is not.

I will often look at a word while reading, one that is very common in everyday language, and it will look as foreign as though it were Russian. When I am writing I will try to think of a word's spelling, and I do not have the foggiest idea how it is spelled. This makes it even impossible to use my Mr. Webster to help find it.

My frustrations with cognitive skills continue to haunt me. In conversations I will reverse syllables of words, not realizing what I said. For example, I was speaking to a friend about an individual who appeared to be unhappy, and said "He appears to be happyun right now with his life." It amazes me how the brain works and how something so simple can get completely reversed. I had no idea what I had said until I saw a smile come over my friend's face. Then I had to ask if I really said what I thought I had said. This happens frequently, and I often catch myself saying something backwards and trying desperately to cover it up.

Spelling is very troublesome for me at times. Even the simplest of words are not familiar. I took a trip to Milwaukee the summer after my accident to visit my mentor and dear friend, Mary Prange. She also happens to have been my fifth grade teacher and coach. She still teaches fifth grade. I was helping her in her classroom one day, preparing for the start of the school year. The new textbooks were lying on the desks, so I picked one up, for old times sake. I was stunned when I recognized I could spell only one out of every ten words on a page. I was embarrassed to admit this to my friend and former teacher.

Things like this stir up a great deal of anxiety within me. It is hard to swallow a regression of intelligence. Each time I recognize these deficits, I need to remind myself this is not just a coincidence. This brain injury is real.

Before I realized and accepted what was causing these deficits, I was extremely frustrated. Physically my body was fine. I could still run, ride, and swim long distances very comfortably, but I could not get my brain to do tasks requiring concentration. Cognitive therapy helped me with these areas. If it were solely for the value of recognition and acceptance of these deficits, therapy was invaluable. But it wasn't. It was also to help me learn how to overcome these deficits and learn to do things differently, using an undamaged part of my brain.

For each deficiency I've described, Cindy had a method of retraining my brain. She read paragraphs and essays to me and I had to work to concentrate, recognize, and repeat information back to her. She pointed out that I would not process all the information appropriately and she'd make suggestions on how I might improve. We worked in a quiet environment initially and then she added distraction, significantly increasing the difficulty for me.

I worked on a computer, trying to learn to identify words and the correct spelling of words. Word finding was my most difficult challenge to overcome, along with sequencing. These deficits continue to haunt me, despite being unnoticeable to others.

I had homework each night, which I diligently performed, striving to improve my performance. One of my assignments was to play video games, such as Pacman, which would help my reaction time with decision making. I knew how much it could help and thus turned what used to be my physical training time into brain training time. I had to focus all my energy on my game of life, as opposed to recreational games and races.

Eleven years prior to this, in my senior year of high school, I was asked to give our graduation speech for our honors ceremony. I don't believe it is a coincidence I chose to speak on how life is so much like a game. I spoke of how our parents and teachers are our coaches and our friends are our teammates. I used analogies to the game of basketball describing what we were about to encounter as we ventured into the real world. Fourteen years later, during my recovery, an article was written about me and the title was, "Wells in the Game of Her Life." There is a master plan out there in God's hands. I just know there is.

Cindy counseled me on what to anticipate as a survivor of a brain injury. She said statistics show most survivors quit or lose their jobs within three months of their brain injuries. I thought, "This will never happen to me. I'll blaze a new trail for survivors." This seemed more like a challenge than a threat.

Within two months, during my working hours at Munson, I walked out of my office to my car, saying to myself, "I cannot do it anymore, I quit." I looked over to the right of my car, and my boss's car was parked nearby. Ronna had been a big inspiration to me and was so willing to help me in all aspects of my work and recovery. I was overcome by the feeling of letting her down. It felt as though I were betraying her by giving up.

My life has always been primarily motivated by inspirational people and God. I have followed the example of others and the word of our Lord, indebted to them for the time, energy, and grace they have given me. Life seems so much easier if we work together as a team, but we have to be team players. This life is not a single's sport. Therefore, I had to set aside my self-pity and remind myself I wasn't playing alone. There were plenty of others eager to assist me, and even more who had far greater problems than I.

After about twenty minutes of tears I walked back to my office and returned to work. I could not give up. I had never been a quitter, and my game was not over yet.

Headaches and dizziness continued to bother me. The pain was very sharp and centered around my eyes. It felt as though my eyeballs were going to pop out from extreme pressure behind them. At these periods of intensity, I felt dizzy and nauseated. I had to hold my head, try to relax, and let the intensity subside. The higher periods of intensity lasted thirty seconds to a minute, but then left me feeling very wiped out. Most of my pain and discomfort came from the left side of my head. I experienced similar pain in my left ear, but not as often as my eye.

One day, while in therapy with Cindy, I bent over to pick up papers on the floor and fluid came flowing out of my nose. I became very dizzy and felt as if I were going to pass out. Cindy asked me to sit down for a few minutes. When the pain didn't diminish, she called the emergency room. She requested a wheelchair and someone to take me to emergency.

More CT scans were run, but the results came back normal. I did not bother mentioning the fluid that had come from my nose. It seemed trivial compared to how my head was feeling. I had noticed when I bent over that the pressure in my head increased, but at this point I was not thinking clearly enough to suggest there was a connection.

It seemed as though this saga was never going to end. While Cindy was able to clearly pinpoint the location and degree of damage to my brain, what seemed like the more definitive type of test, the CT scan, always came back normal. It never made sense to me that these evaluations could be at two different ends of the spectrum.

But even though I struggled with the understanding of what happened to me and the acceptance of reality, I still managed never to ask the question, "Why me?" The question "Why not me?" precluded me from asking this question.

I came into this world with nothing. Everything I have acquired since then has been a gift. I have deserved nothing, yet God loves me anyway. Why wouldn't I expect bad things to happen to me and every other person on this earth? People often think they are deserving of good things. I felt very grateful for God's grace and mercy, and his willingness to help me through this tragedy. My foundation of faith prevailed, through the good and the bad, but now my injury was opening the door for me to build on this foundation. Something I should have done long before this time, but nonetheless each day slowly shaped my life, just as flowing water shapes a stone.

I refused to accept the notion this injury had the power to ruin my life. I didn't care what the statistics were, I wasn't going to be one of them.

Cindy had told me that most marriages, where one spouse survives a brain injury, end in divorce, even at a much higher percentage than the normal fifty percent. Never for a moment did I see myself being threatened by these issues. God was beaming light on my path, guiding me, and protecting me, not allowing this injury to destroy my life. Nor was I going to allow this to happen.

I never lost sight of the promises God has given us, "Trust in the Lord with all your heart, and lean not on your own understanding; in all your ways acknowledge Him, and He will make your paths straight." (Proverbs 3:5-6 NIV) But I did try to lean on my own understanding numerous times. I believe it is humanly impossible to completely relinquish the desire to have control, especially for those of us who have lived within the competitive arena. It's an instinctual survival technique, reinforced by one's previous competitive success. I have tried to take matters into my own hands numerous times. However, I always return to praying, "Not my will, but Thy will be done." I certainly was ready and willing to compromise, but God wanted to do everything His way.

God's methods and plans are not always in line with what I want, but who am I to say what should happen with this life He has given me? "And we know that in all things God works for the good of those who love Him, who have been called according to His purpose." (Romans 8:28 NIV) My faith tells me, God has a plan for me. I have a purpose, my injury has a purpose, and so does God.

Dag Hammarskjold quotes, "Life only demands from you the strength that you possess. Only one feat is possible-not to have run away." While I have often felt as though running away might be the easier path to take, I know deep down this is not how I operate, nor how God would want me to respond. It's at these moments, when one must walk closer to fear, a flash of turning the other direction crosses one's mind.

I always felt that God would not give me any more than I could handle. Eventually, I turned this around and added, He will not give me any more than *He and I* can handle. There are reasons for everything, even though we may never know exactly what His plans are, or have the answers to "Why me?" and "How much more?" God does not send us direct answers to our suffering, instead He takes it upon Himself. Just like He did at the age of thirty-three, when He suffered and died for our sins. As I sit here, writing a part of this book at the age of thirty-three, I think of the suffering I have had to endure throughout this year. Age thirty-three, it was a tough year for Jesus and a tough one for me. But my suffering is not even a tiny fraction of the weight of the world our Savior endured. In fact, boy do I have it easy because of His tough year. Thank-you Lord! Thus, I need to keep praying as if everything depends on God, and work as if everything depends on me.

Four

Rehabilitation—Why Me?

*Then the time came when the risk
it took to remain tight in a bud
was more painful than the risk
it took to blossom.*

ANAIS NIN

I WAS THE FIRST one to deny that I was in denial. This was the first stage of my grieving process. I had no memory of the accident and thus it was hard to believe it was real. I kept attempting to do all the things I had done prior to my accident, thinking I was okay. My standard reply to those who asked how I was doing was to say, "I'm fine." I actually wondered why I was getting so much attention from a little bike crash. I convinced myself nothing was wrong, even though I knew I was struggling.

All I needed to do was listen to myself speak and common sense would have told me something was wrong. When I talked with someone, it would take what seemed like forever for me to find the next word I wanted to say. I had to pause in-between each word, trying to think of the next word. Thus, I found myself not wanting to talk, because of the difficulty and embarrassment. I preferred to isolate myself, not wanting to admit there was something seriously wrong with the speech compartment in my brain. I did not want to take ownership of the damage that had occurred in my brain. Yet, each time I would speak or struggle to perform something simple (which was no longer simple), reality sank a little deeper.

Cindy is an exceptional individual and therapist. She became my confidant in recovery. When she was assigned to my case, she definitely had her work cut out for her. I thought there was nothing wrong with me, and thus thought it was ridiculous to be involved in a therapy program. Cindy never once failed to recognize where I was coming from or how I was feeling. She did not always agree with what I did, nor did I agree with what she was trying to do, but at this point we could agree to disagree.

While in rehab, the advice of two dear friends helped tremendously. The first came from my basketball coach at Michigan State University, Karen Langeland, whom I deeply admire and respect. She once said to me, "K-Dub, always remember, there are two ways to do everything," meaning do not believe yours is the only way. This road of life we travel can take us in many directions. Even though there are often road signs to point our way, there are also roads which are harder to travel than others. There are occasional barricades to detour us, but there are ways to maneuver around them. The second piece of advice came from one of my assistant coaches and close friend Nancy Dreffs. Nancy told me to always remember, "The harder you fall, the higher you bounce." Things get messed up now and then, but it will all work out for the best.

I remembered both of these quotes each time I'd feel myself doubting Cindy's help or when I felt down in the trenches. Cindy also helped motivate and inspire me to continue with my therapy. She is one of the most kindhearted people I've met, having a heart of gold. I could immediately sense, even through my stubbornness, she truly cared about my recovery. This was not just a job for her and I was not just a patient. I was an important person to her. I felt valued, despite her evaluation of my deficits. She never made me feel inferior because of my injury. In fact, she made me feel good about the things I could still do very well. The focus was on what I could do, rather than what I could not do. I liked this, being the positive person that I am.

For me to understand the importance of her guidance and orders, Cindy had to be very firm with me. There were times when it felt like I was back in sixth grade, being told by the teacher that I had not followed all the rules. Things needed to be spelled out very clearly to me in order for it to register in my memory. We learned the most effective forms of communication. In order to remember things I needed them written down, and if I was the one writing, she had to talk slowly, repeat, and rephrase things. For me to communicate, the most important thing was for me to lay down my fears. If I worried about what and how I was going to say something, I would never be able to get my point across.

It was easy for Cindy to sense my frustration when I tried to perform what used to be simple tasks. She seemed to always find very challenging assignments, constantly monitoring my progress and level of performance. She was most interested in assisting me with my return to work efforts. She came to my office one day and observed me while I was working, so she could make suggestions as to how I might work more efficiently. She also asked me if I would agree to invite my two supervisors to one of my therapy sessions, so they could watch me and see what things I was struggling with. I agreed. Both Ronna and Marianne Foster came to one of my sessions. I will never forget that session. Again I was scared to death this would jeopardize my employment. It did not.

They watched me work on the computer. One task was to work on my reaction time. After the session Ronna commented, "I was shocked at how long it took you to push the button once the box appeared on the screen. I thought to myself, 'When is she going to push it?'"

Ronna's observation was another confirmation that my deficits were real. The more it was verified, the closer I moved to accepting reality.

During this session with my supervisors, we also demonstrated how my attention and listening abilities were negatively affected by distracting noise of any kind. The difference in my ability to perform in a silent room versus a room filled with noise was dramatic. While I am not sure how Marianne felt, I know Ronna was very glad she was allowed to attend the session. The more information she had regarding my deficits, the more she believed she could help me. This proved to be very beneficial.

D R. STAFFORD WAS very supportive of my cognitive rehabilitation and kept close contact with Cindy and I to chart my progress. During the first three months after my accident a lot was taking place in my life, although it felt as though life was standing still. Amidst numerous trips to the doctor I went with my husband, Jerry, and parents to New England for a trip we had planned all summer. My friend Nancy Dreffs was getting married and I didn't want to miss it, despite feeling terrible. I don't have much memory of this trip since it was within the first month after my injury. I do remember how hard I had to work to hide the pain of my headache. I wanted to make sure no one knew anything was wrong with me, including my family. I knew my parents would be devastated if they knew the degree of my injury.

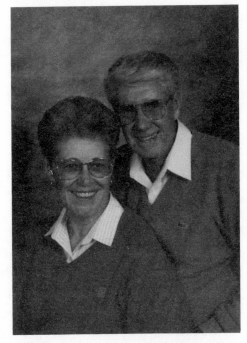

My parents, Dorothy and Bill Wells.

If I could not come to accept it, how could they? I desperately wanted to spare them the pain, never thinking they could be a great source of strength.

Meanwhile I continued to take Darvocet, the pain killer Dr. Stafford had prescribed. It didn't seem to help much, but I figured if I didn't take it I'd feel much worse. Dr. Stafford also continued working very hard to dry up the fluid in my sinuses, which was thought to be the cause of my severe headache. We tried Ceclor, Bactrim, Keflex, and other antibiotics, with no success. Finally, he decided to refer me to an ear, nose and throat specialist, an otynlaryngologist.

He gave me the name of Dr. Harry Borovik, who he described as a fine doctor who might be able to give us some insight on treating my problem.

I was fortunate to be able to see Dr. Borovik within a week, and arrived at his office feeling as though I was being shuffled around by doctors. My case seemed to have taken on a more challenging perspective the longer my pain persisted.

My first examination by Dr. Borovik was quite memorable. I'll never forget the eight-inch steel rod he pulled from his instrument case, as he prepared to look into my nose. My neck had never stretched so far in my life, as it did when he inserted the steel rod up a nostril to take a peek. I was certain he had the entire instrument up my nose and into my head. Tears flowed down my cheeks from the discomfort. It was obvious he wanted to go even further than he was able from the way he kept moving it around and pushing further. He finally gave up, convinced there was an obstruction in the left sinus cavity, and unsure of what it was and why. He ordered another CT scan, which included a view of my sinuses.

I returned to his office the day after being scanned, to get the results and to talk to Dr. Borovik about what was next. Results showed I had a broken left turbinate and fluid buildup in my left maxillary sinus. He indicated the only way to repair this damage was with surgery. Suddenly I pictured myself with scars on my face. He then described the method of surgery and the approach he would take through my mouth and nose. The only incision would be under my lip, above my teeth. I consented to the surgery and it was scheduled for the following week.

I asked Dr. Borovik if he thought this had any connection to my accident. His response was indecisive. I felt there was a direct connection, since I never had sinus problems prior to my accident. It seemed even more conclusive, since everything was pointing to the reason for my headache, which began immediately following my injury.

My dear friend Joy Schmuckal, who is an operating room nurse, was very concerned about me having this surgery. Having seen patients undergo this type of surgery she encouraged me to get a second opinion. Following her advise, I saw another otynlaryngologist in Traverse City, Dr. Nelson. He had a very different idea on how to treat it, and he was considerably less aggressive than Dr. Borovik. He would have continued the same modes of treatment Dr. Stafford had been trying for two-and-a-half months, namely antibiotics. Surgery is always a last resort, but since the other methods weren't helping me, I decided it was time for surgery. Dr. Stafford agreed it was time to be more aggressive and so I went ahead with Dr. Borovik's recommendation.

The thought of having surgery was a little difficult to handle, but I was still relieved it was not brain surgery. Surgery in my sinuses, where he could go through my mouth to enter the cavity, did not seem as invasive to me. I was more relieved than worried. If there was a chance of getting some relief from my headache, it was well worth the risk. The headache was disabling me at an increasing rate.

My hopes were high going into this surgery. I was sure this would take care of my headache and I would be back to my old self again. My perception was that once my headache was gone I wouldn't have any of the cognitive problems either. I had the feeling I was going to be completely healed by this surgery.

The surgery went very smoothly. I awoke to a very sore mouth. I did not know what to expect upon waking in recovery. Waking up to the unknown is always the scariest part of surgery for me. Dr. Borovik had told me he might need to pack my nose after surgery, to stop bleeding, and I could expect to have difficulty breathing through my nose. I was, therefore, surprised to find I could breathe through my nose and that he did not need to pack it.

I found myself very tense upon waking, but was relieved to hear a familiar voice in the room. I heard Steve Hall, R.N., a recovery room nurse and one of the first employees I met after starting to work at Munson Medical Center (where I was now having surgery). As soon as he saw that I was awake, he came to my side to check on me. It was very comforting to have him there. I didn't feel so alone.

Due to a shortage of beds available in the hospital, I was moved to the chemotherapy room for the night. The funniest thing that came out of this experience happened in the middle of the night. They had given me pain medication, so it should have been easy for me to sleep. There was, however, a woman in the next bed who snored louder than a freight train. I tossed and turned for hours. Finally, she awoke. There was silence. I began thanking God I could now finally get some sleep. She got up and walked past my bed to the rest room. She must have noticed I was awake and asked if I was having trouble sleeping. I replied, "Yes, I am usually a light sleeper and you are snoring very loud."

She looked horrified. "I was? That is why I am here. I had surgery today to correct my snoring problem."

The next morning Dr. Borovik came in to check on me. I told him about not getting much sleep because the woman next to me was snoring so loudly. Suddenly he displayed the same horrified look as the woman had. He explained that he had operated on her to correct the problem. He then told me he had removed the middle turbinate of my left maxillary sinus, as well as the fluid that filled the sinus. He was confident this would take care of my headache. I would, however, have temporary numbness in my upper lip, where the incision had been made.

I returned to see Dr. Borovik two weeks later, for a follow-up visit. My lip numbness was still prevalent, making eating, smiling, and speaking some words difficult. I had experienced no change in my headache and fluid was still flowing out of my nose. Dr. Borovik informed me the lab had tested the fluid he had removed from my sinuses. "There was no sign of infection," he stated. This was a relief.

"What was the fluid, then?" I asked.

"It was clear liquid and blood," he replied.

He proceeded to look in my nose with his handy-dandy eight-inch steel scope. Just the sight of this instrument brought tears into my eyes. I must have grown two inches the first time he used it on me.

He found my sinuses had filled up again. He was baffled. How could this be? He had removed the fluid, opened up the obstruction, so it should have been working fine. But it was not. He said he wanted to try to remove the fluid with a needle, in the emergency room. This did not sound pleasant. I felt as though this guy enjoyed seeing patients squirm in their seats.

I walked back to Munson, stopping by Ronna's office on my way to the emergency room, so she would know where I was. (I had planned to return to my office after my appointment.) She saw I was whiter than a ghost and offered to go with me, for which I was very grateful. I felt very weak. My whole body was trembling. I felt as though I could pass out at any minute. I had no idea what to expect, and once again fear of the unknown was haunting me.

In the ER they asked me to sit in a chair, much like a dentist's chair, similar to the one in Dr. Borovik's office. They brought in their equipment. Sure enough, once again the steel rod appeared, along with a long needle syringe. This looked as though it were going to be painful. Dr. Borovik took the syringe and inserted it in my mouth above my gum line. He punched it through the wall of my sinus, removing only a small amount of fluid, nothing significant. He made repeated attempts, but was unsuccessful each time. My knuckles were white as my hands had a death grip on the arms of the chair. He still could not understand why there was fluid again in this area. He then suggested more surgery.

Within a week I was back in the operating room for more sinus surgery. This time he reported scar tissue had formed near the location of the first surgery. He removed the tissue and fluid. It was apparently causing an additional obstruction, similar to the first.

The morning following surgery, Dr. Borovik came into my room to discharge me. He was quick to ask how I slept, having remembered my previous experience with his snoring patient. I had no problem sleeping this time, and he was very pleased. He then explained he had performed another surgery to correct snoring on the woman who was now my roommate. We shared a laugh. I never realized there were so many women who snored.

I recovered from the surgery quite easily, having only a bit of soreness in my mouth. The most difficult part was the numbness which engulfed my entire upper lip. This was a result of him having to work around the nerves which control the feeling and movements of this area. He said the feeling would most likely return in a few months. I said a prayer that it would, because it was challenging to eat and drink, similar to after visiting the dentist.

Soon after surgery, I returned to my previous schedule of cognitive rehab, and was disheartened by the fact that even two surgeries had not changed my skill level. Nor had they alleviated the intense pain of my headache. So I returned once again to Dr. Borovik's office to report that my headache, once thought to be sinus related, was still beating me up. He looked in my sinuses again with his infamous tool, and said he saw no evidence of any problem. He told me I should return to my primary care physician for additional treatment.

M EANWHILE, I CONTINUED riding mountain bikes with my friends Karen Ferguson and Joy Schmuckal, trying to maintain my normal routine. Although it was no longer physical training for racing, it was, nonetheless, intense activity. I had always been the stronger athlete. Even a few months after my head injury, my body was still in excellent condition, though my head was still severely injured. However, not wanting them to see my pain, and the strain it took for me to perform at my previous level, I pushed myself hard enough to stay in front of them. I'd ride ahead so I could stop, rest, and hold my head, while waiting for them to catch up.

There were times I'd stop and feel an incredible pressure in my head, as though it were going to explode. The pain pierced through my eyes. The earth felt as though it was rotating in circles under me, as trees and flashes of light became a blur. I'd vomit as I heard voices coming down the path. Then, before they reached me, I'd quickly wash my mouth out with a squirt of water and plaster a smile on my face. We'd talk as they rested, before starting this series of "having fun" over again.

The price was high, but I wasn't about to miss the opportunity to be with my friends. They were my support system. We shared countless hours together, common goals, and a wonderful friendship. I needed them more than they knew. Instead of telling them, I silently immersed myself in their warmth, laughter, and support. I didn't know how to tell them how I felt. I didn't know how I felt.

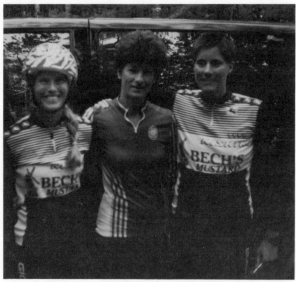

Karen Ferguson, Joy Schmuckal, and author.

Five

Good Grief

Minds are like parachutes,
they function only when they are open.

ANONYMOUS

I RETURNED TO DR. Stafford, as Dr. Borovik had advised, since it was now going on six months post-injury and I did not like the fact I was still struggling. I recalled very clearly my notes from a conversation with Cindy, when she said, "It may take you six months, rather than three, to feel better again." I was ready to get back to my old life-style. I had had enough of the headache, and I thought I had plenty of rehab.

Dr. Stafford began trying a variation of pain killers to help make me more comfortable. He also suggested I see Dr. James MacKenzie, a Physical Medicine and Rehabilitation Specialist, who works with survivors of head injuries. I was beginning to wonder if any of these physicians knew what they were doing. My first thought, when Dr. Stafford recommended I see James MacKenzie M.D. was, "Not another doctor." It felt as if there were a lot a people out there ready to cook dinner, but no one had the recipe. But I had nothing to lose by seeing one more. I was feeling as though I was up against a major barricade in my recovery. I could not see any detours to help keep me moving forward. So I followed Dr. Stafford's recommendation, and made an appointment to see Dr. MacKenzie.

Upon talking with Dr. MacKenzie for the first time, I knew I was in good hands and finally heading in a positive direction. I did not realize at this time, however, how important he would become in managing my rehabilitation and recovery. To this very day, he is priceless. If ever someone would ask me to point to a model doctor, one who treats and cares for his patients as friends, has a warm and caring touch, and goes one step further then most physicians to help a patient, my recommendation would be James MacKenzie, M.D.

Dr. MacKenzie would not only be my physician, he would eventually be my link to other physicians who would return more wholeness to my life. He began to control and coordinate my care, and show a genuine interest in my recovery.

He started treating me by suggesting various medications that might lessen the intensity of my headache, as well as help my insomnia. The first six months after my injury I averaged eighteen hours of sleep per day, but by the time I saw Dr. MacKenzie, I was having a difficult time falling asleep and thus not sleeping much at all. He first prescribed Desyrel, but without success. Next, we tried a low dose of Elavil, an antidepressant. In low doses it has the side effect of sedation. He prescribed 50mg of Elavil before bedtime.

The first night I took it, I fell asleep very quickly. In fact, I did not wake up until noon the next day, and then it was only because I had to go to the bathroom. I returned to bed and quickly fell back to sleep. I slept around the clock for three days. What was supposed to be a low dose was too high for me. Dr. MacKenzie called and told me to reduce the dose 25mg. It was much better. It was still very difficult for me to get up in the morning, but with extra effort I could manage. This was Dr. MacKenzie's lesson on how sensitive I was to medications.

After starting to use Elavil, I had no problem sleeping. In fact, the medication helped my body relax enough to feel its fatigue. Prior to this I was strung on nervous energy. With Elavil, I'd fall asleep, so tired that when I realized I should get up, my mind did not allow me to open my eyes. I was fully aware of what was happening around me. I knew if someone had walked into the room, but it was physically impossible for me to open my eyes. This was a very strange sensation.

Dr. MacKenzie attempted to medicate my headache with the use of a low-dose calcium channel blocker, Verapimil. This, too, was unsuccessful.

Dr. MacKenzie suspected I might be having intermittent seizure activity, so he wanted me to have an EEG and hearing tests to verify. My first EEG showed a mild abnormality, thus prompting him to suspect my headache pain was a form of seizure. Therefore, he prescribed Tegretol, an anti-convulsant, to see if it would relieve my pain. After my blood level reached the therapeutic dose of Tegretol, it seemed to help reduce the sharp stabs, but I still had a constant intense ache behind my eyes.

Hearing tests, to detect whether I had suffered any losses to my hearing or damage to this part of my brain, came back negative.

Dr. MacKenzie was very thorough in his evaluation and recommendations for my recovery. Contrary to what many of my family and friends believed, Dr. MacKenzie's number one prescription was to maintain my exercise routine. He said it was vitally important to try to maintain my fitness level, which would help reduce my ongoing fatigue, keep me healthy, and reduce stress. We discussed my previous level of fitness and what I was currently doing for exercise. He agreed my self-prescribed exercise program was adequate for my current needs.

It's very common for people to automatically assume you should not exercise with an injury. It must come from the old theory that when you are sick, with a heart attack or arthritis for example, you should stay in bed. This is quite the opposite of what new research has found regarding the need for exercise in rehabilitation. Or maybe it comes from the theory that when, as a child, you were too sick to go to school, you couldn't do anything fun that day either. Regardless, there are very few situations when you should *not* continue efforts to enhance your physical fitness level.

Some people came right out and asked me, "Does your doctor say you can exercise?" Others said nothing and assumed I wasn't following my doctor's orders. I resented their feelings, as it was a reflection of the type of person they thought I was. I didn't feel I had to justify my actions. Why didn't they trust me? Why would I want to jeopardize my recovery?

I came to the conclusion that those who doubted me were probably not doubting Karen, their daughter, sister, or friend, rather they were most likely doubting my competitive self. After all, I most likely had a stronger competitive inner drive than anyone else they knew. Thus, I came to resent people who asked me about my exercise and then doubted my word.

The next step on Dr. MacKenzie's protocol for therapy was a neuropsychological assessment by Neuropsychologist Glen Johnson Ph.D. He said it would be similar to the testing I had with Cindy, but more detailed.

I made an appointment with Dr. Johnson. Even if my HMO was not going to pay for it, I believed it was important enough to do. The assessment was more intense than Cindy's. Again I had the feeling I had done very well, but had a rude awakening when given the results.

Each time I went through this type of testing, my brain felt as though it had been hit by a truck. It completely drained my energy and intensified my pain. I began to understand why it was so difficult for me to perform daily cognitive skills. Even when cognitive tasks were not in a concentrated period of time, like the testing process, my resources were depleted.

I met with Dr. Johnson about a week following his assessment to review the results. My biggest deficit was in the area of verbal skills. It was especially noted when compared to my visual skills. My visual skills were at the 93rd percentile, my verbal skills were at the 20th percentile. As I began hearing the results of my evaluation, my head injury became more and more real to me. My fears were increasing at a very fast rate.

He explained that the damaged areas would not return to normal. I would, however, be able to retrain my brain to do things differently, but at this point it would take months of rehabilitation. I was already on the right path with cognitive rehabilitation, and months turned into years.

Dr. MacKenzie, Cindy Monroe, and Dr. Johnson each recommended I begin counseling. They knew I had to go through all of the stages of grief in order to accept my injury. This would only be possible with assistance. Cindy asked me if there were any counselors I felt comfortable seeing. The only person I would consider at that time was Margo Million, M.S.W. I met Margo when she worked at Munson, but then she went into private practice shortly thereafter. She is a very kind and gentle person, always exhibiting a caring touch. The friendship I developed with Margo was special, but I was confident it wouldn't interfere with my therapy. I knew it would only help because of my deep sense of trust in her.

During the first year following my accident, I had become very attached to and dependent on Cindy, often seeking emotional support and guidance from her. Now it was time to reduce the frequency of my sessions, and time to enter psychological therapy/emotional rehab.

I was apprehensive about reducing my sessions with Cindy, not sure I could fly on my own. When the going gets tough, some people grow wings, while others buy crutches. I thanked Cindy for helping me to fly and giving me a push. I had to be willing to risk and to learn from my experiences. I could not let fear stand in my way. My biggest fear was fear itself. It was a new feeling for me to experience, and I was quite uncomfortable with it.

David McNally states in his book *Even Eagles Need A Push*, "Success begins the moment we understand that life is about growing; it is about acquiring the knowledge and skills we need to live more fully and effectively." I needed to recognize that life was a continuum of growth. There are no finish lines to learning. Just because one graduates with a diploma or degree does not mean they are finished with learning. I needed to learn everything beyond the sixth grade again. Maybe this time around I would appreciate it more. Considering the most important things one learns after sixth grade, like values and morals, were still intact in my brain, the hard part would be the three R's... reading, writing, and recall (memory).

I continued to see Cindy occasionally. She always had encouraging words, while being very understanding of what I was struggling with. I have always expected a great deal from myself, much more than I should. Cindy helped me to keep my focus realistic and positive. She always put things back into perspective.

Knowing my level of denial, Cindy took me to a Head Injury Alliance banquet one evening. I believe she knew what my reaction would be, even though I was totally oblivious to everything. As I observed those in attendance, people who had suffered closed head injuries, I did not include myself as a member of this group. Many were easily recognized as having head injuries by their physical impairments. I am sure others had head injuries I did not recognize, because they were like me. To the casual observer, I did not look any different than before my injury.

I kept thinking to myself, "Why am I here?" I introduced myself to many people, stating only that I was an employee of Munson Medical Center. I was not ready to say, "I have a head injury."

This evening helped in many ways, despite my denial. This was the first time I was in a crowded room and tried to converse since my injury. The room was filled with a very loud hum, from everyone's conversations. I could pick out a word every now and then, but by that time I had lost the whole topic of conversation. I remember leaving there very confused.

Cindy and I discussed my experience at the banquet. While I still did not want to admit I was *one of them*, I knew Cindy's perspective was accurate. I was in denial, which was taking me very quickly to the next stage of grieving: anger. It was not a question of how could anything like this ever happen to me. I took full responsibility from the very beginning. I knew it had been my choice to ride in the race on July 9, 1989. I never blamed the rider who crashed in front of me, nor did I blame God. The anger was directed more toward my inability to cope with the effects of what happened, and my dysfunction in performing cognitive skills. I got angry when I forgot things and when I couldn't think of the words I wanted to say. It was no longer easy to perform some of the most simple functions. I couldn't listen to numbers and record them in the right order. This made it very difficult to make a correct phone call. I suddenly felt very inadequate, quite a contrast from being successful at most anything I tried.

My frustration grew as I recognized I could not do some tasks correctly. When my headache stood in the way of doing my work and physical training, I held a great deal of anger towards the pain. I did not realize then that anger was my biggest disability.

I BEGAN WORKING with Margo Million, M.S.W. during my first year of recovery, mostly to follow the recommendations of Dr. MacKenzie, Cindy, and Dr. Johnson. During my first session with Margo, I was extremely nervous. I tried to put on a front of "everything's fine." After all, if she thought I wasn't fine I'd probably end up in the psyche ward at Munson. This was my irrational way of thinking. As time passed, Margo helped me feel more at ease talking with her, and I allowed myself to believe she really could help me. There was still a subconscious need to present myself in a strong and determined way. I believed showing fear, sadness, anger, or pain was a display of weakness, and thus I suppressed them.

During one session, Margo asked me to write in my journal about the anger I was experiencing. When I sat down to do so, I actually had to look it up in *Webster's Dictionary* to find its definition. It said, "A violent, revengeful emotion, excited by an injury to oneself or others." I didn't place myself in this category, although, I knew at some level, there were feelings of anger present. It seemed as though my boiling point came more from my lack of patience rather than anger about my injury. No one seemed to have any answers for me regarding what I was experiencing or what I could expect to experience from my injury. Anytime it was suggested this injury would change my life, my buttons were pushed.

I became angry at myself for not having the drive and determination I once possessed. I felt as though I could not even meet this challenge half way. Before my accident, whenever the going had gotten tough, the tough in me had always got going. But I guess the going was never this tough. Now, before I can get going, I usually have to take a nap!

I can laugh now at a statement I wrote in my journal five months after the accident. "It has been five months since I have felt human, strong, and healthy. Isn't this long enough to be suffering from a little knock on the head?"

My innocence helped me during this stage of grief. I didn't have any idea of the extent of my injury, otherwise it might have taken a lot longer to move through the anger. I still needed time to heal, but eventually I was able to relinquish my anger to God. Five years later, I would be more at peace with myself, even after having experienced two brain surgeries and knowing at least one more was necessary, because I had turned everything over to God.

What I didn't know earlier in my recovery certainly did not hurt me. I thank the Lord we don't know His plans. I cannot honestly say I always felt this way. There were countless circumstances when I was distressed because I didn't know what was coming next. For the most part, however, and given the things I experienced, I can say I am happy I did not foresee the future. It would then have appeared like hell, despite being beauty in disguise.

I moved away from anger by beginning to have more commentary with God. Up until this point I continued to live with God like I always had, knowing He was within me but not taking the time to feel His true presence. I simply went through the motions of being a Christian, living my life according to God's Word, but never embracing it.

I began to release my anger to God, letting go of that which I had no control. This took me into the bargaining stage. I started to pray more. "God, if I promise not to be as competitive, will you take this burden away from me? I will never race again. You have my word." I knew God was the only one who could free me of the pain and frustration. Deep down I knew it would take a miracle to return to my pre-injury self. But what I failed to do, even at this time, was to truly lean on Him. I was ready to release my anger to Him but nothing else. And I wanted something in return. I didn't recognize I had zero control. I was still trying to stay in the driver's seat by bargaining.

Many of these characteristics come from my competitive background. Just like being on the starting line of a bike race or on the basketball court, I always felt a need to push through the pain without revealing any feelings. It never occurred to me that by not allowing myself to feel the pain or fear, I would never know the true beauty of the other end of the spectrum, peace and happiness.

Margo was very instrumental in leading me through this process. I looked forward to our sessions, knowing I was going to always come away from them feeling better about myself and my recovery. She was very sensitive to my lack of understanding of feelings and emotions, teaching me, being my mentor. Once I overcame denial, Margo led me to new heights of awareness.

She asked me to keep a daily journal and to draw pictures of what I was feeling. My cognitive deficits included word finding difficulties. It was hard for me to find the words to describe what I felt. Rather than reveal my deficits, I often chose to remain quiet both with Margo and with others. I knew what I wanted to say, but it often seemed like a guessing game. When I couldn't connect a word to my thoughts, Margo tried to fill in the blanks. While the journal seemed like an easy thing to do, I still had difficulty with words. Writing wasn't nearly as easy as it once was for me. I was a little uneasy about the thought of drawing pictures, but I had to be open to all of Margo's suggestions. I trusted her recommendations.

The very first drawing I created was a picture of a sailboat washed ashore. The sails were lifeless. The bow was damaged. There were foot prints walking away from the boat. A lightning bolt was the identification on both the sail and the boat. There were many other sailboats out in the water, sailing through the calm waters behind the boat, as well as in the rough waters ahead of it. Two sea gulls sat on piers, watching me from behind. Mountains could be seen in the distance, in the direction I was heading. Stars covered the sky where I had been along with the sun, and a rainbow, ever so small, swept across the sky. (Figure 1)

I saw myself as the beached sailboat, sitting lifeless with a bruised head. The sails that used to power me forward weakly flapped in the wind. The lightning bolt was my personal symbol.

The picture I drew also included footprints in the sand, walking away. This may have a double meaning. One might think I was walking away

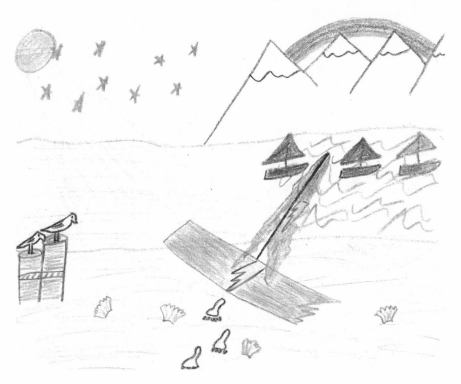

Art Therapy (Figure 1)

from my challenge, giving up, ready to quit. Or it could be viewed as walking away from my former life, in need of finding a new self but not knowing where to turn. I believe it means the latter. It's never been my nature to give up.

The sea gulls were my parents, watching their daughter from a distance, terrified of the future. The mountains had always been a symbol of challenge for me. It was apparent there were many to come. The countless stars filling the sky behind me characterized all the accomplishments and successes I had previously experienced. But the rainbow and the sun, they would hold the key to my recovery. While the sun represented the Son of God, the rainbow was the symbol God gave us for hope. It is a constant reminder of the grace of our Lord and Savior. Each time I see or think of a rainbow, I remember there is always hope, even in the face of the most darkest storm.

I began to look for more rainbows, signs from God that everything was going to be okay. My heart was slowly opening, searching for ways to be comforted.

This picture proved enlightening for both Margo and me. We discovered I was wanting to fight to survive, while at the same time desiring to run from my injury. She said this was very common. It was all a part of the recovery and grieving process. She knew me well enough to know I was definitely going to fight this one with all my might. I'd learn to blow into my own sails. I was not a quitter.

My drawing stimulated many discussions and brought to the surface my need to grieve my losses. I never thought of grieving as being a part of healing from physical injury, but I was certainly going through all the textbook stages of grief. Margo helped facilitate the work I needed to do to heal.

In addition to drawing, writing became a very helpful release of my pent-up emotions. Since high school I had done a lot of creative writing. It was always a nice way for me to express what was deep within my emotions. Those who have read my work often comment on the exceptional depth of my emotional expression.

Journal writing is a good way to regurgitate both the ugly stuff inside, as well as my deepest emotions. One can ramble on and on forever in a journal, without fear of being judged or criticized. It is also a way of reflecting on the past, so as to measure progress in one's life.

Creative writing, on the other hand, has been more helpful in truly analyzing my deepest thoughts and feelings. When I use my right brain to express myself, the more emotional hemisphere of the brain, it brings out more questions about what I am feeling. It actually stimulates more discussion within me, as if the right brain is conversing with the left brain, the more analytical side. This helps me to go deeper and deeper into my emotions, opening doors I never knew existed.

It took a long time after my accident before I became motivated and capable of writing creatively. The first ten months of my recovery, I was only capable of journal writing. I am not sure if it was fatigue that became my biggest barricade or if it was still an emotional block of some kind. I tend to believe it was the latter.

Similarly, I had not had any dreams since the accident. It was as if my brain was put on ice for awhile, until it healed enough to handle its daily operations. This is most likely one of God's ways of helping us cope.

There may have also been some fear of writing. I know how much writing facilitates the release of deep emotions, and at this point, I was scared to see them, scared to feel them. I did not know for sure what might come out or how much. I was afraid of the unfamiliar territory my injury had created. It was like a deep, dark black hole, a bottomless pit. I was trying to protect myself from something. Most likely it was from reality, the reality of my new physical self and the emotions tied to it.

I needed desperately to break free of the shame in feeling and expressing some of these emotions. I knew the hole I was peering into was outlined in fear and sadness. I was trying to cap it with courage, not recognizing that climbing in and exploring it would demonstrate more courage. Until I was ready, however, I avoided writing creatively. Writing a journal brought me close enough to the unfamiliar territory. It became a very valuable tool in my recovery process.

RECOVERY WAS A new and very unfamiliar road for me to travel. Until my accident, as I demonstrated in my picture of the sailboat washed ashore, the waters I had sailed were very smooth. Suddenly, there was a change in sailing conditions. The waters were now very choppy ahead, and I was still washed ashore. In a discussion with a friend about my first drawing, she shared with me some encouraging words. She promised me the tide would come back, and I'd be sailing again in no time. The tide signified life, and thus my return after a temporary delay.

There were many other feelings inside of me and I did not really know how to express them other than to draw another picture. I drew a picture of a river with a bridge going across. The bridge was broken and impassable. There were stones in the river large enough to walk on. The person crossing the river was trying to step on each stone to get safely to the other side without getting wet. (Figure 2)

Here I was. My biggest goal was to get safely beyond this challenging part of my life; life with a brain injury. It seemed to be a water issue again, only this time I was avoiding the water. Did I not want to sail the rough seas? Nonetheless, I did not want to risk getting my feet wet and thus searched for stepping stones, or ways to get over this major obstacle in my life. My usual path, the bridge, was not accessible. Life used to be very easy for me. Now I was challenged, but by nothing I could not easily overcome.

Just look at this last statement. "*I* was challenged, but by nothing *I* could not overcome." It is not hard to see who the focus was on at this stage of my recovery. Much of my frustration and anger stemmed from *my* inability to recover. Meanwhile, there was a huge lesson waiting to be learned. God certainly demonstrated His patience with me as it took a long time for me to figure things out.

A big insight came when I discussed the picture with Margo. She asked, "What is wrong with getting your feet wet? What is in the water you are avoiding?" I did not know, until she suggested it might be emotions. I began to speak of the emotions I felt in years past...excitement, satisfaction, happiness, love, and pride. I called these positive or good emotions, feeling as though I rarely felt negative or bad emotions. I would not allow myself to feel pain, anger, sadness, or frustration. Margo questioned why I called them negative and positive emotions. I explained this was the way I was taught to live. I grew up this way. Mom and Dad never showed these "bad" emotions. This moment proved to be a turning point for me.

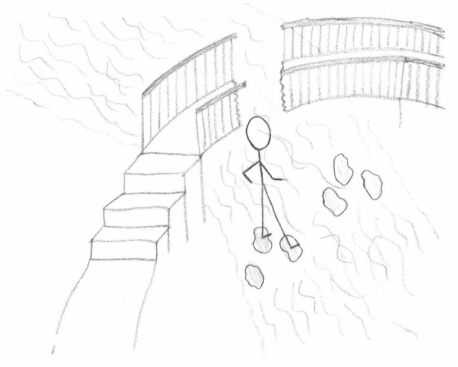

Art Therapy (Figure 2)

I began to recognize, indeed, there were many more emotions floating around inside me than I was allowing myself to feel. Working through the emotional pain became even more challenging than the physical pain. I started to feel an overwhelming rush of emotions and did not know how to react to them. My first instinct was to try to hide them, afraid to show a weakness. I thought I had to be strong. I showed my strength by not revealing my pain, fear, and sadness. I thought courage meant never crying. Fear had to be overcome in a valiant way.

During this time I felt an instinctual need to hide everything I was experiencing. If I revealed my abnormal behaviors, I would be vulnerable to what other people might think of me. I never told anyone that sometimes I would get lost in very familiar places. I would drive around Traverse City and have no idea where I was or how to get home. I had to stop and ask someone, pretending to be a tourist. One day, I found myself driving

thirty miles south of Traverse City, with no idea how I got there. On another day, I was running in the woods on my favorite trail. Suddenly, I
came to a spot where I had to choose to go right or left. I didn't know
which way to go or where I was in relation to where I had been. I had
planned to run for thirty minutes; three-and-a-half hours later I emerged
from the woods and finally found my car.

Rather than ask someone to teach me how to use items, like a can
opener or garden hose, I'd ask them to do a task for me, then I'd casually
observe them, to see how to do it. I would know the concept of what to
do, but I'd be missing one key factor, like turning the faucet on where the
hose was attached.

I'd avoid conversation whenever possible, sticking to one word answers and minimal questions. When I was engaged in a conversation, the
energy it required was comparable to how I felt after leaving the GRE
exam for entrance into graduate school: mentally exhausting.

People would tell me things I needed to remember, but I was too
proud to say, "Wait a minute. Let me write it down." Instead, I chose to
appear competent, knowing I'd forget and later would appear nonchalant.
I did a nice job of hiding my deficits, but for no greater gain than to stroke
my ego. Where was this instinct to hide coming from?

While I was growing up, my father had a back injury that caused him a
great deal of pain. He was a model to me. He never showed his pain. I
would see him lying on the floor flat on his back and ask him what was
wrong. He would reply, "I am just resting my eyes." I knew he must be in
pain, otherwise he would have been outside working. But he never showed
it or talked about it. I viewed my father as a very strong man, and connected this tolerance of pain with strength. I admired him a great deal for
many things and one of them was his ability to handle pain and keep going.
So why would I not want to follow his example?

It was still around the ten month mark of my recovery, when struggling to be valiantly courageous, that I learned something very critical to
my recovery. I learned bravery is demonstrated by those who let the tears
flow where they may, and those who acknowledge fear as a meaningful
emotion. Our souls would not have rainbows if our eyes did not have
tears. It was hard to let the tears flow, while trying so hard to be strong. It

was like a duck. Ducks always remain cool and calm above water, even while paddling like mad below water. I eventually realized that allowing my tears to flow would be the only way to cleanse my heart and to water the seeds of my determination.

In order to let the tears flow, I had to relinquish my control, control I never had in the first place. I gave it to God. In order to allow oneself to cry, one must trust God. We must trust that the beautiful garden God has planted within us will grow from being watered by our tears.

These emotions seemed like major mountains to climb. I often times would rather have fast forwarded this part of my life. I attempted to do this one evening, when I was supposed to attend an office Christmas party. Before leaving, my headache reached an all-time high. I panicked. I took off driving in the car, trying to run from the pain. I knew I could not go to a party in this condition. I needed to be alone. I was really trying to run away from having to deal with the situation and also scared of what was happening to me. I was not thinking clearly and I cannot even recall where I drove. When I didn't show up at the party, those expecting me began to worry. Upon arriving home and learning of their terrified concern, I learned I could not run as I had. It was not fair to others, and it was not fair to me. It did not help my pain go away. I couldn't run from it.

Much of my fear stemmed from not knowing why I was in pain and what would happen next, fear of the unknown. No one truly knows what will come next. I believe this is a gift from God, a buffer to our worries. Therefore, we must trust in our Lord. Everything will be okay. "Trust in the Lord with all your heart, and lean not on your own understanding." (Proverbs 3:5)

Looking back, the only way I was able to keep riding in this race called life was to feel the pain. Life is just like an athletic race. We constantly monitor our physical efforts by levels of discomfort and pain. Life hurts, and it will continue hurting. Fortunately all things on earth are temporary. What we have to look forward to is reaching the highest mountain peak, the greatest finish line of all, the gates of heaven. Only then can we coast. For now, we must keep moving. We must keep living. God will tell us when it is time to check our bags and head to His home. I love the verses John 14:1-4 NIV. It is as if God is writing a note to us and leaving it on the counter top, "Gone to Father's house to prepare a place—will be back for you soon." Signed Jesus.

God grants us strength to keep moving forward. He keeps telling me, "Keep Pedaling." I only need to look back on the past to appreciate today. I have really never had to ask, "Do I have what it takes to get through this?" I always knew God would be there to help me throughout my life, and once I began turning to Him with an open heart I was even more confident.

"I can do everything through Him who gives me strength." (Phil. 4:13) God strengthens my faith with each step I take, while holding His hand. Even though He needs to carry me often, He never lets go. He continues to guide me through experiences, which leave me in awe of His presence and devoted love. As author Barbara Johnson said, "Hope can mend your broken heart—if you give God ALL the pieces." Not just the broken ones, but all of them. I learned to relinquish my pain and joy to God, and pray not so much for a lighter load, but for greater strength.

During the initial stages of my recovery, a friend sent me a poem. It was most appropriate, given I was a cyclist and my life was being challenged in a way which could easily be compared to the challenges of cycling.

THE ROAD OF LIFE

At first, I saw God as my observer, my judge,
keeping track of the things I did wrong,
so as to know whether I merited heaven
or hell when I died.
He was out there sort of like a president. I
recognized His picture when I saw it, but
I really didn't know Him.
But later on, when I met Christ, it seemed
as though life were rather like a bike
ride. But it was a tandem bike, and I
noticed that Christ was in the back
helping me pedal.
I don't know just when it was that He
suggested we change places, but life

has not been the same since.
When I had control, I knew the way. It
was rather boring, but predictable...
it was the shortest distance between
two points.
But when He took the lead, He knew delightful
long cuts, up mountains, and through rocky
places at breakneck speeds. It was all I
could do to hang on! Even though it
looked like madness, He said, "Pedal."
I worried and was anxious and asked, "Where
are you taking me?" He laughed and
didn't answer, and I started to learn to
trust. I forgot my boring life and entered
into the adventure. And when I'd say, "I'm scared,"
He'd lean back and touch my hand. He took
me to people with gifts that I needed,
gifts of healing, acceptance, and joy.
They gave me gifts to take on my journey,
my Lord's and mine.
And we were off again. He said, "Give the
gifts away, they are extra baggage, too
much weight." So I did, to the people
we met, and I found that in giving, I
received, and still our burden was light.
I did not trust Him at first in control of
my life, I thought He'd wreck it. But
He knows bike secrets; knows how to
make it bend to take sharp corners; knows
how to jump to clear high rocks; knows
how to fly to shorten scary passages.
And I am learning to shut up and pedal in
the strangest places. And I'm beginning
to enjoy the view and the cool breeze on
my face with my delightful, constant

companion, Jesus Christ.
And when I'm sure I just can't do anymore,
He just smiles, and says, "Pedal."

Author Unknown

I know when God and I traded places on our tandem. Unfortunately it was not on the day of my accident. It took me a couple of years of gradual change and spiritual growth before I would finally agree to give up my driver's seat and let God take over. Prior to this, I wanted to be in control. Yes, life was predictable. During a long period of time after my accident, I still wanted control. While I never doubted God's ability to get me through the mountains, I wanted the recognition of being the pilot, the one who overcame adversity. Then I recognized I really needed to lean on Him more than anything. I could never pedal solo through this life. He needed to always be my pilot. All I needed to do was pedal. He would do the rest.

Six

Planting Smiles

Humor is not only to see myself as others see me.
It is even more than seeing myself as only I can see me.
It is seeing myself and my circumstances as God sees me.

GEORGE SHEEHAN

I THINK IT MIGHT be easier if pain were predictable, if we knew how long it would last. Unfortunately, it's an unknown. My headache pain was so intense at times, I had to curl up in bed and cover my head to protect it from any light or noise. Often times I cried myself to sleep in the middle of the day, woke up after four or five hours, put my pajamas on and went to bed for the night. I was beginning to wear down. I had no idea how much longer I'd have to endure the pain.

The first year after my injury I averaged eighteen hours of sleep per day. I lost thirty pounds. As an Exercise Physiologist, I could not fathom this. Doctors explained that my brain was utilizing three to four times the amount of energy it used to, just to heal. It was frightening to other people to see me melt away. They often blamed me for not eating or they thought I was trying to lose weight. This was hardly the case, but it took awhile before it clicked in my brain what and why this was happening.

In fact, one morning as I was getting dressed, I reached for a pair of sweats that had recently been altered three sizes smaller. When I put the pants on, I found they were huge on me. I drew the drawstring tighter, trying to hide the obvious, though it hardly did the job. I glanced towards the floor, only to find they were also too long. I panicked. I thought for sure I was shrinking. As I put the top on, I realized the arm length was four inches too long. My only thought was, "What is happening to me?" It was frightening. Suddenly it registered, I had put on my husband's sweat suit! My husband was 6'5". What a relief! I was not shrinking after all. But how frustrating to even have thought I was shrinking in the first place.

It took time before I was able to laugh at things I did that were amusing. I remembered the story of Norman Cousins, and his use of laughter as a healer. I soon recognized the value of laughing at myself. When I said things like *byegood* or I thought I was shrinking, I found it most appropriate to laugh. There were many things that my brain used to do automatically that I took for granted. Things it doesn't do so well, even now.

At times it is disappointing, but somehow I find the humor, knowing the only alternative is to cry. I am fortunate that I am eventually aware of the silly things I do and am able to laugh at them. At the split second that I clue into what I have done or said, an overwhelming amount of laughter fills my heart.

Sometimes, when I speak, an oddball word will pop into my speech, such as happened one morning when someone asked me what I had for breakfast. I quickly replied, "Bran cereal and a hot dog." I have not had a hot dog in twenty-five years, and everyone knows how nutritious minded I am. Where did that answer come from? Something must have short circuited in my brain. I really had bran cereal and a bagel. I knew the second after I said it, that my brain had misfired. Everyone within earshot was overcome with laughter. (I was the first one to break the moment of silence.) Simple tasks were oh so difficult to perform sometimes.

Thoughts of my bloopers are often recalled at the most unpredictable times, arousing hysterical laughter once again. It's most embarrassing when it hits me someplace like church. Containing uncontrollable laughter is quite challenging. But then again, I am sure God does not mind us sharing in the laughter He is experiencing. I can imagine He has quite a few more laughs than we do about our behavior. I look forward to the day when I can sit by His side in heaven and share a "Remember when..." conversation.

One could easily be angry at such nonsense, but why? I see it as adding fun and joy into life. I have always enjoyed making people laugh and this adds a whole new dimension to my personality.

There are many occasions when I fail to put my new cognitive therapy skills to work, and laughter appropriately fills the void of what to do next. It is then that I really enjoy sharing with others the stories of the humbling events that occurred while on my recovery roller coaster.

Laughter massages the heart, frees the mind, and plants smiles. My theory is, when someone laughs, they immediately regain control of whatever it is they have lost control of. If someone is lucky, they might even lose control of their laughter, making the need for control seem quite senseless.

I laugh at myself often. It is hard not to, especially when I find my running shoes neatly placed in the refrigerator, or the milk souring at the foot of my closet. A day does not go by without me doing something odd and humorous. It sure adds spice to my life.

One day I was really proud of myself for watering all of my indoor house plants. This was a major accomplishment. I was not so thrilled, however, when I realized I had watered them with root beer. Oh well, maybe it helped their roots.

In the beginning, it was easier for me to laugh than it was for others to laugh at me. I had to communicate to them it was okay to laugh at me and with me.

One day when I was playing tennis with my husband, the ball came sailing over the net at full speed. He had just launched one of his hardest tennis serves. I stood in the ready position, waiting to return the serve. I held my racquet in a place where it could most easily reach for the ball. The ball was coming directly at my face. My reaction was extremely slow. Nothing connected in my brain to tell me to move my racquet, or my body. At the last possible second, before the ball hit my face...I ducked. I could feel the ball whistle over my head, brushing my hair. It was the fastest slow motion experience I have had. My reaction time was definitely delayed. A smile broke out on my face and my husband was trying to hold his back, until we both realized how funny it was. We laughed uncontrollably. We laughed about it for many days to come.

I continued trying to carry on with my life as if nothing had happened.

In addition to riding mountain bikes, I played tennis, basketball, and ran. I had no memory of my accident, and thus very little fear of getting back on a bike. Seeing crashes on television of other races, however, did send chills up my spine.

Laughter became an important part of my recovery process, but it didn't stop me from going through the dreaded stage of grief: depression.

ONCE I RECOGNIZED God wanted to do things His way, and that bargaining was not an option, depression set in. While people around me would say I have always been upbeat and have remained positive throughout my recovery, there was a time when I hit rock bottom. It began at the one year anniversary date of my accident.

Initially after my accident, doctors and therapists told me, "It will take at least three months before you are back to *normal* again." When it got closer and closer to this time, they began saying six months. Once six months came, they said one year. For some reason I thought the one year point would be a magical day for me and everything related to my injury would be behind me. I had made plans of returning to racing that summer and had been invited to the Olympic Training Center for cycling. When this time drew closer and closer, reality began sinking deeper and deeper. I knew there was no way I would be able to begin training, let alone race. Once again, my Olympic dream came to a screeching halt. It felt as if I had lost my best friend. Competition was such a big part of my life. If I could no longer compete, I wouldn't know which way to turn. It was not only the competition that attracted me, this was a major part of my social life as well. Most of my friends were active in racing and I thought my absence would mean I would not see them as often. This was not the case, but to me the future was looking very bleak.

During this period of depression, recovery seemed very far away. I spent more and more time in bed, not just because of the headache, but also as an escape from reality. I lost my desire to have fun. My job became a chore. As an Exercise Physiologist I worked with individuals who were wanting to begin exercising to lose weight, reduce stress, or rehabilitate from heart disease. I grew impatient with people who made excuses for not taking care of their bodies, when others like me were struggling with a disabling injury. This wasn't normal for me. Patience while teaching others had once been my strength. It was very atypical for me not to enjoy helping others.

Margo commented on my facial color and solemn expression. She knew I was depressed and worked hard at helping me out of my hole. We talked about Dr. Johnson's description of life as being a spiral path (Figure 3), as opposed to a straight line. One side of the spiral will always have a bright side as we move further up the spiral in our journey of life. However, it is inevitable we will come to the other side in our journey, the dark side, at least half of the time. The most important part to remember is that the satisfaction is in the journey and hope is just around the corner. Life is a journey, not a destination. Even heaven cannot be earned. Jesus took care of that Himself. Thus we need only travel through life glorifying God and living with His promise of our ultimate destination.

We are always moving upward, no matter how dark it might seem. We are always making progress, it is just sometimes very difficult to feel the progress when we look at ourselves day after day. I found that my progress needed to be measured by longer periods of time. If I look at myself today and compare my improvement to one year ago, or even six months ago, it

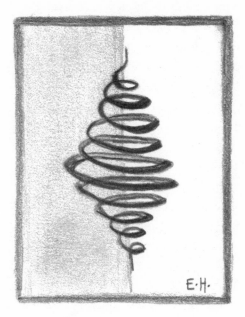

The Spiral of Life (Figure 3)
Illustrated by Emily Helman

is much easier to see my progress. Looking at yesterday may not show a change.

I must keep in mind to live for today. I saw a quote on the wall in a hospital one day, "Yesterday is a dream, tomorrow is a vision, but today well lived, brings yesterday's dreams of happiness and tomorrow's visions of hope." I don't know who wrote this, but it captures life in a nutshell very well.

When Jesus speaks of our journey, He does not say to us, in this world you *may* have trouble or in this world there are *some of you* who will have trouble. He clearly tells us, in this world *you will* have trouble, you *will* have pain, you *will* have problems. He tells us those who endure *will* be saved. The end will come. And we can count on it.

He does not say *if* you succeed you will be saved. Or *if* you come out on top you will be saved. He says if you endure, if you hang in there, if you go the distance. We need only stay in the race, and God will make sure we win by getting home. In other words, keep pedaling. As it says in James 5:11, "As you know, we consider blessed those who have persevered. You have heard of Job's perseverance and have seen what the Lord finally brought about. The Lord is full of compassion and mercy." There were many times I likened myself to Job and prayed that I might be even half as strong.

I was certainly building a great deal of character and perseverance. What I did not know was that I would continue to build more and more, with an increasing amount of suffering during my recovery.

More than a year had passed since my accident and I continued to search for something that would bestow peace upon me. I spent way too much time looking around me, rather than looking within me. As author Max Lucado states, "God comes to your house, steps up to the door, and knocks. But it is up to you to let Him in."

God's peace was within me. He kept knocking at my door throughout my recovery, figuratively saying, "Hello, is anyone in there?"

It would take five years of recovery before I could honestly say, "I am content and truly at peace with God's plans." Up until that time, I kept thinking there must be something *I* could do to change this course of suffering I was on, so as to reach a peaceful state. I kept thinking God must have made a mistake. He did not really mean for me to suffer this injury, did He?

God does not make mistakes. Nor does He send us suffering. If He had it His way, we would all be perfect and not have to endure any suffering. Many people use the saying, "We must pick up our own cross and carry it." In essence, we need to take responsibility for what we do; but because Jesus picked up all of our crosses, and suffered and died for us, we don't have anything that compares to a cross. He paid for everything so that we might live. How much does He love us? Reach both your arms out to your sides as far as you can reach, and picture Jesus nailed to the cross in this position. He loves you that much.

I came through my depression by accepting helplessness. I began to pray the "Serenity Prayer:"

God, grant me the serenity to accept
the things I cannot change, courage to
change the things I can, and wisdom to
know the difference.

I began to hand more and more of my phantom control over to God, until finally I was willing to accept the fact I never had any control. I needed to hand Him *all* the pieces. I divided what God wanted me to control and that which He needed to control.

I knew I could continue working hard at my recovery by going to therapy, exercising to maintain my strength, getting enough rest and sleep, and eating properly. He had blessed me with a body that was magnificent, and it was up to me to keep it operating at maximum efficiency. After all, our bodies are temporary loans God grants us for a lifetime. I only get one, so I needed to take good care of it. In this regard I would pray:

MY BODY

Thank you God, for this body,
For the things it can feel—
The things it can sense,
Thank you for the wondrous things it can do.
For the bright figure of my body at the day's
beginning.

For its weariness at the day's end.
Thank you even for its pain—
If only to sting me into awareness of my own
existence upon earth.
I look upon Your creation in amazement.
For we are indeed fearfully and wonderfully made.
All its secret, silent machinery—
the meshing and churning—
What a miracle of design!
Don't let me hurt it, God.
Or scar it, or spoil it.
Or overindulge or overdrive it.
But don't let me coddle it, either, God.
Let me love my body enough to keep it agile.
And able, and well, and strong.

Author Unknown

I found this prayer when I was in grade school and cut it out of the paper. Even at a young age, I had great respect for the body God had given me. At the age of ten, I began exercising my body to build its strength and endurance, before exercise was even popular. I did this solely based on intuition, and would later learn I was very accurate in my methods of staying healthy and strong. It began reinforcing my desire to keep listening to my intuition. It still is often times right on target.

By praying these two prayers, I began to feel more at peace with my life and the pain. While I needed to go through the initial stages of grief: denial, anger, bargaining, and depression, now I was on my way to acceptance and, eventually, hope. Each of these stages are essential. All of them are good. Grief is very difficult, but it is a part of good healing.

IN ADDITION TO meeting with Margo Million, M.S.W., I began working with Dr. Johnson to deal with my head injury frustrations. Believe it or not, I was coming to like psychotherapy, feeling the tremendous strides I had made. I was becoming more open with my feelings and thought Dr. Johnson's perspective might complement my work with Margo.

In addition to meeting with him individually each week, he also held a monthly survivors support group, which I attended. I began attending this about ten months after my accident. This was another thing I didn't think I needed to do, since I believed my injury wasn't severe. But again, I cooperated with Dr. Johnson's recommendation, remembering how I also thought I didn't need cognitive rehab, but eventually realized I did.

The support group was a wonderful way to meet others who were going through similar experiences. We shared stories and gave one another support. During the first two years I attended, I gained a great deal by listening to others talk of their injuries and subsequent difficulties. During the next two years, I found I was able to give back what I had gained to new members of the group who were seeking information and support, as I had.

There came a time, however, when I became frustrated with the group's dynamics. Our time together would most often end with a dark cloud hanging over us. There were so many negative feelings expressed, it was hard to feel good at the end of the meeting. I found myself constantly searching for ways to bring more positive talk into the conversations, but then ended up feeling like a cheerleader. I did not want anyone to get the impression I was making light of their problems and feelings, but it could have been seen this way, if I was not careful. I decided the time had come to wean myself away from the group. If this was my complaint about attending the meetings, I must have been ready to venture out on my own and seek other ways of gaining support from people.

I became close friends with another survivor, Carrie Mayes. We rarely discussed our ongoing problems with head injury. It was like we knew what each other was feeling. When there was a need to talk about head injury we did; otherwise just having a close friend who understood was wonderful.

Carrie was a very positive person and a joy to be with. She was very insightful and could quickly bring light to any dull and dreary moment. We laughed often and enjoyed each others company. She has been a major influence on me, helping me relax my competitive side and place more value on my relations with people. We entertained ourselves with frequent philosophical conversations, that added a wonderful dimension to our friendship. Carrie also helped me see the normalcy in our lives, which always seemed surrounded by recovery.

I have always cherished my friendships, and have worked hard at stoking the fire of these connections. Previous to my injury, my life was not built entirely around them. Now, I look at my friendships as being the heart of my life. If they ever stop beating, my life will be scarred from love deprivation. My friends fill me up.

During the early days of my recovery, I needed to surround myself with people like Carrie. I also realized the impact I might have in reaching out to others who were carrying a dark cloud. I could possibly help turn their life towards the sunshine. I couldn't do this, however, when there was a chance it might jeopardize my recovery. Balance was essential.

There needed to be a balance in how much I helped myself and how much I helped others. I found I had to organize my time, and truly call it *my* time. There must be a time for work, a time for others, and a time for me, all of which are God's time. If I failed to take time for me, I became agitated, and if I failed to take time for others, my cup was not replenished. By taking time for others I helped myself. I had two framed poems sitting on my desk at work for many years. One of them addresses my thoughts on helping others. It was written by Amanda Bradley.

Lord, Help Me to Help Others

Please help me think of all the nicest words that I can say, The nicest favors I can do to brighten up a day. Please help me be as gentle and as kind as I can be, whenever someone turns for warmth and thoughtfulness to me. Please help me gladly listen, and help me truly care whenever someone turns to me with special things to share. Please help me be deserving of lasting faith and trust. Help me to be generous, always fair and just. Whenever someone turns to me, please help me to come through...The way that You come through for me each time I turn to You.

Each time I think about helping others, how good it makes me feel, and the importance of it, I think of this poem and remember how God is always there for us. We need to follow His example.

The second poem is about taking time for important things. We live in such a fast-paced society, it is often difficult to take the time, or at least we find many excuses why we cannot take time.

Take Time

Take time to think...It is the source of power.

Take time to play...It is the secret of perpetual youth.

Take time to read...It is the fountain of wisdom.

Take time to pray...It is a God-given privilege.

Take time to love and be loved...It is the greatest power on earth.

Take time to laugh...It is the music of the soul.

Take time to be friendly...It is the road to happiness.

Take time to give...It is too short a day to be selfish.

Take time to work...It is the price of success.

Author Unknown

It is sad we have to remind ourselves of each of these. If only human nature could over-ride our learned behaviors of *busyness* and competitiveness. Is that why *busyness*, according to spelling rules should really be spelled business? This is exactly why I had these two poems on my desk at work. Business should never mean too much *busyness* leading one away from taking time to help others. I was fortunate to have an occupation where it was my job to help others and to always take time. Unfortunately, even this can be taken to an extreme, to the detriment of other aspects of life.

It is such a marvelous feeling to know I have assisted someone in some way, whether it be physically, emotionally, or spiritually. Just as Barbara Johnson said, "There is no better exercise for the heart, than reaching down and lifting someone up." A time remains for each element of life.

There is a time for everything, and a season for every activity under heaven: a time to be born and a time to die, a time to plant and a time to uproot, a time to kill and a time to heal, a time to tear down and a time to build, a time to weep and a time to laugh, a time to

mourn and a time to dance, a time to scatter stones and a time to·
gather them, a time to embrace and a time to refrain, a time to search
and a time to give up, a time to keep and a time to throw away, a time
to tear and a time to mend, a time to be silent and a time to speak, a
time to love and a time to hate, a time for war and a time for peace.
(Eccl. 3:1-8)

While I recognized the importance of surrounding myself with friends,
I eventually learned to be alone with myself and at peace. Being alone was
more difficult than it first seemed. I often kept moving, to distract myself
from the fact I was alone. Ultimately, I was attempting (subconsciously) to
escape this world. I needed to truly be at peace with myself while alone. In
order to find peace I had to lay aside the pettiness and prejudice which all
of us inherit. I had to open my mind and rise above material things. When
I was finally at peace being alone, I recognized it was because I wasn't
completely alone, God was with me.

Each of us has a different role and destiny in life. We need to accept
others as equal partners in this human race, and accept the fact humanity is
always growing and will forever be imperfect. Then, we must have enough
confidence in ourselves to recognize that being alone is temporary.

Part of my uneasiness at being alone stemmed from my competitive
nature and drive to always be working towards a destination. Dr. Johnson
helped me tremendously. He helped me to recognize that the path I was
on, the road of recovery, did not have a finish line. No matter how fast I
traveled, I was not going to get to my destination: complete recovery. Nor
would I be able to return to my previous life-style. I would see continual
progress, some days more than others, but I would keep learning.

Dr. Johnson and I had several discussions about how the significant
people in my life were handling my injury. We spoke of my parents, brother,
sister, husband, friends, and coworkers. At first, my husband refused to
attend the support group for family members of survivors. He would not
say why he chose not to attend, and he was very adamant about not going.
It took more than a year before he finally went. I'm not quite sure why he
changed his mind. I guess it was only to please me, rather than to help us.

Not only did Jerry not have the capacity to acknowledge his feelings and verbalize them, he never showed interest in learning more about my feelings. I wrote poems expressing my feelings and was asked to give speeches about my head injury, yet Jerry never expressed a desire to read them or hear them. I was very disappointed in his reaction, because this was something very important to me. He didn't attend the first Head Injury Seminar for survivors and family members, which was especially disappointing, since I was a presenter. It was quite awkward to answer questions concerning my husband's whereabouts, as most spouses attended the conference.

During cognitive rehab, Cindy told me that statistically most marriages end in divorce when one individual survives a head injury. She also said most employed individuals who survive a head injury lose their jobs within six months. I was certain I would not become a statistic.

As a result of the distance between Jerry and me, I experienced a great deal of emotional pain. Prior to my accident, we spent our free time playing together, as one would with a childhood playmate. Jerry and I never built a foundation for our marriage. We never shared what I would call heart-to-heart moments. The closest thing to heart-to-heart moments was when both of our hearts would be beating rapidly from chasing one another up a hill on our bikes, or when I would dish a pass to him under the basket while playing basketball. These felt like connections. Not only did Jerry not have the ability to recognize and talk about his feelings, I was too caught up in my competitive life-style to see a need for it.

All we cared about was how fast we could move on our bikes, whether I could keep up with him while cycling or running, or what other thrilling activities we could be involved in. I believe I have had the ability to feel deeply most of my life. I have experienced many heart-to-heart moments with people close to me, but never placed enough value on this portion of my life to take the time to feel its strength.

I was always ready to try anything. My husband, on the other hand, would only participate in things he knew he could perform well. He was not adventurous. He hated change. This would be the final break in our marriage. Change was inescapable. Our fairy tale lives were not allowing us to be open to this reality.

While I was going through recovery, Jerry kept trying to get me to return to my previous level of activity. When we went running together, he would ultimately end up running four feet in front of me, trying to get me to pick up my pace, knowing my competitive instinct. Then, he would tempt me to run an interval, by taking off into a sprint, knowing how hard it would be for me to resist chasing him. The worse I felt, the easier it was to just hold onto the pace I was running. Rather than fueling my competitiveness, he was fueling my resentment toward him. I not only felt physically left behind, but also emotionally alone.

Now, when I think of this analogy, I can see that Jerry was actually being left behind and alone. I was growing emotionally and spiritually, and he was staying exactly where he had been all of his life. He was perfectly content there. I couldn't be. My life had moved forward.

The more I recognized our separation the more frustrated and alone I felt. This man was supposed to be by my side in sickness and in health, and to death do us part. Unfortunately, it took an injury for me to acknowledge we were worlds apart. Suddenly, in the face of almost losing my life, other pieces of my life became more important to me.

No longer was it a priority to compete in races. I began training for recovery, to build my emotional and spiritual well-being up to a healthy level, while regaining physical strength to enhance my healing.

This type of training was just as challenging as any physical training I had ever done. It was easier to hide my feelings rather than to express them. When opening the doors of your inner being, you become vulnerable. I began by opening a few windows, to get just a touch of the fresh air. What I found was remarkable. Within no time, people showed great interest in what was behind the determination and perseverance of Karen. Their response encouraged me enough to open my doors. In doing so, I revealed my wholeness and my centeredness, characteristics of me I never knew existed. This, however, was not all. I also revealed my fears and weaknesses, attributes I had always tried to hide. This was the real me, uncovered by my head injury. Yes, I was real.

What stimulated this change? Was it the head injury alone? No, it was not. It was a multitude of experiences and *Godincidences*. One experience I will never forget happened within the first two weeks after my accident, before I was able to do any physical activity. My dear friend and cycling partner, Karen Ferguson came to visit me. She brought a friend with her, whom she eventually married, Kerry. We sat on my deck in the bright sunshine, talking about the accident and how I was feeling. After a short time, Kerry said they had brought a book for me, and he would like to read it to me, if I would let him. The name of the book was *The Velveteen Rabbit.*

I was not very familiar with children's stories, and did not remember having read this one at all. He read *The Velveteen Rabbit* to me with great expression and feeling, knowing there was an underlying message that was very appropriate for me at this time. At first, I thought it strange for him to be doing this. But once Kerry reached the part of the book where the Skin Horse is explaining to the rabbit what is real, I connected myself to the feelings expressed in the story.

This is what the Skin Horse said:

> Real is not how you are made, it is a thing that happens to you. When someone loves you for a long, long time, not just to play with, but REALLY loves you, then you become Real." "Does it hurt?" asked the Rabbit. "Sometimes," said the Skin Horse, "When you are Real you don't mind being hurt." "Does it happen all at once, like being wound up, or bit by bit?" asked the rabbit. "It doesn't happen all at once, you become, it takes a long time. That's why it doesn't often happen to people who break easily, or have sharp edges, or who have to be carefully kept. Generally, by the time you are Real, most of your hair has been loved off, and your eyes drop out and you get loose in the joints and very shabby. But these things don't matter at all, because once you are Real you can't be ugly, except to people who don't understand.

It wasn't until several days later that I realized there were several messages within this story that were touching me in a very special way. At this point, Karen and Kerry knew more about me than I did. They expressed their thoughts and feelings in a very loving, compassionate, and delicate way. I was in awe of how these dear friends had reached out to me. In the midst of worrying about not being able to go bike riding with them, I felt an inner peacefulness with this different type of connection we had made.

It put our friendship on a totally different level, one which I will cherish for a lifetime.

Having this experience gave me a desire to open up and *be real*, with myself and with others. Yes, it might hurt now and then, but when you are real, it does not matter. You cannot be ugly once you are real, except to people who don't understand.

There were many individuals who did not understand. Some thought they did, or tried to, but really did not. It took a long time before I could forgive these individuals for not understanding. I learned to let go of my feelings of disappointment and hurt. It was hard for me to understand how they felt watching a relative or friend go through such pain. I knew their struggle had nothing to do with the real me. I had to recognize I was not responsible for how they viewed my life. I could only pray for their support and willingness to walk along with me on the path God had paved for me.

At first, I thought everyone should understand, and thus, be sympathetic. But, often times even those closest to me did not understand. My husband didn't. He observed me more than anyone, watching as I attempted to move forward in my life. He saw me as I bumped into walls, fell over while standing still, slept endless hours, and vomited routinely. Sometimes I'd be up most of the night, vomiting in the bathroom. Eventually, I'd fall asleep on the bathroom floor, while Jerry remained sound asleep, in bed. At this point, neither of us understood, but at least one of us was trying to understand.

I felt like a sponge, taking in every fragment of information about head injuries that I could find. I talked with people, read articles and books, and did anything that could help me grasp the complexity of this challenge.

My parents thought they understood, though they really didn't. They tried to understand as much as they could, but it was difficult with the added component that I was their daughter. It was someone who they had watched grow and become a very successful individual, someone for whom they were proud.

Comprehending the impact this injury would have on all of our lives was impossible. They wanted to deny the reality of the injury; sometimes more than I did. "This could not possibly have happened to our daughter," they would think.

My parents watched me as I attempted to maintain the momentum of my life. They knew exactly how competitive I was and how determined I was to not let the accident slow me down. The last thing I wanted to hear from them was, "Maybe this is what you needed to finally slow down."

They had a great deal of admiration for Jerry. My father was worried I wouldn't find a man to marry who could keep up with me. Jerry definitely kept up with me. What they never knew was that Jerry was the fuel to the fire of my determination to return to physical training and competition. A part of me knew that our sports activities were the foundation of our marriage. If I was not able to compete, what would happen to our marriage?

Physical activity was also a way for me to escape the stress caused by Jerry's lack of participation in my recovery. If I remained busy enough, I could ignore this heartache.

It felt as though my parents, on the other hand, began to blame me for my slow recovery. Just as I thought my injury would heal in three months, they too wondered why I was not back to work full-time and feeling wonderful. Because I attempted to protect them from the truth, brain damage, they had no chance of understanding and fully supporting me from the very beginning.

They thought I was doing too much and not following my doctors' orders, when in fact I was faithfully following my doctors' recommendations. My doctors admired my determination to keep my body physically fit, knowing it was paying off in my recovery. I was doing what most survivors did not, exercising and increasing my endurance. It was part of the protocol for rehabilitation.

My endurance was low enough as it was. Had I chosen to sit around and wait for my brain to heal, my body would have surely weakened more, and my mental health would have deteriorated. The less time I had to think and worry about my condition the better off I was.

I did, however, end up working too much. My employer was very understanding of my need for accommodations, which was the only way I could continue working. I began to rechannel my energy into building my department, a health promotion program. The program had been cut back recently, and I was left with the entire department under my coordination. It was my nature to want to see things grow, so I went to work developing new programs and services. I knew if I did not continue working, I would surely lose my job.

Within one year, the department went from losing $70,000 to breaking even. Within two more years it would begin making money for the hospital, and in five years, under my direction, the department doubled its revenue from the previous year. I was able to hire more staff to assist me, as the demand for services increased. The program became very well-known in the community and I became recognized for its success. Seeing the momentum of the program and the success of my efforts stimulated my desire to work throughout my recovery. (I was also scared of the prospects of losing my job, given the national statistics of survivors losing jobs.)

This was all surrounded by my rehabilitation, severe headaches, fatigue, and frustration. The headaches alone caused extreme exhaustion. They were constant, with periods of time when they were completely disabling. They accompanied me wherever I went and in whatever I did. The only way I can attempt to describe them is to say they felt like I was being hit by a baseball bat at full swing. It felt as though the left side of my head was shattered.

Even today, pain medications hardly help. The strongest narcotics do not give me relief. When the headache intensifies, all I can do is bury my head in a pillow, with an ice pack on it, and cry myself to sleep. I expend a ton of energy trying to hide the pain, just like at the starting line of a race, afraid to show a weakness. At times I feel like a wimp, thinking I should be able to handle the pain and work through it. I know I have an extremely high tolerance for pain, but this is beyond tolerance. It is hardest to handle the pain in the morning upon waking. You would think the pain would be less after a good night's sleep. It is not. Feeling the pain even before lifting my head off the pillow is the most discouraging moment of every day. When will it go away?

I know people still do not understand the pain I am in, and this is okay. I do not always understand the pain they are in either. I need to seek first to understand, then to be understood. No matter what someone is struggling with, whether it be pain, stress, fear, depression, or loneliness, the level of importance will always be significant. There are no insignificant problems. One person's burden might be another's joy, but it will always be significant to the one who is challenged. It does help to look around and view other people's challenges, to put our own in perspective.

It's just like riding a bike. After completing a 170-mile race, all other rides shorter than this distance seem easy. Everything is relative. Perceptions are significant measures. While they are very different between individuals, what a person perceives is always real to that person.

At this stage of my recovery, just over one year, most other problems seemed insignificant to me. This was my perception. If I encountered something that attempted to pull me back into my previous life-style, values, perceptions, and perspectives, all I needed to do was remind myself of where I had been and how I had survived. I couldn't help but say, "What a wonderful world."

As time evolved, both family and friends began to slowly understand. Many understood certain aspects of my head injury, while misunderstanding others. It used to really hurt when people said to me, "I forget things all the time too, and I don't even have a head injury." Or, "I do screwy stuff like that too. You have nothing to worry about." At first, these statements really bothered me. It seemed as though people were trying to diminish what I was going through. In reality, however, they were searching for something to say and that was what came out of their mouths.

One day while we were playing tennis, my own brother made a comment that devastated me. I was serving, and had missed two balls entirely. I knew my reaction time was bad, so I laughed. He barked across the net, while laughing, "I know you are head injured, but I didn't know you were brain injured." He didn't realize what he had said. If he had used his uninjured brain, he would not have said it. It was clear he had no idea what those words meant. Yes, I have a head injury, which also means I have a brain injury. There are parts of me that will never heal or be the same. This comment was part of his shortcoming, not mine. I forgave his lack of understanding.

Forgiveness is very hard for some people to practice. It is easy to hold onto feelings begrudgingly, especially when you are hurt by someone's words or actions. It is easier, however, to move on with life once you forgive, freeing yourself of the pain. To forgive is to let go of the responsibility of harboring this emotion which inflicts pain on yourself.

You might think that pain would be more prevalent in the person who needs to be forgiven, but it is often the opposite. Those who fail to forgive often experience a greater amount of pain.

To not forgive is like choosing to carry a bag of rocks on our backs, constantly feeling the weight and increasing fatigue. It can literally tear us down. Forgiving and handing the rocks over to God, however, frees our life and lightens our load. I feel sorry for those who have difficulty forgiving. Their burdens are countless.

A comment like my brother's was not about me, nor my responsibility. I felt the initial hurt, then moved beyond it.

I found the only people who really understand are the ones who have walked in the same shoes, other survivors. They don't have to be a survivor of a head injury. Survivors of any major challenge have the tools to understand to a given degree. I do not believe it is possible to understand, unless you have been there and done it. This does not lessen the value of those who try to understand. I believe there are many layers of potential understanding, and all those who seek to understand look at one another not only with eyes, but more importantly, with connected hearts.

Seven

Visions of Reality

*Once suffering is completely accepted,
it ceases in a sense to be suffering.*

M. SCOTT PECK, M.D.

I N THE FALL OF 1990, I was askED TO SPEAK at a Head Injury Seminar in
Traverse City. Cindy, my cognitive therapist, was one of the coordina-
tors. The seminar would be directed toward survivors, family members of survivors, and health care professionals working with survivors. I
was very excited about this opportunity, as public speaking was one of the
favorite elements of my career.

This experience would be different, however, as I now struggled with
my speech. My word finding capabilities were diminished when talking
with *one* person, and I surmised they would be even more pronounced
when speaking to two hundred people.

Writing the speech helped me turn another corner in my recovery. It
motivated me to begin writing again, which had always been a vital way for
me to release my feelings. Fearful that I would forget what to say, I decided to use slides. Since my visual memory was so strong, I knew this
would help.

These were the types of adjustments I was learning to make in therapy.
I was beginning to see the benefits.

On this day, I revealed to others that I am a survivor of a head injury.
This was the first time many of my colleagues from the hospital had heard

this. I literally blew my cover. They knew I had an accident, but many did not know the extent of my injury. I had hid it rather well.

Writing and presenting this speech brought me to a new level of consciousness. Standing before two hundred people and revealing my secrets felt as if I were standing before them stark-naked. It opened doors within me I never knew existed. Emotions flooded my heart and overflowed my tear ducts. I was afraid it would be difficult to say what I had written, without crying. Yet, it was a risk I was now ready to take. I choked up several times during my speech, the whole audience was in tears, and it felt wonderful. One-and-a-half years prior to this I would have been totally out of my comfort zone. I was still out of my comfort zone, but there was no longer a need to be in it. This was the beginning of a major transformation.

What I experienced after speaking was a true inspiration. People surrounded me immediately, expressing their thankfulness for my courage and willingness to share my feelings. They wanted to share their stories and pain, recognizing my depth of understanding, not realizing they were filling my cup with energy too. This carried me through the next six months, as a day didn't go by without someone saying how much they appreciated my speech.

This day seemed like a milestone to me, similar to the anniversary of my accident. I thought I had finally accepted my injury. I felt as though I was looking into a rear view mirror, seeing the past and ready to go forward with my *normal life.*

Unfortunately, the road to recovery does not have little mirrors, preparing us for what lies around the corner. I had a false sense of recovery victory. I thought I was at the finish line, not realizing there are no finish lines while we live.

Acceptance of my head injury was incredibly difficult. After the injury, my strength was my visual capability. Yet, I could not *see* my injury. I could only *feel* its effects. I looked into the mirror each day and saw only the outside of my head, not what was going on inside. Head injuries are usually very hard to recognize. The vision of reality is very dim. You cannot see them, and often times the deficits can be covered up, so as not to appear foolish.

When you look at a survivor of a head injury, you might not always see what it truly means, until you become more involved with the individual who is injured. Just like when you look at an optical illusion (Figure 4), at first you see black objects that mean nothing at all. After you study the picture for awhile, then you begin to see what it truly represents. From that point on, you will always see the words within this illusion. They will be with you for the rest of your life, just like a head injury is with me for the rest of my life. You can only begin to learn what it signifies. You'll never come to completely understand it. Even survivors of head injuries never fully understand.

My experiences often make me feel like an expert on head injuries, but not even the doctors and professionals working with me know everything about head injuries. They seemed to be learning as we traveled down the road of my recovery. They are health care providers, not health cure providers. I had to accept their limits, and recognize this was a joint effort.

As I traveled this road, I chose to share with others my experiences, as well as the hope I found for a *normal life*, with some inconveniences and adjustments. I found a great deal of satisfaction from helping others make it through their own set of challenges. Rather than feel like I had to take on my challenge like a tiger, I realized the need to turn to God to take on this challenge. God rebuilds our heart in Matthew 5:3-10 when he says: "Blessed are the poor in spirit, for theirs is the kingdom of heaven. Blessed are those who mourn, for they will be comforted. Blessed are the meek, for they will inherit the earth. Blessed are those who hunger and thirst for righteousness, for they will be filled. Blessed are the merciful, for they will be shown mercy. Blessed are the pure in heart, for they will see God. Blessed are the peacemakers, for they will be called sons of God. Blessed are those who are persecuted because of righteousness, for theirs is the kingdom of heaven."

Eventually I came to feel God's presence beside me and within me. In fact, I could feel I was resting in the palm of His hand. I needed to be reminded by these words that it was okay to mourn, to be meek, and pure in heart. God would surely continue to bless me. There was no reason to fight like a tiger, to remain courageous when meekness is what is going to build strength.

Not knowing God's plans makes it difficult, especially when doubting

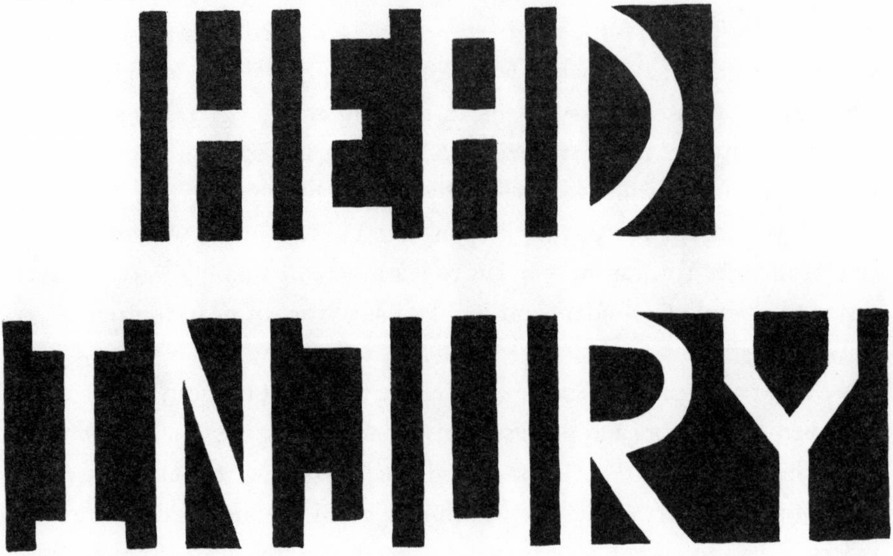

HEAD INJURY

Figure 4

Him. My faith was weak, I wanted to do things my way because I was confident in myself. Through my success in competition I had built my self-esteem and thus felt assured of traveling the right path. Regardless of my success and confidence, I would have never made it onto the right path had I gone my way.

> For I know the plans I have for you. Plans to prosper you and not to harm you, plans to give you hope and a future. Then you will call upon me and come and pray to me, and I will listen to you. You will seek me and find me when you seek me with all your heart. I will be found by you.   Jer. 29:11-14 NIV

While I believed all my life Jesus was there beside me and within me, I recognized now that I did not take notice with my whole heart. Instead of opening doors to let Him in, I merely left my windows ajar. Unfortunately, it usually takes a tragedy or crisis to open up everything. It would be nice if everyone could have this feeling without having to be awakened.

Our lack of trust becomes a big issue. We doubt His presence and thus think we must take control. Even when faced with challenges, we do not always turn immediately to Him for help and comfort. This is depicted in my favorite poem "Footprints." I read it often, as a reminder of God's presence.

Footprints

One night a man had a dream. He
dreamed he was walking along the beach
with the Lord. Across the sky flashed
scenes from his life. For each scene,
he noticed two sets of footprints in the
sand: one belonging to him, and the other
to the Lord.

When the last scene of his life flashed
before him, he looked back at the footprints
in the sand. He noticed that many times
along the path of his life there was only
one set of footprints. He also noticed that
it happened at the very lowest and saddest
times in his life.

This really bothered him and he
questioned the Lord about it. "Lord, you '
said that once I decided to follow you,
you'd walk with me all the way. But I have
noticed that during the most troublesome
times in my life, there is only one set of
footprints.

I don't understand why when I needed
you the most you would leave me.
The Lord replied, "My son, My precious
child, I love you and would never leave you.
During your times of trial and suffering,
when you see only one set of footprints,
it was then that I carried you."

—Margaret Fishback Powers

Reading this reminded me I was currently being carried. It made it so much easier to handle the suffering and pain I was experiencing. Jesus says, "I will not forget you! See, I have engraved you on the palms of my hands." (Isaiah 49:15-16 NIV)

Fear often gets the best of us, though. The uncertainty of the future is breathtaking. Barbara Johnson says, "Fear is the darkroom where negatives are developed. To remain positive we must turn to the *Bible* where we will find 354 'fear nots.' Almost one for every day of the year."

I now know why people say the biggest fear in life is fear itself. It can tear you apart. Unfortunately, we often wait too long and end up asking God to sew us back together, rather than hand Him our fears ahead of time. As quoted in *God's Little Instruction Book*, "Sorrow looks back, worry looks around, and faith looks up." I spent a lot of my waking moments looking around, missing the whole point of being here on earth.

I never looked back, except to take with me what I learned from past experiences. My primary focus was on the future and what goal I could achieve next, commonly called an over-achiever. Yet through it all I managed to remain sensitive to other pieces of my life that I valued: my family and friends. The difference between now and then is I wasn't maximizing my potential in these relationships. They were important, but they weren't my priority.

O NE OF THE many things my mother taught me at a very young age, was to smile, even when it was the last thing I wanted to do. In the midst of anger, fear, and sadness, she plastered a smile across her face. I could not help but smile, even when I tried very hard not to. My mother's smile, displayed through me, has been recognized more times than she will ever realize. She taught me to wear it wherever I go. A smile will definitely give the message to anyone who see's it, someone is home.

I never realized how much I smiled, until one day when Tina Krah, our assistant women's basketball coach at Michigan State, said, "K-Dub, whatever you do, don't lose that smile of yours." There were times during my recovery when I felt as though I had lost it, until I thought of Mom. I know her smile is one of God's billboards.

People have said how wonderful it is to always see a smile on my face, despite my insurmountable challenges. In the midst of the toughest times, I retained my smile, knowing its importance. I recognize some people must be too tired to smile, so I give them one of mine. They seem to be the ones in need of it most.

I enjoy watching the reactions that smiles bring. I can be walking down a crowded mall, and those who catch my smile will say, "Hi," to me. My companions will ask if I know all these people, and I say, "No, all I am doing is smiling at them."

Smiles can uplift people who are discouraged. They break through the clouds of sadness. A smile is a valuable commodity; it cannot be bought, borrowed, or stolen. The true value is in giving it away. While it only takes but a moment to give, it often lasts forever as a memory.

Smiles enrich whoever receives them. We cannot get along without them, no matter who we are. They stimulate more giving, because just as soon as you receive a smile, it is hard not to give one away in return.

M Y ACCEPTANCE OF my head injury would evolve over a long period of time, as it blended into the final stage of grief: hope. As I continued with my cognitive therapy, I could see gradual improvement in my ability to remember. In order to use my intact skills more effectively, I had to increase my awareness of my needs and alter my environment and the way I did things. I came to understand that the damaged parts of my brain would never regain their original working capacity, but I could see other parts of my brain learning to compensate and takeover the work load. This inspired new hope for a brighter future.

I began feeling the hope of recovery the day a friend said to me, "Karen, you are telling stories again." I hadn't noticed the absence of this part of my personality, but it was true. I hadn't told stories since my head injury.

I take after my father and grandfather. They too have a love of story telling. After my accident, my story telling came to a halt. It might have been because of my reduced ability to remember. It was difficult for me to repeat things. This could have been compounded by my difficulty with speech. Nonetheless, it took me about fifteen months to begin telling stories again.

It was a compliment to have someone notice this change and say, "It is nice to have a part of the old Karen back again. It blends nicely with the new Karen."

It felt good to be able to remember something and to repeat it to another person. There was hope my new memory skills would help me be *normal* again. My parents always said that as a kid I had a very good memory. My long-term and short-term memory seemed to be stronger than most. My fear was that this had changed, but now there was hope. When I began to tell stories again, I felt it was a sign of good things to come.

I love to tell stories. It is entertaining. I know I always enjoy other people's stories when they are of interest or funny. Even to listen to a story of no interest or one I've heard before is neat, because I know how great it feels to be the storyteller. It's fun to share the joy of others.

I also began to dream again, or at least I started to remember dreams upon awaking. My sleep patterns had been severely disrupted, so this was welcomed, since I had a history of dreaming every night. I enjoyed the creativity dreams brought into my life. There was quite an emptiness in my life without them.

In my dreams, interestingly enough, I always played the part of someone with a head injury. This helped validate that I was beginning to accept my injury.

I distinctly remember the first dream I had following my accident. I dreamed I was walking around in the mountains and I was lost. I did not know where to go or which way to turn. All the paths looked equally difficult and nearly impossible to travel. I was tired and in pain, though I had the determination of a mule. There was no way I was going to stop and rest. I felt a dire need to keep moving, even at the risk of hurting myself more. The harder I worked, the worse my situation became. The path I chose kept getting tougher and tougher. It seemed I had chosen the steepest mountain to climb. The alternate paths were diminishing. I was alone. I was scared. Physically I was strong, but emotionally I was weakening.

When I woke up and recalled what I had dreamed, I recognized the significance. This dream mimicked my life. I was wandering aimlessly, surrounded by what seemed like the biggest challenges in the world. I was confused about how to get over these obstacles. As I continued to motor forward, thinking this was best, my decisions were actually making my life more difficult.

One of the greatest dreams I ever had came during this period of time. In the dream I was at my parent's cabin at Houghton Lake, where we vacationed during the summers as a family. The cabin was handed down to my mother from her parents, my grandfather and grandmother Boettcher. I never knew my Grandfather Boettcher. He died before I was born. I do not remember my Grandmother Boettcher; I was less than two years old when she died.

In my dream, I was twenty-eight years old. I was waiting at the cabin for my grandparents' arrival. There was great anticipation amongst all of us. Everyone in my family had known them, except me. They were very excited about my opportunity to finally meet Grandma and Grandpa. I was extremely nervous and excited. They were two very important people in my life, and I had never had the pleasure of meeting them.

As they drove into the driveway, my mother announced their arrival. I was in the bedroom. As I walked out of the room, there stood my grandparents, just like I had seen them in photos. Grandma wore a navy blue polka-dotted dress and an old-fashioned hat. Grandpa wore a brown suit.

Grandma came up to me and gave me a big, long hug. She said, "It's so good to see you again. We are so proud of you and we love you." Grandpa stood at a distance, but reached out and patted me on the back. "I've waited a long time for this. It's nice to meet you finally," he said.

I woke up and felt as though I had just been given a very special gift. The dream was very real to me. It truly felt as though I had finally met my grandparents, after twenty-eight years.

I called Mom immediately and told her about my dream. She choked up. When I described to her how they each acted towards me and what they said, she was amazed. She had never described their personalities to me before, yet my description characterized them perfectly. I could tell this was special for her too. Throughout all these years, she must have felt an emptiness because her youngest daughter had not known her own parents; and her parents had not known me. Now, at this point in time, it was as though I had met them. I do not know why I had the dream, but I'd guess it was one of God's ways of saying, "Have hope in tomorrow. I've given you eternity."

During the first fifteen months after my accident, hope was sparse. But because of God's guidance in my recovery, the light at the end of the tunnel was getting bigger.

Another picture I drew early in therapy (Figure 5), was a picture of a road going through a dark tunnel. There was a very tiny light at the other end and a road sign saying "reduce speed." I felt my recovery was going extremely slow at the time, and the light seemed very far away. The light was only at the end of the tunnel, not by me or in me. This was before I recognized the vastness of God's light surrounding me and within me during my entire journey. The comfort of His presence helped me turn the corner of acceptance into hope. It helped me look at suffering in a very different way, a more positive way. I felt as though I had accepted my injury, but didn't have any idea of what the future held. Acceptance without hope is very depressing. I had been a person who focused on the future, and thus, finding hope eventually restored new life. It didn't happen overnight. It evolved over time, as I had to continually be reminded of hope.

D ESPITE HAVING BEEN tested to be at a sixth grade level, I was now confident I could learn all over again. I knew the second time around would probably be easier, given the right attitude. My attitude was going to determine my altitude. I would have no chance of soaring higher if I failed to keep things in perspective and remain positive. In the middle of every difficulty there lies an opportunity. My brain injury created many big opportunities for me. I found myself in a position to witness God's love to others more frequently.

There were also more opportunities for personal growth. Any form of tragedy or suffering can open doors, if looked at and reacted to in the proper way. This must be one reason why we suffer. It is the ultimate means to a brighter, wiser tomorrow.

The trick is to see suffering in such a way and to react accordingly. Instead of following a path or stereotype myth of a closed head injury, I have tried to go where there are no paths; to make trails. While this may not have sped up my recovery, it sure has made me feel better, knowing I am taking an active role in my recovery.

Suffering is not always a bad thing. It is painful, but it is there to give

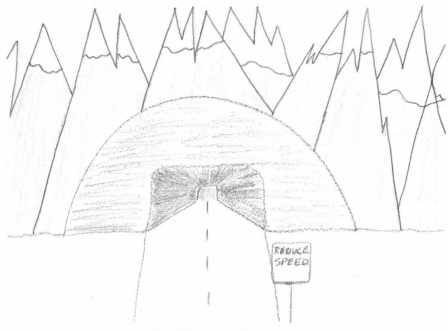

Art Therapy (Figure 5)

us a message. Physical pain and suffering tell us that something is wrong with our body, whether it is injured, sick, diseased, or broken. Therefore, with emotional suffering and pain, we must hear a similar message. The message of suffering begins the lesson of healing; healing our minds and tending to our souls.

While healing is a natural process of our extraordinary physical selves, most times our intellectual selves and learned behaviors get in the way. Suffering creates an optimal environment in which we may learn, but only if we open our eyes to the possibilities. It's very easy to miss a brilliant rainbow in the sky if we are looking down on our sorrows. Through suffering, we learn to focus on that which is positive, a critical element to healing.

Other people were often more aware of my suffering than I was, or they merely had an entirely different view of it. The hurricane appears more threatening, dark, and hopeless when viewed from outside its perimeter. When peering through positive lens, the view from within the eye of the storm appears calm, with blue sky overhead.

Suffering had to become extremely intense before it got my attention, but once it did, nothing else mattered. I had to focus only on the rainbow. This helped me to overcome fear and find greater peace. Whether in the eye of a storm or walking through life, it's best to carry your own personal rainbow of hope. I kept looking up, and will continue looking up, knowing there's a rainbow of hope for me.

Anytime someone says to me, "What's up?" my heart giggles, because everything is up. Have you ever noticed how much we use the word up in everyday conversation? We wake up, look up a phone number, write up a report, open up a gift, and get dressed up, along with a great deal more. We instinctively are a society who seeks hope in every corner of life, often without recognizing it.

Acceptance was a difficult pill to swallow, but hope washed it down very nicely. My life is never going to be the same. What I had yet to discover at this point, was the fact my life was really becoming more rewarding than ever before. It was exhilarating to turn weakness into strength and fear into faith. I found this feeling to be very fruitful. Taking hold of suffering was painful, but once I accepted it, I found amazing strength. Wearing impatience in my heart, instead of acceptance, would have assuredly had a negative impact on my recovery.

There was a dire need to let go of the past. I could not hold onto my memories of yesterday while painting today. Life is like a canvas. We have beautiful colors to work with, and no matter how fast we paint, we will never know how tomorrow will look until tomorrow is today. With each stroke God helps us paint, we are closer to the finished product. Only God knows when we are ready for display. We are His works of art.

God was leading me down this path. I was following, with only a subconscious understanding of why. He says, "My sheep listen to my voice; I know them, and they follow me." (John 10:27 NIV)

Hope is a pretty nifty thing. Jon Secada sings, "In the midst of the most hopeless storm, rainbows shine over me." There were many moments of despair that were showered with many rainbows, filling me with hope. I was finally on the right path.

D RAWING PICTURES PROVED to be effective in helping me discover what was going on inside my head. Therefore, I knew that writing would do even more for me, especially since creative writing had always been my way of digging deep into my heart and soul, and pulling out my heartfelt feelings. My brain demonstrated it was ready to dream and tell stories again, so I knew it was time to put a pen in my hand and to write more than just a daily journal.

It felt risky, not knowing what I would find in the deep dark hole of my emotions. Yet writing was a valuable tool in my recovery. Once I started writing there was no turning back. I was convinced it was necessary to my recovery, and I was thrilled by what I found.

I used the first picture I had drawn for Margo as a tool to get me started with writing. I wrote about waiting for the tide to rise, so my sailboat, that had washed ashore, could once again float free of obstacles. While I saw myself being in God's hands, I believed my injury was a test. I knew at this time I needed His help to float free.

The first piece I wrote was a poem I titled "Life In The Fast Lane." It depicts my old inner drive to keep moving fast, no matter what might try to stand in my way.

My Life In The Fast Lane

Jog, run, sprint,
Pick it up, pick it up;
Spin, push, hammer,
Pick it up, pick it up.

The schedule says now,
Go fast, go hard;
Don't let up 'til the end,
No matter the distance, no matter how far.

This is the pace,
Of my life thus far;
No speed limit set,
For this human car.

Don't put off 'til tomorrow,

What you can do today;
There's always time,
If future plans you lay.

Do unto others,
As they would do unto you;
Be the best you can be,
You've been given the tools.
Plan ahead, be on top,
Pick it up, pick it up;
Give more than you got,
Pick it up, pick it up.

A few hurdles here and there,
Never breaking stride;
What's life without a challenge,
To overcome gives one pride.

Pushing to the very limit,
No matter the energy given;
Beyond the point of stress and pain,
Reaching for my goals, I'm driven.

Words like NO,
And SHOULD are lost;
YES, I WILL, at any cost.
Give a little,
Then some more;
There's plenty there,
Nothing to save for.

Painting a picture of my life,
Past, future, and present;
Would tell a story in itself,
Of who I represent.

The stars in the sky,
Mark the dreams come true;
The memories shining bright,
Boy how those days flew.

The tide is out,

And here I rest;
On the shore abandoned,
This may be a test.

My sails are empty,
Even as the wind blows;
Calm waters behind me,
Ahead rough waters flow.
Boats waiting in the distance,
Keeping eyes on me;
Key people have assisted,
Alone I cannot be.

A blur from the distance,
The past was a fast pace;
Only to be halted,
By one incident in a race.

The moon shines bright,
Sparkling on the sea;
Controlling the tide,
And watching over me.

Footprints in the sand,
Escaping reality first;
The Lord allows me to go,
My decisions make things worse.

Returning to the boat,
One set of steps I see;
This is where I needed help,
He rescues and carries me.

Seashells in the sand,
Dreams waiting to be found;
Some are big, some are small,
Some are sharp, some round.

Many lie within the reach,
While others lie beyond;
I'll never watch them wash away,
As long as I'm here upon...

The shore that breaks my stride,
Slowing me, making me still;
For when the tide returns,
I'll sail again until...

I find these dreams,
So meaningful to life;
As the mountains challenge the way,
Towards the rainbow I will fight.

The lightning bolt reminds me,
To appreciate what we're given;
Don't take life for granted,
Each second is worth livin'.

Just as quick as lightning,
It could be taken away;
No matter how strong we are,
We are vulnerable each and every day.

So as I sit here waiting for the tide,
I'm learning many lessons today;
While I may never know the reason why,
It's given me a chance to weigh...

My priorities put to order,
For they may have been misconstrued;
Life has so many distractions,
It's hard to find our way through.

The energy is building now,
Waiting to be let go;
Once the tide has risen,
My life can never be slow.
I'll charge forward with new appreciation,
For the brain inside my head;
Remembering I'm the lucky one,
While some end up in bed.

Lord give me strength to endure this test,
It's one of the toughest yet;
I cannot by my own brut strength,

Float free, this challenge I've met.

Give me patience and understanding,
To listen to what You say;
For my heart belongs to You,
And in Your hands I lay.   (Written: March 1990)

I was so delighted with the outcome of my first poem, I continued writing. It felt good to uncover the feelings I so diligently stashed away. I allowed myself to open my doors wider, prompting a flood of emotions.

The second poem I wrote expressed more of the pain I was enduring. It became apparent there were many questions about my brain injury that nagged me. I realized there was a giant lesson to be learned from experiencing such a tragic injury. This was the beginning of me taking what had happened and turning it into an opportunity, rather than just seeing it as a tragedy.

Broken Thoughts

Pain, give me darkness,
The light intensifies;
Be still, little movement,
What happened to me and why?

Words won't link together,
Thoughts are very slow;
The struggle to communicate,
Not like it used to flow.

I hesitate between each word,
And have to think it through;
I feel as though in a drunken state,
No control and very confused.

No memory of the accident,
No vision can be seen;
As if a frame of time was snatched,
Oh Lord, what does this mean?

Could there be damage to this brain,
That will affect my life;
Will I struggle for words and never know,

The thoughts I have to fight.

Fears begin to grow inside,
For my future and career;
Seems so distant from reality,
I'm fine when looking in the mirror.

One day soon I'll just wake up,
And the nightmare will be gone;
This really never happened,
The empty night will turn to dawn.

The picture begins to be painted,
Of the bruise inside my brain;
Short term memory and attention,
Thoughts will not be the same.

Admitting all my weaknesses,
Took great courage from deep within;
For I pride myself on being on top,
And never willing to give in.

It's hard to say to myself and others,
I'm not working with a full deck;
I'm something less than normal,
My thoughts I must double check.

Will I be able to function in my career,
At the quality I used to know;
What will happen when I'm lost for words,
My audience listens, no where to go.

You'll never know until you try,
And force the words through;
Twice the energy it'll take,
To respond the speed I knew.

Just like competition,
We push through the pain;
No matter what it takes,
We'll perform just the same.

There's obviously a change,

In the way my brain is used;
Fear lingers with each thought,
It's so unknown, complex, confused.

I still look forward to the day,
When I can look back and say;
I learned from this a very good lesson,
The brain's price we cannot weigh.   (Written: March 1990)

Writing the poems brought my feelings to the surface. It helped me acknowledge each feeling as being real. My vision of reality had been blurred by my competitive drive to live as I had before my brain injury. I was denying its existence. Writing introduced me to reality, as I allowed myself to sit amidst all of my feelings, rather than run from them.

I also needed to swallow my pride and lean on someone for a change. Thus far I had always relied heavily on myself, seeking very little assistance from others. My initial way of leaning on people was to share these poems with a few select friends. I wasn't sure how they would respond. Their responses were undoubtedly favorable, bringing down many of the unspoken barriers between us, creating greater depth in our friendships.

In addition to Margo and Dr. Johnson, Ronna was someone I trusted enough to share my feelings. I shared with her my drawings and she too had good insight to their meaning. Her response to my writing was very much the same. She encouraged me to express my feelings and helped me to understand their value within my life. Ronna had a clear understanding of the whole picture of my brain injury. This is not to say she understood what I was going through. She simply saw the complexity of all the variables to my injury.

Meetings were routinely held with all of my health care providers in attendance, including: Dr. MacKenzie; Dr. Johnson; Cindy Monroe; my boss, Ronna; my husband, Jerry; and myself. These meetings took place monthly to review what each health care professional was doing with me, how my progress was coming, and what needed to take place for additional rehabilitation. It provided Jerry and Ronna an opportunity to learn more about my case, so they could help me in my work and personal lives.

At this time, our biggest challenge was finding a way to manage my work schedule without hindering my recovery. Ronna was able to give valuable input regarding my work conditions, necessary accommodations, and work hours. The challenge was not trying to get me to work. On the contrary, it was trying to get me to reduce work hours. Inevitably, I would work far too many hours than I should. My competitiveness was still a significant force.

I had built the health promotion program at the hospital to a level most people never thought possible. I was very proud of my success, and knew the amount of work the program required to maintain this level. I was not, however, ready to let go of this success.

I was too much of a perfectionist. I felt if I let down even just a little, everything would wash down the drain. My greatest fear was defeat. I measured winning and losing by career achievements, hence my fear of losing my job. Nothing else mattered, even my health. I denied the fact that I could jeopardize my recovery by working, when subconsciously I knew the truth.

I told my health care professionals that work kept me from worrying about my injury and about my job not getting done. I said it was a stress reducer. (In essence it was, but the negative impact by far out weighed the positive.)

I didn't see reality. I was well on my way to defeat, not only with my job, but also with my recovery. My energy was focused in the wrong direction. I thought that my career success during recovery would demonstrate recovery success. I was too caught up in winning. It was an addiction, a barrier on my road to recovery.

Eight

Inevitable Change

Life only demands from you the strength that you possess.
Only one feat is possible—not to have run away.

DAG HAMMARSKJOLD

HERE WERE MANY AFTERNOONS when I'd curl up in bed for a nap and wake up five hours later. It felt like a time warp. Sometimes the pain was so intense in my head that it would make me very nauseated, causing me to vomit. Then I'd lay in bed with an ice pack on my head and cry myself to sleep.

An example of some of the disappointments I experienced while trying to live a normal life-style, is the evening Jerry and I went to see a Kenny Rogers concert at the Interlochen Arts Academy. We were on our way in the van, when I was suddenly overcome with a tremendous pain shooting through my head. I immediately felt the effects in my stomach. After parking the van, we discussed whether we should go inside. We didn't have to make a decision. I got sick by the side of the van. I felt so awful I could hardly communicate to Jerry my desire to go home. I laid down on the back seat, and we returned home without seeing the concert.

The Tegretol helped the pain somewhat, but not completely. Then, within six months of starting Tegretol, I developed a skin rash, a possible allergic reaction to the drug. Dr. MacKenzie suggested that I taper the medication to see if the rash went away. It did. Within a few days of the Tegretol being out of my system, Jerry found me passed out on the floor of

107

our bedroom. He called Dr. MacKenzie at home, and was told to bring me into emergency. Dr. MacKenzie would meet us there.

CT scans were taken, and found to be normal. It was implied by the emergency room physicians and Dr. MacKenzie that I might have had a seizure. They could not know for sure, however, since it was not witnessed.

To further explore the issues of post traumatic seizure disorder, Dr. MacKenzie referred me to Diane Cornillier M.D., a neurologist. My first appointment with Dr. Cornillier rekindled feelings of depression. "When will this end?" I wondered. I was with yet another doctor. My confidence that any of them, except for Dr. MacKenzie, knew what they were doing, was dwindling. After Dr. Cornillier performed a neurological evaluation on me, she scheduled another EEG to be performed in her office.

The day before I was to have the EEG, I was playing basketball in a men's city league game. I tried to catch a pass while the defender intercepted it. His strength prevailed. He overpowered me and pulled the ball in his direction. I continued to hang onto the ball, fell to the floor, and once again, struck my head. I quickly got back on my feet (they said), but then I blacked out. I went into a grand mal generalized seizure.

I was taken to the emergency room at Munson Medical Center in the rescue unit. Gary, the EMT, sat by my side in the back of the unit. I was confused. I did not know what had happened. Midway through his explanation, I went into another seizure.

I remember very little about my arrival at Munson Medical Center, somewhat like my accident. They said I had three seizures within 45 minutes. My husband met us in the emergency room, even though he had not been at the game. One of the players on our team had called Jerry and told him I was on my way to Munson.

In the ER, they began injecting me with Dilantin to stop me from having more seizures. I remember trying to make sure all of my extremities moved voluntarily. I was experiencing tingling in my hands and feet. I didn't know what was causing this, but I was scared.

Dr. Stafford admitted me. I did not sleep all night. Each time I almost fell asleep, my legs or arms twitched and woke me up. These were stronger and more frequent than ordinary twitches. Each time I jerked, I was terrified I was going to have another seizure. I was scared to close my eyes. It took ten days before I went forty-eight hours without a seizure.

Even with my extensive background in physiology, I never would have imagined anything could take so much energy. The marathons I had run seemed easy compared to these seizures. They literally drained all the strength and energy from my body.

When I experienced my first five or six seizures I had no idea what was happening to me. After I regained consciousness, I felt like I had been beaten up. Eventually, I recognized that the feelings after every seizure were the same, and I no longer had to ask, "What happened to me?"

The nurses and doctors kept asking if I had an aura—or warning— prior to my seizures. Initially, I didn't know what they meant, but the more seizures I had, the more I was able to recognize some patterns. Before each seizure I would feel a tingling sensation in my right hand and foot. It was a feeling similar to when an extremity falls asleep, like pins and needles poking me. I also felt a change in my stomach, similar to what I would experience before a race, like butterflies floating in my stomach.

Once I recognize these feelings, I'm instantly alarmed. I know I'm going to have a seizure, though there are still a lot of unknowns. I only have 15-30 seconds before the onset of the seizure. Many emotions race through my head, fear being the strongest. Sometimes I have enough time to say, "Help me," and to lay on the floor. Sometimes I am not so lucky.

No one warned me of the possible onset of seizures. Dr. MacKenzie didn't tell me that most seizure disorders caused by brain injury don't occur until ten to twelve months later. It was one year and four months post-accident; when I thought I had the major pieces of my injury behind me and under control, before I had my first seizure. It seemed as though each time I reached acceptance, something more resulted from my brain injury. I found myself asking, "God, how much more must I endure?"

The chance of having a seizure was terrifying. I didn't want to leave my home. At first, I despised this defect in my brain. It was like having a little monster inside my head that could go off at any time or any place. The loss of control was most difficult to handle. This disorder was totally unacceptable. Having a damaged brain that no one could see was one thing. But now I felt like a freak.

Fortunately, with a more positive outlook, my feelings began to change. I started working hard at accepting my post traumatic seizure disorder the day my friend Jean Greene brought me a teddy bear in the hospital. I named the teddy Seizure, because I knew he and I were going to have to become friends. Gradually, I embraced this additional change in my life, but not without fear. I accepted it as a piece of me, but by no means the whole. I was damaged, but not broken.

My fear rested with the unknown of where and when I might have a seizure. One seizure occurred while I was sitting in a meeting at work. I suddenly became terrified, when I sensed my pre-seizure warning, my aura. All I had time to do was whisper to the coworker next to me, "Help me." I fled for the door, making it one step into the hallway before a grand mal seizure battered my body.

Diane Wendt, my friend and coworker whom I had whispered "Help me," to, and Ronna both followed me out of the room. There I was, in my business suit, convulsing on the floor in a highly-traveled hallway. I imagine it was not a pretty sight. I regained consciousness, finding myself face down, surrounded by health care professionals. By this time, I could recognize immediately what happened based on how I felt and where I was: exhausted and, most often, on the floor.

Eventually, they moved me into Ronna's office. I continued to fade in and out. I was exhausted. I remember feeling very scared, tears ran down my cheeks. Diane and Ronna didn't know what I was feeling, but they knew whatever it was, it hurt. The hurt was not physical, it was emotional. I was terrified of life. They asked what I needed. Asking for the only thing I thought might help, I asked them to hold me. On the floor of her office, Ronna cradled me like a baby, as I continued to cry. If ever there is something in life which makes you feel a longing to return to your mother's womb, it is this experience. You just want to feel the warmth, safety, and security of the one who will always love you.

Those who have weathered these storms with me have responded with tender hearts, never allowing me to be alone in the pain and fear. It is most comforting to be held in their arms, feeling their presence, love, and protection. These friends replicate the love of God, the comfort and peace of knowing we are held firmly in His arms.

Unfortunately, I have also experienced seizures while alone. When regaining consciousness, the feeling is one of loneliness. I am without strength to alter my position. Fear lingers longer and more intensely when I am alone. As with all seizures, I end up sleeping until I can ambulate again.

Like thieves in the night, the seizures come with little, and sometimes no, warning. They rob me of all energy like nothing else does. They leave me hammered, helpless, and in pain; emotional pain. At first, I despised this seizure disorder, not willing to accept it as a part of my life. The fear of cohabitation is like the fear of surrendering to the enemy. I found it best to negotiate. I would take my medication, if the seizures would keep a low profile.

I still wrestle with its presence, but I have learned to love the enemy, for it is a part of me. As for my question, "How much more shall I endure?" the apostle Paul wrote in his letter to the Romans: "We also rejoice in our sufferings, because we know that suffering produces perseverance, perseverance character; and character, hope. And hope does not disappoint us, because God has poured out his love into our hearts by the Holy Spirit, whom he has given us." (Romans 5:3-5 NIV)

God does not like to see us suffer. If we could see His face when we are amidst disharmony in our life, it would replicate the pain in our own face. For every tear we shed, God sheds two tears. He takes on our suffering as if it were His own. This is why we are able to hold onto so much hope. Because He suffered and died, we know our suffering will be minimal, and is only temporary. He died so we can live without true fear.

It's difficult for many people to see this perspective. It often feels as though God is punishing us for something we did or did not do. Events in life can be seen in countless ways. One of the individuals who helped me relearn this concept was Sherri Helman, M.S.W., C.S.W. A member of my psychotherapy team, she was very valuable in my recovery. Sherri helped me understand how individuals see things in many different ways. She teaches through analogies, and used a motor vehicle accident to explain this phenomenon. There may be three witnesses to an accident, who were all looking from three different angles. Each of them will probably describe the same accident in a very different way.

It depends on what set of lenses we peer through each day. The lenses change as we gain new insights. Take my accident for an example. One may see it as a catastrophic event, that disabled me and ruined my life. Others may look through a different set of lenses and see a very painful event, that was also a blessing.

I began my recovery peering through the former set of lenses, I now use the latter. Perceptions are the cornerstones of hope. It isn't what happens to us that is important, but how we respond to it. Faith in God allows us to look through positive eyes. The choice is ours, misery is optional.

It is tempting to say God is either testing me right now or trying to teach me something. God is *not* the one who sends trouble our way. The devil and our sinful nature are the reasons we face adversity. If God would have had it His way, this world would be perfect. We screwed it up, and are paying part of the price. Jesus paid the rest. God cares so much for us, "...He gave His one and only Son, that whoever believes in Him shall not perish, but have eternal life." (John 3:16 NIV)

As Max Lucado said, "He would rather go to hell for you, than go to heaven without you." What an incredible, priceless gift!

On a Christmas card it is written: "If our greatest need had been information, God would have sent an educator. If our greatest need had been technology, God would have sent us a scientist. If our greatest need had been money, God would have sent us an economist. But since our greatest need was forgiveness, God sent us a Savior."

We are born with love in our hearts. It is competition, fear, and limitation that are learned behaviors. We lose sight of love and our spiritual journey while fighting to stay on top. This stood in my way of carrying out one of my missions in life: to love one another. It stood in my way of feeling the hope that is ours forever. Thus, when faced with tragedy, I initially struggled to see and feel that which would carry me, my Heavenly Father.

Soon after the onset of my seizure disorder, in January of 1991, I wrote a poem depicting the feelings I was encountering. I was struggling to see hope. It felt as though I was on a roller coaster, wanting desperately to get off, but knowing very well I was buckled in for the duration.

The Battle Within

Think.
Think faster.
I know there's a word there.
They're waiting.
They're listening.
Silence.
My brain is spinning.
Thinking fast.
Going no where.
Spinning its wheels.
The silence lasts forever.
For one simple word.
For one simple thought.

I blew it.
This is frustrating.
What causes this to happen?
There's an......emptiness.
There's a......... gap.
The....link....is....s..l..o..w.

There it is.
I knew what to say.
Now it's too late.
Now I lost my thought.
Now they'll never know.

Thoughts are scattered.
Sometimes they come.
Sometimes they go.
Why is this so difficult?
How I struggle!
No one will ever know.

I hate this feeling.
It doesn't feel right.
To struggle with conversation.
Wondering if I've said it right.

The pieces don't always fit.
What a puzzle it is.

Think ahead.
How will the conversation go?
I can say what I feel.
If I really know.
Until I have to reply.

Remember.
Visualize the picture.
Keep listening.
Write it down.
What did they say?
I forgot.

Listen.
Concentrate.
Minimize distraction.
Wait a minute, I didn't hear it.
Respond.
How?

When did they say that?
I don't have a clue.
They must think I'm a fool.
An empty space in time.
An empty space in my head.
I can never reveal.

I can wing it.
I've done it before.
Just listen for clues.
They'll never know.
My only hope is,
I can listen this time through.

It takes so much to communicate.
My energy slowly drains.
Sometimes I'm just not ready.
It may appear that I'm in a fog.

I really am.
100 miles away.

Back to work.
Down to earth.
Put your feet back on the ground.
My brain still works.
It just takes more,
Patience and time.

Hear the number, 1208.
Write the number, 28.
That's not right.
Please repeat, 1208.
Write the number 1082.
No. Repeat.
Slower please.
Repeat again.
This is bull—.

Write the word, c-h-o-i-c-e.
H-o-i-c-e.
NO!
Skipped a letter!
Write the word.
Get it right!
I knew the spelling.
But what happened to the "c"?
It got lost, the link was...severed.

Stay on task.
This is hard to do.
Others are around.
There's too much stimulus.
An overload.
What was I saying?
What did I do?
It's lost, I am too.

Frustration.
Exhaustion.

They keep hitting me hard.
This doesn't seem fair.
The harder I work...
The more I fatigue.
And the harder it gets.

My head hurts.
It hurts really bad.
Just hang in there.
I'm tired.
It'll be okay.
How long?
I don't know.

There's more to do.
I have to keep going.
No, I must rest.
No, keep going.
It won't get done...
Unless you do.
It won't be how I want it...
Unless I keep going.
Just keep going!

The chance of seizures.
Fear is always there.
Where am I now.
What would I do.
Is it safe?
Am I in danger?

I can't let it happen...
Where I'd be embarrassed.
I'll limit the places I go.
No I can't live in a bubble.
I'd never be happy.
I'm used to taking risks.
This is just one more.

Risks are challenges.

They can be overcome.
It's bound to happen.
I'll survive.
It's not as bad as I think.
It sure feels like a nightmare though.

The invader is coming.
A seizure, Russian Roulette.
Will it happen this time?
No, please, no............
I'm confused.
Is someone here?
I hear my name.

And sometimes there is silence.
My God, what happened?
Someone talk to me.
Someone hold me.

I don't want to be alone.
I'm scared to death.
Where am I?
Am I in public?
Is this for real?

I'm on the floor.
I can hardly move.
I feel wasted.
I feel numb and weak.
I feel nauseated.
I just want to sleep.

I was totally out of control.
How will I speak?
Is this like the others?
Will I always come out of these the same?
Is there more that I don't know?
What do these drugs really do?

It's coming again.
What will this one be like?

Not this time please.
Just leave me alone.
You're invading my body.
One step closer.

I wish they understood how I feel.
Don't tell me I'll be fine.
Don't tell me I'm strong,
Or that I'm a survivor.
I know.
It doesn't help.

I'm struggling
I'm weak.
I'm frustrated.
And there's so many other things I feel.

But it helps to know others understand.
It helps to feel their love.
They give me strength.
They give me hope.
And the will to keep moving on.

I know I won't lose the battle.
I know I won't let it get me down.
I'll ride the coaster 'til it's over.
And sail away, on and on.   (Written: January 1991)

Living a life with a seizure disorder is like gambling and riding a roller coaster at the same time. Seizures can occur in public, while alone, at work, and with friends.

I was leaving a luncheon meeting at a restaurant with a coworker and had a seizure in the parking lot. Cindy Neilson was able to take care of me. Not wanting to take me back to work, she took me to my in-law's house, near the hospital. I had no idea whether Cindy had seen a seizure before, let alone taken care of someone seizing. It never occurred to me to discuss this with her before we left the hospital together. Cindy did a great job, but I know I scared her half to death (like anyone else who has ever seen someone seizing).

I learned from this experience to make sure I discussed with others my susceptibility to seizures. I needed to address the issue, while not making it a major one.

Dr. Cornellier had prescribed anti-convulsant medication to control the seizures. She started with Dilantin, which did not work. She added Depokote to the Dilantin. Eventually, it was discovered that the Depokote blood levels could not come up to the therapeutic level with the Dilantin in my system. Thus, she gradually decreased the Dilantin and increased the Depokote. Finally we gained more control of my seizures once I reached 3500mg/day of Depokote. This was an extremely high dose, but it seemed to work very well for me. After this, I had breakthrough seizures very infrequently.

I developed a few side effects of the Depokote, including hair loss. Fortunately, this was a temporary side effect.

I also began to notice difficulty with breathing, especially when I was running. I went from being able to run six miles at a seven-minute-mile pace, to having to walk every other mile, because I was short of breath. This was extremely unusual. I mentioned it to Dr. MacKenzie. He was not aware that Depokote caused breathing problems, so he advised me to speak with Dr. Stafford about it.

Dr. Stafford ordered a pulmonary function test, which revealed I was suffering from asthma. This was a shock to me. I had never had asthma in my life. I was convinced the Depokote was the cause.

One day while driving back from down state, I began laughing in the car. My laughter stimulated an asthma attack. I could not stop coughing and wheezing. I was taken to Dr. Stafford's office. He had me try a Proventil inhaler. This stopped the wheezing within thirty seconds. He then prescribed Proventil four times each day, and as needed during attacks. I left his office thinking no way am I taking this. I didn't believe I had asthma. I wanted to get off the Depokote and see what happened.

Of course, Dr. MacKenzie and Dr. Cornellier were not thrilled with the idea of taking me off Depokote. Eventually I talked them into at least reducing the dose. On a lower dose of the Depokote, the asthma problems lessened, but I began to have stomach problems. This prompted my doctors to change drugs entirely. Once I was off the Depokote, the asthma disappeared and I no longer had breathing problems. It was a side effect of the Depokote after all, even though it is not listed as one in the *Physician's Desk Reference.*

I tried Dilantin again, hoping it would control the seizures. Immediately, I developed a skin rash, similar to the effects of the Tegretol. Therefore, my doctors prescribed the oldest anti-convulsant around, Phenobarbital. Dr. MacKenzie was worried about its sedating effects, but I did not experience any added fatigue. I am generally a high energy person, so unlike the many other drugs that knocked my socks off, the side effects of Phenobarbital were tolerable.

I can use the saying "This is my brain, this is my brain on drugs." It is quite different than the fried egg in the commercial. This picture (Figure 6) shows my brain without anti-convulsants, while in the midst of a seizure. The picture below it shows my brain on drugs (anti-convulsants), no seizures. I have no choice. I must use these drugs.

It was difficult to accept the idea of having to rely on drugs. There's little doubt I'll need them the remainder of my life. It became easier, however, when I recognized that if I failed to take them I would have seizures and possibly damage my brain. Taking drugs is easy, considering the alternatives.

I had to accept this part of my journey, picturing myself handing the bag of stones I was carrying on my back over to God. I needed to believe this seizure disorder was only a piece of me, by no means the whole. I put it into God's hands and accepted the birth of my new self, one with post traumatic epilepsy. Seizures were interrupting my life, I was not about to let them control it.

At first I felt like they *had* taken control. I was always afraid, and felt a need to be protected by others. There were too many risks involved. How could I go swimming and be safe? How could I sit in a chair lift at a ski resort and be safe?

Michigan law states that a person must be seizure free for six months before driving again. I lost my sense of independence. It took me one and a half years to reach this milestone. During this time, I had to rely on friends and family to drive me everywhere. It was not as difficult as it first seemed. It was more inconvenient than anything else. I did not like these

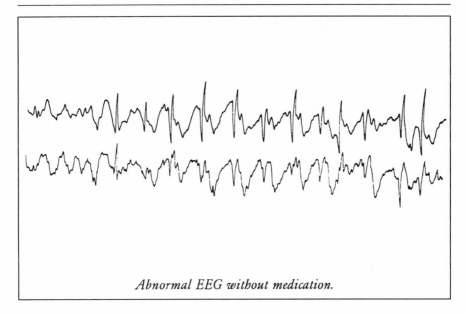

Abnormal EEG without medication.

Figure 6

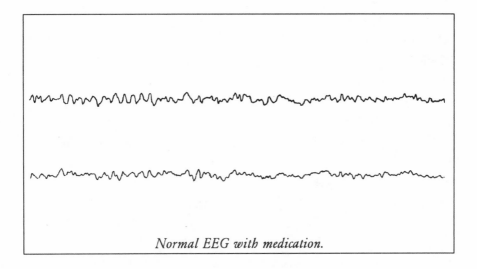

Normal EEG with medication.

changes at all; they were an intrusion. I had to be super-organized and plan well in advance for each venture away from home.

My friends Paul and Diane Fetter offered to take me with them to their church, Feast of Victory Lutheran. They knew I couldn't drive and knew the importance of me staying connected spiritually, especially during this time of trial. I really enjoyed attending Feast of Victory. The people of the congregation were exceptionally friendly. I instantly felt like I belonged. I gained a great deal of spiritual strength when I worshipped with them and it always seemed as though every sermon was written just for me. Becoming involved with this church stimulated a greater interest in studying God's word. It also provided lifelong friendships, building the network of my spiritual support. The pastor of Feast of Victory, Jim Helman, was a spiritual inspiration to me. At a time when I felt like a lost sheep, he became my shepherd.

My mother-in-law and sister-in-law were most helpful in getting me to and from work. It helped that my husband also worked at the hospital, though our schedules did not always coincide. I was not working a full day, and he was working the afternoon shift. Thus, I needed others to take me both to and from work each day.

During the summer months, once I was strong enough to ride my bike, I rode to work. I sent my clothes in with my husband, so I could shower and change once I arrived at work. This really helped fill my need for independence. I began running again that summer, and gradually increased my endurance so that I could run to work as well. I could only do this one way, however, since it was a distance of eight miles. I would arrange for someone to give me a ride home.

Once I was able to run this distance, I got the itch to try a running race again. In June 1991, there was a half marathon race in Ludington, Michigan. My friend Paul Fetter was planning to run in it. Diane Fetter went with us as our support crew. I decided since Paul's pace was normally slower than mine, it would be safe if I ran the race with him. This way my competitive instinct would not get me in trouble physically.

I started the race with Paul, and felt very strong. When we approached the sand dune area, someone on the side of the path called out that I was the fourth woman. This meant there were only three ahead of me.

My deep-rooted competitive nature suddenly took over. I wanted to try to catch the other women. I had plenty of energy left, since I had been running slower than I normally would. My legs felt great. Along the lake shore I started to pick up the pace. Paul could not stay with me. I kept looking back, hoping he would also pick it up, but he couldn't. I had to make a decision. Do I stay with Paul and keep my promise to run with him or do I take off and see what my legs could do? I opted for the latter.

I caught the next woman ahead of me pretty quickly, but was not close enough to see another. I kept increasing my speed, however, and sank into my old running stride. I felt a rush of adrenaline. I was back. I desperately wanted to believe I was back to normal again, although this time I accepted reality. My body was back to my previous level of conditioning, while my brain remained damaged. It felt terrific to run at this level again. I never thought I would see the day when I could run like this. I could not hold back my tears. They blended in with my sweat. I began to praise the Lord and thank Him for such blessings. Not only was I running again, but I was running with a new appreciation for my life, my body, and more importantly, my faith. I was now running with God.

Even though a touch of my old competitiveness came through during this race, it was not like before. I did not need to win the race, rather I wanted to acknowledge my recovery and unwillingness to let an injury beat me. I was running this race for God, and just like in my recovery, He probably was saying, "Go for it, Karen. You are learning the lesson well. One lesson of many I have yet to teach you."

It seemed as though every emotion passed within me as I ran. I replayed the events following my brain injury. I was thankful for every stride I took.

I finally came upon the second place woman two miles from the finish line. I passed her with ease and cruised to the finish line for a second place finish overall, first in my age group. What a feeling! I had overcome great odds. This was certainly going to boost my confidence for the challenges yet to come. I had a big case of perm-a-grin plastered on my face the entire time I was running, and for many hours thereafter. It seemed a perfect way to show the triumph inside me, a way to show the presence of the Holy Spirit within me.

I was not celebrating a return to my former life-style. I will never be able, nor would I want, to return to the past. I was celebrating my ability to overcome the challenges that first appeared to have destroyed my love for life. The flame of this love was still burning bright. I could feel its warmth within me as I ran this race. This race was only a mechanism that helped me measure where I stood with myself in my life. Like blood circulating, replenishing oxygen as I run, so too does the Holy Spirit flow within me, inflating my positive sense of well-being, the feeling of hope.

A NOTHER TRIUMPHANT FEELING occurred on the first day I was able to drive again. It had been a year and a half. I was not sure I was going to remember what to do. On the first day, I drove myself to work. I could not bear the thought of having to go to work, so I took the long route to work. I drove to Munson, via Suttons Bay, which is twenty miles in the opposite direction. I needed to feel and enjoy my freedom.

I was excited to be free again. I felt this day would be magical, just like the one year anniversary of my accident, and when I gave my speech. I somehow thought this would put everything behind me. I was wrong. My headache went with me as I drove.

I had set aside my desire of returning to my old life-style, but the prevailing competitive instinct was still hoping everything would return. (This stems from our innate desire to remain in our comfort zone.) The Karen at the time of my accident was never coming back. I needed to accept the self which had been uncovered and realize I was very much alive and could live a very fulfilling life, albeit in a very different way; a way that was more pleasing to God, and me.

Three days after my driving debut, I was very excited as I left the house. It felt great not having to rely on someone to chauffeur me. I was not used to this routine yet—I went into the garage, jumped into the passenger seat of my Camero, and suddenly realized, I was on the wrong side of the car. There is hardly a feeling to match laughing alone. It is a personal pleasure.

I CONTINUED TRYING to carry on with my life as if nothing had happened. I played tennis, basketball, ran, and believe it or not, rode bikes. When I returned to ride with my group of training friends, I struggled with a few things. I couldn't convince myself it was okay to ride behind another cyclist, since this was the cause of my accident. It also bothered me when someone new showed up to ride with us and didn't wear a helmet. I felt compelled to lecture them on the necessity of wearing a helmet. All I needed to say was, "Let me tell you about the last year of my life." Even if what I said didn't have an impact, I couldn't live with myself unless I said something.

I started getting requests from newspaper, radio, and television reporters for interviews and public appearances concerning helmets and bike safety. This really made me feel like there was a purpose for my head injury. I kept wondering what God had in mind for my future, and tried to capitalize on whatever circumstances arose.

Everyone who inquired about my story seemed surprised at the severity and complexity of my injury. I always get the question, "Did you have a helmet on?" Upon finding out I did have a helmet on, I can tell they want to say something about the ineffectiveness of helmets and why they do not need to wear one. I've even been asked if I am going to sue the helmet company. Why would I want to sue a company when its product saved my life? Telling others I would not be here if I did not have that helmet on has a dramatic impact. You would think it would immediately convince others to wear a helmet. It doesn't. If my story doesn't, I don't know what will.

Because my accident and injury drew so much attention, I couldn't go anywhere without someone stopping me and asking me about it. I was in the video store one day and another customer came running up to me and said, "I know you. I saw you on television a couple weeks ago." I don't mind this one bit. If one person begins to wear a helmet because of me, the publicity is worth it. I already know of one individual who began wearing a helmet after hearing my story. Shortly thereafter she had an accident and hit her head. She is fine. The helmet definitely saved her from a brain injury. Thus, I will share my story with anyone wanting to hear it, and take as much time as they want answering questions, no matter how many painful memories it brings back.

Nine

Valuable Discovery

*What lies behind us and what lies
before us are tiny matters
compared to what lies within us.*

MORROW

I BEGAN TO WONDER if there might be more damage to my head than had been diagnosed. My headaches persisted, and after talking with others at the head injury support group, I decided to check with my dentist to see if something might have happened to my teeth or jaw during the accident. I had seen my dentist since the accident, but I was not sure he had thoroughly checked for possible damage.

I explained my symptoms to my dentist, primarily my headache and the occasional hot and cold sensitivity on the right side of my mouth. He still didn't detect any damage, but referred me to a specialist, who in the event I would need a root canal, would be the one to diagnose and perform the procedure.

I was able to see the specialist within a week. His assistant performed extensive tests on my teeth, focusing on the area of suspicion. When the physician came in and examined my teeth, the first thing he said was, "Wow, you really shattered your back molar. The entire enamel is shattered." I had no idea what this meant, but immediately hoped this would be the beginning of ridding me of my headache.

He explained that there was little he could do to fix this problem. A root canal was not an option (which relieved me of my anxieties stemming from horror stories from friends who have endured root canals). He spoke of possibly putting a crown on the tooth, but was not in a hurry to do so. He recommended waiting and watching the tooth, to see if the symptoms persisted. While I was in total agreement with his desire to be conservative, this did not provide me with a solution to my pain.

I was amazed that my dentist, who was always very thorough, had missed something that seemed obvious to this specialist. This reemphasized the fact that physicians are human and can easily make errors. What was more astonishing to me, however, was the fact that more than two years had passed since my injury and I was still discovering damage to my head. Unfortunately, this was not the end of my discovery.

Dr. MacKenzie encouraged me to return to Dr. Borovik, who had performed my sinus surgery. He thought Dr. Borovik might have additional insight as to why my headache was still so severe.

Dr. MacKenzie had exhausted his ideas on how to alleviate my pain, and was becoming frustrated. He had prescribed Darvocet, a mild narcotic, because aspirin, acetaminophen, and nonsteroidal anti-inflammatories were not strong enough to take away my pain. The Darvocet didn't take the pain away either, so he prescribed Vicodin, followed by Percocet, a class two, stronger narcotic. It decreased the intensity slightly, but didn't relieve me of pain. This was after we had tried several other drugs, such as Calan and Midrin.

I SAW DR. Borovik again in September of 1992, a little over three years after my accident. After he examined me with my favorite instrument, the steel rod, also known as a scope, he said, "I do not see anything wrong with your sinuses. What is it you are complaining about?"

I stood up, bent over at the waist to touch my toes, returned to a standing position, and fluid flowed out my nose. As I caught the clear fluid in the palm of my hand, I said, "This is one problem."

His eyes got as big as saucers. He exclaimed with shock, "Wow! That looks like spinal fluid to me."

I could not believe what I was hearing. How could I go three years without anyone diagnosing that the liquid from my nose was spinal fluid? Spinal fluid is the central nervous system's cushion. Our whole nervous system floats in cerebrospinal fluid. No wonder my headaches had been so bad. The tissues surrounding and attached to my brain were straining. It was as if someone had pulled the drain plug. My brain was sinking into the base of my skull, without a protective cushion.

After each sinus surgery, I had asked Dr. Borovik specifically what the fluid was; and he had always stated it was clear liquid and blood. He had only had the fluid tested for possible infections, not to determine if it was spinal fluid.

This news shed a whole new light on my injury. It was the missing piece to the puzzle of my recovery.

After leaving Dr. Borovik's office, I immediately called Dr. MacKenzie. He was amazed at this new insight. It made perfect sense to both of us; no wonder I had such an excruciating headache. If spinal fluid was leaking out of my head, it meant there was not enough cushion for my brain to float. The sinking of the brain puts unnecessary strain on the tissues surrounding the brain, thus causing pain. A typical spinal headache is characterized by pain in the eyes, which is what I had been complaining of for three years.

Dr. MacKenzie quickly spoke with John Cilluffo, M.D., a neurosurgeon in the Traverse City area, to find out what we needed to do next. Dr. Cilluffo wanted to see me in his office right away.

Barbara, Dr. MacKenzie's nurse, made an appointment for me to see Dr. Cilluffo the next day. I was a bit nervous as I didn't know Dr. Cilluffo, nor did I know the ramifications of a cerebrospinal fluid (CSF) leak.

My husband was supposed to meet me in Dr. Cillufo's waiting room, but he never showed. I knew Jerry had a dentist appointment after work, but we didn't think it would take longer than an hour. Jerry should have had plenty of time to get to Dr. Cilluffo's office, which was just across the street. We both knew my appointment was critical.

With a few exceptions, my husband didn't go to doctor's appointments with me. He took me to my first neurosurgeon's appointment, when I was going to receive the results of my MRI. He also attended the group appointments. This appointment, however, seemed more critical than the others, so I asked Jerry to be there with me. I did not want to be alone.

Despite my request, I ended up being alone. I was scared of what Dr. Cilluffo was going to say, scared of the unknown. I was terrified.

Dr. Cilluffo spent a great deal of time asking me questions about my accident and subsequent symptoms and problems. After giving him my history, he asked me to try to produce the fluid. I said, "I not only can try, but I am certain I will be able to demonstrate this for you." I bent over and, like always, upon lifting my head, the clear fluid poured out of my nose and into the palm of my hand.

Dr. Cilluffo was shocked. He could not believe his eyes. He jumped nervously towards the Kleenex box, knocking over a mannequin head that sat beside it. He quickly handed me the box and said, "Wow, I have never seen a spinal fluid leak like that before."

This was a very bittersweet moment for me. I was sitting in the office of a well-known, experienced neurosurgeon, who had never seen a CSF leak like mine. At the same time, I was excited about the prospects of resolving my headache problem.

The next twenty minutes were emotionally painful. Dr. Cilluffo proceeded to tell me a few stories of other patients of his who had CSF leaks, all of whom had major complications with meningitis. "One individual had meningitis eight times before I was finally able to stop the leak. It's hard for me to believe you haven't had meningitis, given the suspected mammoth size leak. If fluid can come out, then infection or a virus can go in," he said. He then told me how complicated meningitis is, and how deadly.

Next came reality. This was not going to be something as easy to fix as a fractured foot. He pulled out a head and brain mannequin, and placed it in front of me. There were removable parts. He pointed to his own head and said, "I will need to cut you from ear to ear," as he made a motion forming a head band across his skull. Then, he pulled the front of the mannequin's skull off, and stated, "I will cut a piece of your skull away, so I can work underneath the brain." He lifted up the mannequin's brain and pointed to the base of the skull. "This is most likely the area which is fractured and leaking fluid into your sinuses. I will need to take fat from somewhere on your body, if I can find some, and lay it down over the fractured area. Stopping these leaks is often times like stopping a leak in your basement.

"I will put a drain in your head and in your back to keep the pressure low. By doing so, hopefully a new leak will not form once the old leak is stopped. The drain in your back will be permanent, while the drain in your head can be removed in a few days."

He continued. Statistically, only five percent of all survivors of head injury end up with CSF leaks, he explained, and of those, all but five percent close spontaneously on their own, without intervention. Not only was I within the first very low percentage group, I also fell in the next very small group of survivors. How did I get so lucky?

I couldn't believe what I was hearing. I had to remove myself from the discussion. If I thought of myself as the one he would cut, I surely would have passed out. Instead, as Dr. Cilluffo spoke, I imagined it was someone else we were discussing, not me. This might have been a little easier if someone had been with me for support. But, since that did not happen, I dealt with it the best way I knew how: denial.

I left Dr. Cilluffo's office and returned to my own office at Munson. I was in a daze. I did not know what to do. I felt on the brink of panic, which most certainly included crying at any moment.

I picked up the phone and called the person whom I confide in the most, the person who I know will always be there for me, my sister, Kay. Lucky for me, she was home. I did not know how to describe to her what happened. I did not want to scare her, and I most certainly did not want to describe what was going to happen as insensitively as Dr. Cilluffo had. When I began to talk about it to Kay, my tears flowed. It was suddenly real to me. I was the patient.

Kay was shocked. No matter how gently I said, "I need brain surgery," it was disturbing.

I cannot recall very many details of our conversation. Most of our time was spent in silence. Neither of us knew what to say to the other. It is very rare for either of us to be at a loss for words.

Kay did not want to leave me alone, but I did not have an option. It was late at night and my office was not located near the night shift employee offices. At some point, we had to say good-bye. Unexpectedly, while I was still on the phone, my sister-in-law, Kathy, walked into my office. She had never been to my office before. Why she chose to visit on this night, I do not know. I'm sure God directed her. Kay was so glad when I told her Kathy had just walked in. She said "I love you. I'll call you again tonight, to make sure you're okay."

I began repeating the details to Kathy, and once again I cried. She wondered where Jerry was. It obviously seemed odd he was not with me. I updated her on what had happened the previous night at the gym. While playing basketball, Jerry had been hit in the mouth and broken several teeth. He was supposed to go to the dentist after work, and then meet me at Dr. Cilluffo's office, but he never showed.

Seeing my state of despair, Kathy suggested that I go with her to my in-law's home. I was glad she made this suggestion, because my ability for decision making had been temporarily impaired. The horror of brain surgery was overwhelming me.

After telling the story of my husband's teeth to his parents, they inquired how I was doing. I began repeating the story of my encounter with Dr. Cilluffo. I started to realize the more I relayed the details, the more it was sinking into my emotions. I was scared to death. This was unlike anything I had ever experienced. There is no comparison for someone telling you that they are going to cut into your head and touch your brain. I thought this was only something that happened to people who had severe damage to their heads. I didn't feel I qualified.

All the feelings I had when I underwent sinus surgery three years ago resurfaced. At that time, I was so thankful my head injury was not severe enough to require brain surgery. I truly thought I was in the clear, since I did not need brain surgery during the first few weeks after my accident.

You can never be prepared for something like this. If it would have happened within the first few weeks after my accident, I would not have been as equipped emotionally to handle the feelings. Three years later, I was at a higher level of consciousness, emotionally and spiritually. Maybe this is why God waited until this point in my recovery to put me in the hands of a brain surgeon.

It still was very difficult, but with faith in God, I knew this was not more than He and I could handle. This is a life of give and take. God would not give me any more than I could take, and I was confident that I could take what I was given.

As I told my in-laws what I was told by Dr. Cilluffo, I cried again. My father-in-law needed to leave the room. He could not emotionally handle the details. Kathy began to cry as well. My mother-in-law came to me and held me in her arms. I sobbed. All of the feelings I had experienced since my accident were flooding me.

It felt as though I was coming closer and closer to something I had feared the most in my life, physical disability. I was terrified. I knew the risks of brain surgery. I could become paralyzed, blind, more cognitively impaired, end up in a coma, or die. I was not afraid to die, only to leave my loved ones behind. I was not afraid of pain, I was used to it. I could not imagine that the pain of surgery would be much greater than the pain of my headache. I wasn't even afraid of having my head shaved, this was the least of my worries. I was terrified of disability.

My athletic endeavors trained me to redirect my pain. This training came in handy, but not nearly as much as my spiritual training. My faith in God our Father guided me to relinquish my pain to Him.

At this point in my life, I thought of myself as a strong person, one who trusted in God with all my heart. "Trust in the Lord with all your heart..." (Proverbs 3:5 NIV)

Throughout my life and recovery, however, I was not paying attention to the remainder of this verse, "...and lean not on your own understanding; in all your ways acknowledge Him, and He will make your paths straight." (Proverbs 3:5-6 NIV) I was trying to lean on my own understanding. It did not work, for the simple reason I did not have an understanding. There was no way for me to know why this was happening. I had no answers of my own, only God's word and faith.

I tell you the truth, you will weep and mourn while the world rejoices. You will grieve, but your grief will turn to joy...Now is your time of grief, but I will see you again and you will rejoice, and no one will take away your joy. In that day you will no longer ask me anything. I tell you the truth, my Father will give you whatever you ask in my name.

Until now you have not asked for anything in my name. Ask and you
will receive, and your joy will be complete. (John 16:20-23 NIV)

Even though I had faith, I needed to learn to give all the pieces to
God, not just the broken ones. I needed to pray and ask for help. I did not
spend idle time with God. My life became so busy at times, I did not take
time to just be with God. I wonder how much God weeps because of our
busyness, just as a parent longs for their children to spend more time with
them as they grow older? Eventually, I learned to free myself and recognize the value of spending time with my heavenly Father.

On this evening, I am sure my in-laws felt helpless. It was comforting
to know I could be consoled by them. I only wished my parents would
have lived closer to me, so I could have first been comforted by them.

After I settled down, I told them my next step was a myelogram, which
would help Dr. Cilluffo locate the leak. Today was Friday, and the
myelogram was scheduled for Monday morning.

Throughout my recovery, everything major seemed to happen on a
Friday. It is very difficult to wait through the weekend to take the next
step or to find out more information. I am always more comfortable with
myself if I know what is coming next and when, even if I do not know the
outcome. The unknown is very difficult for me.

These weekends taught me to be more at peace with the unknown.
Recovery, and ultimately life, is built around unknowns. God does not
give us road maps.

I drove home expecting to find my husband already there. We drove
in the driveway at the same time. Jerry first told me about his five hours in
the dentist's chair. He was desperately trying to justify why he had not
shown up at my doctor's appointment. He very descriptively told me about
the x-rays of his lower teeth and the multiple fractures. He showed me the
wires holding his lower teeth together. After telling me how frustrating it
was for him to sit in the chair for so long, and how painful it was, he asked
how my doctor's appointment went. At this point, I had very little sympathy for him; and, I suspected he would have difficulty being sensitive to my
feelings, too.

I told him the details of my appointment. He was speechless. All he could say was, "Wow, I guess that makes my time in the chair look easy." He said nothing more the remainder of the night. He just went to bed.

We never talked at great length about my surgery. He never asked how I was handling the feeling of having to have brain surgery, nor did he share with me his feelings as my spouse. It was as if I was going to have minor surgery. I wanted to talk with him, to share with Jerry how scared I was, but I was more afraid of being hurt by his response or lack thereof. I knew I could talk until I was blue in the face and Jerry would not have the emotional capacity to help me. It was a very lonely feeling.

I DIDN'T KNOW how to tell my parents. They just recently began speaking to me after three months of silence. We were at different ends of the spectrum, as far as understanding one another's feelings. They didn't have a clue what I was experiencing as a survivor of head injury, and I wasn't sensitive to their feelings as my parents. It was as though we were tossed in a raging river and each of us were fighting to survive independently.

Instead of being open in our communication, I focused only on their criticism of the way I was handling my recovery. There was so much tension between us, it was best to remain separate, even though it tore all of our hearts in two. While I felt abandoned during the most critical part of my life, I'm sure they felt much of the same emotional pain as I did, if not more.

Mom broke the silence the day she called to tell me my grandfather had been admitted to the hospital. Things were still tense, but at least we were in contact. I still felt very distant from them, while deep inside my heart I was screaming, "M-O-M, D-A-D, I need you." It's unfortunate that pride prevented me from breaking the barrier between us.

I knew, despite our petty differences, my parents were not going to handle the news of my surgery well. I also knew I would probably never know how they were truly feeling, for two reasons. One, I am not a parent, and I would not be able to relate to the anguish and despair of seeing a child suffer. Secondly, my parents have always hidden their feelings. They show very little emotional and physical pain, trying to "be strong."

It was quite enough to experience my own fear of having this surgery.

I cannot imagine having to watch a daughter go through this surgery. I recognized their potential despair. I was thankful I was the one to have a brain injury and subsequent surgeries, rather than someone I love. I perceived my position as being much easier. Waiting and watching throughout surgery, and having to deal with the power of one's imagination, is the ultimate challenge. Our minds can create enormous fears and anxieties, without reality even touching this part of life.

This, of course, is a perception of mine, which may vary from the perceptions of others. The many ways people view life can often be worlds apart, just as I learned from my conversation with my friend Carol Paxton.

No matter what we face in life, we can look around and always find someone who is struggling more, despite feeling as though we are alone in our suffering. Sometimes we feel that what happened to us is far worse than any problems other people face. We wallow in our own self-pity, until reality strikes.

The day I spoke with Carol, I learned a very important lesson. Carol is a runner and cyclist. One day while Carol was running, a woman drove her car off the road, towards Carol. Carol tried desperately to run away from her, but ended up having her leg pinned between the car and a tree. Carol's leg needed to be amputated. I called Carol soon after the accident, to let her know I was there for her if she needed any help. More than anything, I wanted her to know I was there to listen if she ever needed to talk about her injury.

We discussed how she was handling the loss of her leg, and the physical and emotional scars. She displayed a remarkable, positive outlook for her future. She had already made a connection with a physician who specialized in prosthetics for athletes.

Despite experiencing a very devastating tragedy, Carol asked how my recovery was going. We spoke of the many hurdles we were both facing. I said to Carol, "I cannot even imagine what you are going through. The loss of a limb has been my greatest fear in life. At least with my accident, I did not lose the use of my legs."

Carol's reply astounded me, and immediately put things in perspective. She said, "Karen, the first thing I said to myself after my accident was, I am so thankful I do not have a head injury."

The grass always looks greener on the other side of the fence, but in many cases, on the other side of the fence the sun is not shining. The grass on the other side must be mowed just as often. When struggling with life's toughest challenges, we can always look around and find someone far worse off than ourselves. Carol and I were very thankful we were not struggling with each other's problems. There is a reason for this. God allows only what we can handle to enter our life. It is all in His plans. Having the perception our problem is easy compared to others, helps us hold onto hope. Thankfully, we all view life through a different set of lenses.

T HE NIGHT I learned of my need for surgery, I called my parents. I spoke with my mother first, and told her what I had learned at the doctor's office. She must have been in shock. She replied, "Oh really." She asked a few basic questions, "When will this happen? Who is the doctor?" demonstrating no emotion whatsoever. I did not know what to make of her response. Maybe she had put herself in the "this is not me" mode, as I had done when I first listened to Dr. Cilluffo. Then again, this might have been her "be strong" mode.

I laid awake all night. My mind would not stop thinking of having my head cut open. How could I ever trust this doctor? I had met him only once. How could I place my life, my brain, in his hands? I ran through all the worst possible scenarios. I envisioned how my life would change, all the while feeling so alone in my fear. My husband was sound asleep. How could he sleep? How could he not care? This was hardly like going to the dentist. I needed to talk to someone, so I began to pray.

"God, this seems like an awfully big load to carry. I trust You. I have faith You know what You are doing. I can accept the apparent unfairness of this life, knowing You will even things out in heaven. Please help me to recognize the reasons for this to be happening, and be willing to follow Your ways, fulfilling Your plans. I can do all things with You who strengthens me. I prayed many years ago that if a member of my family must be faced with a major health challenge, that it would be me. I wanted You to choose me to face that challenge. Now it is time. You have indeed answered my prayer, keeping my family healthy, and helping me prepare. So please let me walk Your path with courage and peace."

I had just read a Bible verse that morning, before going to work and to Dr. Cilluffo's office, "You will keep in perfect peace him whose mind is steadfast, because he trusts in you. Trust in the Lord forever, for the Lord, the Lord, is the Rock eternal." (Isaiah 26:3 NIV) Tonight I needed my Rock. I felt so alone. Then I remembered one of my many favorite verses, "Lo I am with you alway, even unto the end of the world." (Matt. 28:20 KJV)

I believe I was somewhat prepared for this tragedy. As I said in my prayer, when I was ten years old, I prayed for God to give the tragic challenge to me, if it were to happen in my family. I would sit by the campfire and imagine what it would be like to suffer, whether it was from a terminal illness or disabling injury. I tried to foresee what my life would be like if I were disabled, and how I would respond.

During this period in my life, I read a book about the story of Jill Kinmont, *The Other Side of the Mountain*. She became a quadriplegic from a skiing accident. The story describes her life and how she handled adversity, as well as how friends and family supported her. I often wondered how my family would handle something like this. I prayed if it were to happen, "Here I am. Send me." (Isaiah 6:8 NIV)

I watched the Muscular Dystrophy and Easter Seals telethons, paying close attention to the up close and personal features. The stories of survivors of challenges inspired me. It was moving to hear how they persevered and to listen to their testimony of faith and hope.

After watching these telethons, I wrote motivational speeches, that I imagined myself giving. Someday I wanted to use whatever challenges and talents God gave me to help others, and to inspire others as many had inspired me. This was all at the age of ten.

Looking back at this time in my life, I can see how God was preparing me for my head injury. He answered my prayers to spare my family from a personal tragedy of their own, but this did not spare them from suffering. In the innocence of my youth I had not considered how suffering occurs to those surrounding the injured. I do not believe we can judge who suffers more. God only knows. I recognize their pain as being equal, if not more, than mine. This was yet another learning experience added to my collection, changing my perceptions for the future.

In the midst of my pain, I sought to lessen the suffering of those around me, knowing their pain was heart-wrenching. It became essential for me to help others feel the comfort of God's everlasting love. Being a good example was an optimal way to lead others to Christ.

My injury may have been inevitable, but He was certainly going to make sure I was prepared, giving me the essential tools to use my injury in a positive way. He had a plan from the very beginning.

"For my thoughts are not your thoughts, neither are your ways my ways," declares the Lord. "As the heavens are higher than the earth, so are my ways higher than your ways and my thoughts than your thoughts." (Isaiah 55:8-9 NIV)

Our acceptance of this plan is a demonstration of our faithfulness to Him. I pray often, "Thy will be done," but in addition to this I pray, "Please Lord, let Thy will become my will." In other words, let me accept what my Lord is giving to me as if it were my own will.

Ten

Dancing On Lemon Drops

When we quiet the mind,
the symphony begins.

ANONYMOUS

AFTER A LONG WEEKEND of anticipation, I arrived at the hospital on Monday morning, for the myelogram that Dr. Cilluffo had ordered. For this test, the doctor does a lumbar puncture: inserts a needle into the spine between vertebrae and takes out a small amount of cerebrospinal fluid (CSF). This is followed by the injection of a dye, Metrizamide, into the spinal fluid. The dye can be seen on a CT scan.

Most of my anxiety stemmed from knowing my father's hurtful experience in having a myelogram for a back injury. He had an extremely bad headache after his test, caused by the dye they injected into the CSF. He said they kept his head elevated, so the dye wouldn't flow into his head and cause a headache or other complications. For my test, however, they had to tip me at an angle so that my head was below the rest of my body. In order to detect my CSF leak, it was necessary for the dye to go into my head. I wasn't looking forward to this.

The spinal tap was performed by Ed Stilwill, M.D., a Radiologist at Munson Medical Center. Once the dye was injected, they tipped the head of the table down. I immediately began leaking fluid out of my nose. At least, I thought, they should get an accurate picture of where the fluid was coming from.

After the first series of CT scans, they left me in the hallway of Radiology, laying on my stomach, still positioned with my head down. Ronna came down from her office to keep me company. We talked about the test and what it was designed to do. Other employees of Munson, who I knew, saw me and wanted to know why I was having more tests. I tried to keep my replies as simple as possible, but as complications arose, it was getting increasingly difficult.

Dr. Stilwill attempted to describe what he was seeing in the scans. It didn't sound good. He said it was difficult for him to see a specific location of the leak. So, he would take thinner slices of the CT scan, to try to isolate it more. After everything was completed, he would give the results to Dr. Cilluffo.

Meanwhile, I was moved to a patient room on the Southwest II floor. The nurses began instructing me on the post lumbar puncture protocol. First, in order to get the dye out of my head, I was to remain at a forty-five degree angle, with my head elevated. This was required for twelve hours. I wouldn't be allowed to get out of bed. For someone who is used to moving vigorously and often, this was a tough task.

It was not, however, half as tough as using the bedpan. To help flush the dye out of my system, the nurses had me drink several huge glasses of water. It worked immediately. My bladder filled almost to the point of bursting, yet I could not use the bedpan. We tried every trick in the book, running the water in the sink and resting my fingers in a pan of water, without success. Eventually, I had to concentrate very hard on visualizing myself sitting on a toilet, while listening to the running water in the sink. At last, I had success and relief. I was not a happy camper having to use the bedpan.

The next day, Dr. Cilluffo came into my room and said the test had not been conclusive. He decided, however, to first put a lumbar-peritoneal shunt in me. His hopes were that, even though it had been over three years since the onset of the CSF leak, the shunt would lower the pressure enough to stop the leak. His theory was that as long as CSF was running through my skull fractures, the bone would not calcify. Like a river creating its own damn, it would not close with elevated pressure. In fact, the longer the CSF was allowed to move through this area, the wider the crack in the skull's fractures would become.

I had to ask him to back up a little in his explanation. Did I hear the words skull fractures? "Yes," he said, "there were two fractures at the base of my skull that were not detected before. This was the area where the fluid was finding its way into my sinuses and out my nose. There also was a tear in the dura, which lines the skull surrounding the brain."

This was déjà vu. Again I was being told information that demonstrated a greater severity of head injury (similar to when I first developed seizures and when I was told about my fractured tooth). Why was it that the severity of these discoveries was increasing? Logic said it should be the other way around.

Dr. Cilluffo said the lumbar shunt was a shot in the dark. The chances of it working, after having a leak for three years was very slim; but worth the effort given the alternative, brain surgery. Although I was willing to try this less-invasive method, I wanted a second opinion.

I asked Dr. MacKenzie for advice. He suggested I see Chris Scheiberger, M.D., another neurosurgeon in the Traverse City area.

I made an appointment to see Dr. Scheiberger a few days later. Dr. Scheiberger was very nice. He looked at my CT scans and told Jerry and I a story about a person who had a CSF leak, which he had repaired. The man had been in an airplane crash and shattered his skull. Dr. Scheiberger had to perform multiple surgeries before he was finally able to stop the leak.

He then asked me if I could produce the fluid. I very confidently bent over and straightened up, filling the palm of my hand with fluid. Dr. Scheiberger's eyes got as big as saucers. He could not believe what he saw. Even the man who had shattered his skull couldn't produce fluid like this.

This provoked a great deal of anxiety in me. I had shown this to four doctors, and every one of them said they had never seen anything like it. I felt as if I was on the down side of my roller coaster, picking up speed, and unable to get off.

Dr. Scheiberger's recommendation was similar to Dr. Cilluffo's. He would do a craniotomy, but unlike Dr. Cilluffo, he wouldn't waste time putting in a shunt. In his opinion the shunt wouldn't help at all.

I did further investigation by talking again with Dr. Zimmerman's nurse, Annelle Kasper, R.N. She had seen the work of all three neurosurgeons at Munson. I respected her advice. In her opinion, Dr. Cilluffo was the expert on head trauma, while Dr. Scheiberger was the expert on backs. She said both neurosurgeons were excellent, and that I was in good hands with Dr. Cilluffo.

So, despite Dr. Scheiberger's recommendation, I decided to go ahead and allow Dr. Cilluffo to put in the lumbar shunt. I figured it was worth a try, since it was so much less-invasive than brain surgery. Even if there was only a one percent chance of it working, I was willing to give it a shot. Then I prayed it would be the only surgery Dr. Cilluffo needed to do.

The shunt surgery was scheduled for ten days later. This gave me some time to get things done at work, in case I was laid up for awhile.

Two days after I was discharged for the myelogram, my mother called to say my grandfather was going in for emergency surgery. When he was being discharged from the hospital, they found his blood pressure plummeting. He was bleeding internally from an ulcer that had perforated his stomach and a major artery.

Jerry and I quickly prepared for the three-hour drive to Flint by throwing our clothes in both cars and arranging for Kathy to take care of our dog, Akita. Although it was difficult to accept, we needed to recognize this trip could be leading us to grandfather's funeral. We briefly discussed our need for good clothes and the need to drive two cars, in case Jerry would have to return to work before me.

During the entire drive my mind was on Grandpa. I truly did not know if I'd see him on this earth again. My fear was that we would arrive too late. I prayed for hours, while driving and crying. Several miles passed without notice, as my thoughts were elsewhere. In spirit I was at Grandpa's side, while worrying of what I'd feel if he died. I wondered how I'd grieve his death and for how long. I envisioned him being in heaven with my grandmother, happier than he had been since her death.

As I drove down the highway alone, I spoke out loud, saying what I'd express if I were giving his eulogy. I could not help but think of my own closeness to death and what I'd feel if I were in heaven with Grandpa soon.

Suddenly, in the face of his death, my medical disaster was not important. Everything falls into perspective when confronted with a loved one's mortality.

My grandfather was a very important man in my life. We had a very special bond. I loved to sit and listen to his stories of growing up in Traverse City. Even though I grew up in Flint, where Grandpa lived most of his life, I had coincidently moved to Traverse City, the home of my ancestors.

Grandpa was a storyteller. I was fascinated by his thoughts, while it warmed my heart to see the excitement in Grandpa's eyes when he told these stories and reminisced. He had a very distinct mischievous grin, which I will never forget.

We were told to go to Grandpa's house first, where my parents, aunt, and uncle were staying. My heart was in my throat when we arrived, not knowing what we'd learn about Grandpa. I knew my prayers had been answered when Mom said, "Grandpa made it through surgery."

My first words were, "Thank-you, God."

My reunion with Mom and Dad was comforting. I hadn't seen or talked with them in over three months. It is a blessing how insignificant issues disappear when critical circumstances arise. It felt so good to be with them. I had missed them so much.

We went to the hospital to see Grandpa, who was still in the Intensive Care Unit (ICU). With his eyes still shut, Mom said to him, "Pop, I brought someone here to see you."

I said, "Hi, Grandpa."

Although his eyes were closed, he immediately knew who I was and said, "Karen, how are you?"

Mom and Dad had been telling him about my doctors' appointments. It was so typical of Grandpa to be fighting for his life and yet be concerned about me. My heart filled with emotion, seeing him like this. He looked so frail and weak. He was on oxygen and it was difficult to understand his words from under his mask. He was still a handsome man in every way. Beauty lies within the heart.

On the day after his surgery, Grandpa's mouth was very dry. He was off the oxygen mask and wanted a piece of his favorite hard candy, a lemon drop. I asked the nurse if he could have something like this. She said yes. To the gift shop I went, to find lemon drops. When I returned to Grandpa, he was very excited to have such a treasure.

He was flat on his back, minus his false teeth. I popped a lemon drop into his mouth, without thinking of how he'd manage it without teeth. It immediately went down the back of his throat and he started to choke. Given my medical training, I knew exactly what to do. I flipped Grandpa over on his side, while striking his back. I shouted, "Spit it out, Grandpa! Spit it out!" Out it came. I sighed a huge sigh of relief and thought to myself, "I can see it now in the papers, 'Granddaughter Kills Grandfather With Lemon Drop.'"

Grandpa was fine, but he still wanted a lemon drop. We discussed how we were going to do this. I thought I could hold the lemon drop under his tongue with my finger, until he felt it and got a grip on it. This might be safer.

He was ready. I was nervous. I placed it under his tongue and asked him if he was ready. He nodded yes. I let it go. Sure enough, it went straight down the back of his throat again. We had a repeat performance. I whipped him on his side, slapped him on the back and shouted, "Spit it out, Grandpa! Spit it out!"

Out it came. We both began to laugh. Grandpa said, with his mischievous grin, "We didn't do so well did we?"

These moments were priceless. Despite the danger, we danced. It was as though we were arm-in-arm, dancing on lemon drops and giggling the entire time.

Grandpa was moved to a regular floor the following day, making it easier for us to visit him. I was able to sit on his bed and listen to more fun stories. I held his hand and he held mine.

My sister, Kay, arrived from Atlanta, Georgia. It was a big relief for her to see Grandpa and to spend time with him. I felt very fortunate to have lived so close to Grandpa and to build a bond with him over the previous eight years.

Every moment of my time with Grandpa was very valuable. I realized these could be my last days with Grandpa before he died. His condition was not improving. Five days after having arrived in Flint, wondering if he was still alive, I had to return to Traverse City. I wanted to stay with Grandpa as long as possible, but it was impossible to know what the future held for him.

Saying good-bye to Grandpa was the hardest thing I had ever done in my life. While you never really know if it is going to be the last time you see someone, I felt quite certain this was our last good-bye.

I stayed in his room as long as I could, in tears and not wanting him to see them. I could not bring myself to say good-bye. My feelings were going rampant on me. What would I ever do without Grandpa? It would truly be a piece of me that left this earth. How long would I have to wait to see him in heaven again? It was selfish of me to want Grandpa to stay here, on earth. He was suffering and would be happier in heaven with Grandma. I needed to pray for what was best for Grandpa, not for me.

I still could not convince myself to say good-bye. This was not a typical, "Good-bye, I will see you tomorrow." This was, "Good-bye, Grandpa. My life with you has been most memorable. I will remember you always. You will forever live in my heart. I'll see you when I get to heaven, too."

Even as I write this many years later, tears fill my eyes and my heart moves into my throat. This may be why we have the saying, "This is a tough one to swallow." Sometimes the lump in your throat created by sadness, seems as big as a softball, and it is tough to swallow. So instead of good-bye, I opted to say, "I love you Grandpa. I'll see you again, soon."

I walked out of his room and sobbed. Feelings I never knew existed flooded me. Nothing else mattered. The world could spin without me for all I cared. Life without Grandpa would leave a major void in my life. He filled a major piece of my heart. I was overwhelmed with emotion. It seemed as though the roller coaster was picking up speed and heading for a deep dark hole. I had no idea what was next.

It seemed enough to deal with my health problems, and to add my grandfather's death on top of this, made it feel as though my plate was heaped very high. I said to myself, over and over again, "God won't give me any more than He and I can handle." I trusted Him, but began doubting myself. I knew God would do His part. I had no idea what in the world was my part. So I began to listen more, paying attention to the incidentals around me.

Prayer is not just one way communication. God answers each and every prayer, not always in the exact way we'd like, but we can be assured they are answered. Answers come in many forms, a thought running through our head, an incident which isn't a coincidence but a Godincidence, or maybe a rainbow in the sky. It's our responsibility to watch and listen.

Too often our minds are running ninety miles per hour and there's no room for us to take information into our brains. There are too many distractions, not only for the injured brain, but for the uninjured as well. God speaks to us daily. I needed to slow down, shut up, and pay attention. Our brain is like an orchestra. When we are quiet we will hear the symphony.

W HILE MY PARENTS had been spending most of their time in Flint with my grandfather, they came to Traverse City the night before my shunt surgery. It felt good to have them with me. I didn't know what to expect from the surgery. I was most worried about having a foreign object permanently placed in my body. I wondered how my body would respond to the shunt, and how it would make me feel. The doctors assured me I wouldn't even know it was there.

The surgery took only one-and-a-half hours. It went as planned. I woke up in recovery to the voice of my friend Steve Hall, R.N., a recovery room nurse. He took me back to my room. I was told to lay flat for twelve hours, before they'd slowly elevate the head of my bed. This enabled me to gradually become used to the change in CSF pressure and reduce the chance of increasing the intensity of my already fierce headache.

I didn't think it was possible for my headache to get worse. I was wrong. I became very impatient during the twelve hours I had to lay flat. I was uncomfortable, simply because of my inability to move around. I had minimal pain, a moderate headache, and soreness in my back, where the shunt originates. That is, until they started elevating the head of my bed.

At this stage of post-op, I might have chosen to lay flat for the rest of my life—if it was an option (and reasonable). As gravity began lowering the spinal fluid pressure in my head, my headache increased dramatically. My pressure had been low, because of the continuous leak of fluid and the reduction of CSF volume. More fluid would now be drained out of my head through the lumbar shunt, creating an even lower pressure.

The pain in my head was unlike any pain I had ever experienced. Until this point, I thought I had become quite tolerant of my headaches. Initially, I could endure less than one minute of having my head above my body. This was not even long enough to drink from a glass, let alone use the rest room.

I knew I was in for a major problem since it was virtually impossible for me to urinate in a bedpan while laying flat. The only way I could urinate was to lift my torso to a sitting position and then tilt my head back as far as my neck would allow. If I could get my head close to a horizontal position, putting CSF back in my head, then I could be up long enough to relieve my bladder. It took every ounce of energy I had. As the hours passed, I found myself getting more exhausted.

Dr. Cilluffo came in to check on me. He wanted to see if I was still leaking CSF. He asked me to sit on the edge of the bed and bend over to see if fluid poured out of my nose. When he requested this I thought I was going to die. I could not imagine myself being able to tolerate the pain this would cause. If I could barely tolerate being upright for one minute, what was it going to feel like to bend forward?

I braced myself for the pain, but an amazing discovery occurred. When I bent over the pain disappeared, just like it did when I laid flat. This was because spinal fluid flowed back in my head in both positions. This discovery helped ease my pain and anxiety during future maneuvers. I always knew if I tilted my head forward or backwards, I could instantly relieve the pain. So what used to be my major challenge during the day, moving to and from the rest room, was not nearly as painful. As long as I kept my head down, it was tolerable.

The first time I bent over for Dr. Cilluffo, fluid did not come out my nose. We both became prematurely excited. He requested a second trial test. Disappointingly, fluid came flowing from my nose, just as it had before shunt surgery. I was amazed that he expected such quick results. He said, "If it is going to work, we'd know right away."

Although I had not put my hopes too high, I was still disappointed. If this had worked, it would have eliminated my need for a craniotomy. Immediately upon seeing the fluid, all hopes were dashed. The road ahead of me looked very long. In fact, it looked endless.

Dr. Cilluffo immediately started talking about how he'd repair the leak with more surgery. He said there was a chance it could be repaired by going through my nose and mouth. This was music to my ears. I'd do anything to avoid having someone cut into my skull. Again, I had to be cautious in getting my hopes up too high. He said he needed to go back down to Radiology to look at the films of my myelogram. He needed to look more closely at the location of the skull fractures. Then he'd be more capable of determining if it was an area that could be reached with a nose and mouth approach.

He returned within the half hour and again shattered my hopes of not having a craniotomy. He had too many doubts about being able to successfully repair it with this less-invasive method. The location of the skull fractures was too far back in my skull to be reached through my mouth. He was not ruling out the possibility, but said it was very unlikely he could make the repairs with this method. He suggested I go to Petoskey (a town sixty miles to the north) to see Dr. Bech, an Otynlarygologist who assisted him in this type of surgery.

After making this referral, Dr. Cilluffo proceeded to talk about a craniotomy and how he'd perform it. This time, I was capable of hearing the information and even asking questions. He spoke more of the specifics of the surgery, describing how he'd take the tissue from my stomach and lay it inside the base of my skull.

He was very concerned about saving my sense of smell, stating how important it was for me to be able to smell. He thought he might be able to save this sense, and impressed upon me the magnitude of losses from severing the olfactory nerve.

He described how he'd use plates to secure my skull back in place. Because of my active life-style, he'd place three plates across the seam of my skull to reinforce the bone.

He discharged me the day after my shunt surgery. I was feeling relatively okay and was eager to get home. Before leaving the hospital, I called Dr. Bech's office in Petoskey to schedule an appointment. I could not believe it was going to take another week before I'd be able to see him.

Everything felt as though it were taking forever. At this stage, I wanted everything to be over as quickly as possible.

This was the beginning of a long process, where it took weeks and sometimes months to see the next doctor or have the next test. Waiting is difficult, even for the most patient individual, and I am not one. The saying goes, "Patience is a virtue." It most certainly is and I commend those who exemplify patience in the most trying times. I started this journey with less than adequate patience. Now I rank my patience in the top one percent of all those I know. It's remarkable how we learn lessons, changing our entire outlook on life.

Jerry picked me up from the hospital and we were home before noon. I went straight to bed. The ride home unpleasant. I started to feel very sick to my stomach and my headache dramatically increased in intensity.

I was not in bed long before I ran to the bathroom and heaved my lunch. While the immediate effect was one of relief, it was not long before I wished someone would put me out of my misery. Every ten minutes I was vomiting, until it turned into the dry heaves. I am not quite sure what was worse. I did know one thing. Something was definitely wrong and we needed to get back to the hospital as soon as possible.

Jerry drove me to the Emergency Room, where they immediately hooked me up to an IV. The ER doctor took the necessary information, and then tried to get in touch with Dr. Cilluffo. He was no longer in the hospital, so Dr. Stafford was called. He came to the ER and examined me. When he lifted up my shirt and started pushing on my abdomen, where the shunt was attached, he found an amazing thing: air had filled my abdomen. We could hear it gush and crackle as he pressed on me. It went all the way up to my armpit. First, Dr. Stafford questioned if this had always been there, even though he was certain it had not. He did not tell me what he thought it was. Instead, he went into the office to discuss it with the ER doctors.

My nausea had subsided with the medication they had given me when I first arrived in the ER. Now I was waiting to find out what would happen next.

Carl Benner, M.D. was called to examine me. I suddenly realized this might be serious. From working at the hospital, I knew the specialty and expertise of all the physicians. Dr. Benner was a general surgeon who happened to also be the hospital's Vice President and Chief of Staff.

Dr. Benner examined me, also pushing on the pockets of air in my abdomen. He reviewed the x-rays that were hanging at the foot of my stretcher. We discussed the shunt surgery and the possibility that the shunt perforated my bowel. While looking at the x-rays, he said it did not appear as though it had, but the symptoms were indicating it had. He said he'd continue to watch me for a few days, while I was in the hospital, to see how I progressed.

I was comforted by the fact that Dr. Benner was taking care of me. He is an excellent physician and very personable. I always had a great deal of admiration for him.

Dr. Cilluffo arrived in the ER shortly after Dr. Benner left. Upon hearing that Dr. Benner was on the case and that they suspected a perforated bowel, Dr. Cilluffo became very defensive. He was most certain he had not perforated the bowel and seemed very angry that anyone had suggested this. I was just the patient. I tried my hardest to stay out of it. I didn't need any of these physicians angry with me. I was at the mercy of their care.

The next six days after being readmitted to the hospital were unbelievable. I could not imagine why I felt so bad, after having felt halfway descent after the surgery. Something must have happened with the shunt, but none of us knew what.

Less than one year later, I would learn that the shunt had completely pulled out of my spine and was dysfunctional. I suspect it happened when I was vomiting at home. The air in my abdomen was probably from a backup of air from vomiting. Air probably went through the leak in my head from the strain of vomiting, and then traveled through my shunt and into the peritoneum, where the shunt empties. The shunt then must have pulled out of my spine from the strain of vomiting and bending over, and thus, produced a spinal fluid leak in my spine as well. This precipitated a horrendous headache over the next six days. The only comfortable position was laying flat or bending my head forward.

Dr. Cilluffo kept saying I'd get used to the headache. I thought he was crazy, but eventually I did. Dr. Benner eventually concluded my bowel had not been perforated. Dr. Cilluffo said everything short of, "I told you so."

With each day that I could not move any farther than the bathroom, I prayed nothing would happen to Grandpa while I was so incapacitated. I could not imagine how I'd manage to go to his funeral, but knew I would never miss it. Even if on my death bed, I would be there. The way I felt, it felt pretty close to a death bed.

It also worked out perfectly for Dr. Bech's appointment to be the following week. Had it been scheduled closer to my first discharge, I wouldn't have been able to see him. As it turned out, I was discharged the day before my appointment.

Eleven

The Run Around

May you live all the days of your life.
JONATHAN SWIFT

THE DAY AFTER I was discharged, Jerry and I traveled to Petoskey to see Dr. Bech, at Burns Clinic. I was not yet used to the CSF pressure change in my head. Prior to the shunt, I didn't think my headache could get any worse. I was wrong. Now that the CSF freely leaked out of my lower spine and skull, the pressure was so low that the pain was only tolerable when I laid down. As long as gravity couldn't push the fluid out, either way, more fluid remained in my head and I was significantly more comfortable. So, I laid in the back of the van during the sixty mile journey.

By the time we arrived at Dr. Bech's office I was quite uncomfortable. Dr. Bech entered the examining room and immediately asked how we knew it was a CSF leak. I did not have any proof, except for the fact that I could bend over and fluid would run out of my nose. Again, it was only a suspicion of the physicians who had seen it.

Before he would commit himself to surgery of any kind, Dr. Bech wanted proof. From what I gathered, he was not confident that a leak of this nature could be stopped by an approach through the mouth and nose. He asked if anyone had tested the fluid to verify it was CSF. No one had. He then requested I collect some of the fluid in a test tube, while I was in his office. I was able to pour a sufficient amount into a tube before leaving.

When I returned to Traverse City, Dr. MacKenzie recommended we do a fluid test at Munson Medical Center, just to make sure it was spinal fluid. I again collected fluid, and dropped it off at Munson's laboratory.

I saw Dr. Cilluffo a few days later. He had spoken with Dr. Bech, and they had decided in order to stop the leak, I would need to have a craniotomy.

Dr. MacKenzie, however, recommended I get a second opinion from a neurosurgeon outside the Traverse City area. I agreed. I would feel more comfortable going into surgery having had another physician confirm my need for a craniotomy. It would feel even better if another physician would say I did not need one at all, although I knew this was pretty unlikely.

I decided to be very open with Dr. Cilluffo. I told him of my desire for a second opinion. He also agreed it was a wise decision, and even suggested a neurosurgeon, Fred Meyer, M.D., at the Mayo Clinic, with whom he had a great deal of respect.

I was not able to schedule an appointment at the Mayo Clinic for another four weeks, so in the meantime Dr. Cilluffo decide he wanted to repeat the myelogram with metrizamide. I had described to him the technique Radiology used to perform the first myelogram, questioning why they hadn't scanned me when my head was positioned downward. We both agreed the test might be more successful if I was scanned in the position I leaked. Dr. Cilluffo said he would come to Radiology himself, to ensure the test was performed correctly.

Dr. Stilwill seemed very upset that I had returned for a second myelogram. It was obvious he didn't like anyone doubting his testing methods or accuracy. Therefore, he was very brief in our discussion and not nearly as friendly as he was during the first test. When I asked Dr. Stilwill about his method of scanning, he was very defensive. Unfortunately, Dr. Cilluffo failed to appear in Radiology, so the test was performed the exact same way it was performed the first time. The results were, again, inconclusive.

THE WEEK FOLLOWING my discharge from Munson Medical Center, after having shunt surgery, I gradually became more tolerant of my CSF pressure. The leak in my lower back, from the shunt pulling out, must have sealed itself. Now my thoughts were on Mayo Clinic and my grandfather.

On November 7, 1992, I awoke at 7:00 a.m., looked at the clock, closed my eyes again, and fell back to sleep. In my dream I heard the phone ring. I answered it. A woman said, "Karen, this is Greta Cummings. I don't have good news." I awoke again and looked at the clock. It was 7:13 a.m. I knew something had happened or was going to happen to my grandfather.

I began to cry. Jerry was sleeping, until my crying awoke him. He asked what was wrong. I told him what I had dreamt. Even though I sensed he thought this was crazy, he held me while I cried. I got out of bed shortly thereafter, and tried to distract myself until I could call my parents in Flint.

I began digging out pictures of Grandpa and our family. I found a wonderful picture of him I had taken while in Florida for Christmas. For some reason I decided I would give this picture to my entire family at Grandpa's funeral. My intuition told me I would not have enough time to get reprints developed, so I began taking pictures of the snapshot. I did not use a tripod. I simply started clicking away, trying to focus and hold the camera as steady as possible. In the back of my mind I kept thinking these would never turn out, considering the haphazard way that I was taking them.

All day I wore a button with Grandpa's picture on it, pinned to my shirt. (We had worn the buttons at Grandpa's 80th birthday party.) I wanted to feel as close to him as I possibly could. I sat and daydreamed of my time with Grandpa and the stories he so enjoyed telling.

Shortly after I finished taking my pictures, my mother called. At the sound of her voice, I began trembling. I was afraid of what she was about to tell me, fearing she didn't have good news. Her first words were, "Karen, I don't have good news. Grandpa's still with us, but things don't look very promising."

Subsequent to Mom and Dad returning to Flint after my surgery, Grandpa had another emergency surgery. Although he suffered terribly, when Mom told him, "I am going to call Karen today," he opened his eyes for the first time since his surgery.

He said, "How is she?" He kept asking if I was going to need another operation. He was so weak, yet he worried about me.

As she continued to speak, my memories overshadowed her words. All I could think of was the precious time I had spent with Grandpa three weeks ago. I recalled how he had cracked jokes, laughed, and showed me his famous mischievous grin, just one more time. I had told him I loved him and he had told me he loved me, as he squeezed my hand tight. I could see us with ice chips, lemon drops, and his wave as I left his room, as if he always knew I would turn and look, one last time.

While still on the phone with Mom, my mind refocused on our conversation. I told her about my dream. Then I asked her to do me a favor. I said, "Please tell Grandpa, 'I'm strong because you are strong Grandpa. I'll be okay. I love you.'"

My mother had no idea what these words meant. It was my secret reminder to Grandpa of a conversation we had several years earlier. Grandpa and I were having dinner together, talking about how hard life was without Grandma. Grandpa had been extremely lonely since her death. I said to Grandpa, "It will be very lonely here without you, Grandpa. I don't know what I will do. But, I know when the time comes, I'll be okay. I can be strong, just like you have been."

After we got off the phone, my mother relayed this message to Grandpa. Despite not having said many words on this day, he turned to Mom and said, "Yes." He knew it was okay. It was time to let go. Grandpa could die in peace. I had been prepared. It was okay.

I took the roll of film to a one hour photo shop. When I picked them up, much to my surprise, they had turned out beautifully. Every one of them was perfect.

As soon as I arrived home, after picking up the photos, my phone rang. It was Mom. I sat down on the couch, with Grandpa's pictures in hand. She told me Grandpa had just passed away. No matter how prepared you think you are, it is still a shock to lose someone so close. I thought I had shed all the tears I needed to that morning. I was wrong. There were many more to come.

Each time I think of Grandpa and the memories we shared, tears flood my eyes. These are priceless memories, that will forever bring him close in mind and heart. I know I will see Grandpa again, and it will probably be sooner than I imagine. It is a comfort to know he is with our Heavenly Father, and no longer lonely or in pain. His funeral was indeed a celebration of his life. He was a wonderful man. Grandpa truly lived every day of his life.

While grieving Grandpa's death, I felt as though I received a message from him several days after he died. My parents were going through his house, sorting his belongings and preparing for an estate sale. They opened the large metal safe, that sat in Grandma and Grandpa's garage for as long as I could remember. Grandpa put all his valuables in the safe. Amongst the items, Mom and Dad found a letter addressed to Grandpa from me. It was dated a few days after Grandma had died. In the letter, I shared my sadness of losing Grandma, and also my sympathy for the grief he was enduring. I could tell he was heartbroken, after having been married sixty-five years. I wanted him to know how much I loved him, and also to reassure him that we would be with Grandma in heaven someday.

To have found this letter in his safe was such a gift. It said to me, "I love you Karen. This letter meant a lot to me, just as you mean the world to me. Thank you for being such a wonderful granddaughter." This was not a coincidence. Grandpa put it there for us to find after he died. God was conducting a symphony of support for me during this difficult time. I knew when I saw the letter, Grandpa was looking down at me from heaven, smiling mischievously.

ONCE DECEMBER ROLLED around, I was extremely anxious to go to the Mayo Clinic, as I had heard it was an exceptional medical institution. I was scheduled to see two doctors, Fred Meyer, M.D., Neurosurgeon, and John McCaffery, M.D., Otynlaryngologist.

We flew into Rochester, Minnesota the day before I had my appointments. We settled in for what we anticipated would be a week-long stay. The Howard Johnson's motel shuttle picked us up at the airport. The shuttle was convenient. If we wanted to go shopping, they took us shopping. If we wanted to go to a restaurant, the shuttle took us. The motel certainly made its Mayo Clinic patients/guests very comfortable. (All of these little things add up when you are in an unfamiliar area for an unpleasant reason.)

When we walked into the Mayo Clinic, both Jerry and I were in awe of the facility. It was huge. I registered at the front desk. They gave me a small pocket folder as an identification. We had time to spare before my first appointment, so we wandered around and explored the layout of the clinic.

We were fascinated by the subways under the clinic. How could this place be so big? It seemed like Rochester itself was not that big. As it turned out, the subways were not what we would consider subways. They were not tunnels for motorized trains. They were actually my kind of subway, where people must use their own motors to walk from place to place. They were simply tunnels that connected the parking garage, Rochester Methodist Hospital, a shopping mall, and a hotel (for the convenience of patients wanting to pay the extra expense of staying within a short walking distance to the clinic).

Ten minutes prior to my scheduled appointment, we ventured upstairs to Dr. McCaffery's office. To our amazement, the waiting room was the size of an auditorium. I walked up to the desk and gave the receptionist my MRIs and CT scan films. It was a relief to hand these over, since they weighed nearly twenty pounds. I had been guarding them with my life since leaving Traverse City. I didn't see too many other people walking around with quite as many films under their arms. My stack was at least three inches thick.

We sat down in the waiting area, along with at least one hundred other patients and family members. I was shocked when I heard patient names announced over a loud speaker, typically five at a time. Ten or more people would then gather near the announcer, who would then escort them away, seemingly never to be seen again.

With great anticipation, we waited for my name to be called. One hour went by, and we were still waiting. It was almost past the second hour, when finally, my name was announced. Jerry and I gathered with the other people who had been called. We followed the leader, like in kindergarten.

I was expecting to be placed in an exam room; instead I was told to sit in another waiting area. We sat for another forty-five minutes before we were lead to an exam room. My anxiety was at its peak. I had used every bit of patience during our extended wait. By this time I was expecting to see God walk into the room. Instead, Dr. McCaffery walked in.

It didn't take long before I wished I had taped all my previous conversations with doctors I had met thus far. I began repeating my medical history. Then Dr. McCaffery asked the big question, "Can you bend over and produce the fluid?"

During the two weeks prior to coming to the Mayo Clinic I had a cold. Unfortunately, during this time, fluid didn't flow as easily out of my nose. I was too stuffed up. I doubted the leak had stopped, though I prayed it had. Before bending over I explained this to Dr. McCaffery. I was unsuccessful in producing fluid.

He continued to examine me (he, too, had a handy dandy eight-inch steel rod). He was very gentle in his approach, but not enough to prevent my eyes from watering. This was the first time Jerry had seen this type of exam. He had heard a very detailed description of it from me, but it was nothing like seeing it in person. His eyes watered, too.

Once Dr. McCaffery was finished with his examination, he told us that he tries to find the location of the leak by using fluorescein, a dye which is injected into the spinal fluid. He then scopes the patient and uses a black light to see where the Fluorescein comes through the walls of the sinuses. His last comment, however, before leaving the exam room was, "We're not going to see anything, though, if you can't produce the fluid."

Dr. Meyer was next. He came down to Dr. McCaffery's office to see me. Dr. Meyer was very prompt and he spent a reasonable amount of time with us. He agreed with Dr. Cilluffo, that a craniotomy was needed. He did not believe the leak could be stopped by approaching it through my mouth and nose, nor would he have performed the lumbar-peritoneal shunt. I told him he was accurate in his diagnosis, as my shunt was unsuccessful.

While I wished Dr. Meyer would have said my repair could be performed through my mouth, it was encouraging to have him agree with Dr. Cilluffo. It certainly increased my trust in Dr. Cilluffo. I had already accepted that surgery was imminent, it was just a matter of deciding how it would be done. The one thing that scared me was Dr. Meyer's comment, "I would not go into your head without knowing where the leak was located. You have to find the leak first." This was frightening, since two myelograms had come back inconclusive.

Dr. Cilluffo was ready to perform surgery and to look for the leak, since no one was successful in finding it through non-invasive methods. I liked Dr. McCaffery's recommendation, however, of using the Fluorescein and scope to find the leak first.

Dr. McCaffery returned to the exam room, after Dr. Meyer left. He wrapped things up by reviewing his conversation with Dr. Meyer. They both agreed there was a need to locate the leak. He wanted me to have a CT scan at the clinic later that day, but that would be the extent of testing.

As we walked out of the exam room and approached the front desk, Dr. McCaffery turned to me, handed me his business card, and rudely said, "Come back when you don't have a cold."

I was floored. Who would ever say anything like this, let alone a well-known surgeon from Mayo Clinic? While walking away, I said to Jerry, "He will never see me again." I was extremely disappointed in the Clinic, because of one physician.

I realized it was difficult for Dr. McCaffery to evaluate my leak when he couldn't see the fluid, however, I had waited five weeks and spent a lot of money to get to Mayo Clinic. Now, I was being told to simply come back when I didn't have a cold.

It's sad to think one impersonal physician could ruin my impression of an excellent medical facility. I tried to give Dr. McCaffery the benefit of the doubt. Maybe he'd had a bad day. Nevertheless, that was no reason to treat a patient, who happened to have had three years of bad days, so rudely. As I said, I didn't know what to expect from such a prestigious medical care clinic, but I had expected to be treated better than that.

After completing the CT scan, Jerry and I packed our bags, rearranged our flights, and returned home the next morning. While I was very discouraged by my interaction with Dr. McCaffery, I focused on my conversation with Dr. Meyer. He agreed with Dr. Cilluffo's recommendations, giving me more confidence. Since I preferred to have surgery at Munson, my second home, my mind was made up. I would have a craniotomy performed by Dr. Cilluffo.

THE DAY AFTER returning home from Rochester, I had an appointment with Dr. Cilluffo to discuss my decision. By this time, he had received the test results from the CSF collection. The results came back positive for protein and glucose, and negative for beta II transferin. Dr. Cilluffo said the typical tests for determining whether fluid is cerebral spinal fluid are protein and glucose. He did not know what the beta II transferin test was. He had never heard of it.

I thought it was very strange that a test was run that Dr. Cilluffo didn't know anything about. I had never heard of beta II transferin, either, but I was new at this game.

Dr. Cilluffo then stated, "I cannot justify doing a craniotomy on you to fix a leak I don't know the location of nor have the evidence to show it is definitely spinal fluid. I know you have a leak and it needs fixing, but until we have more evidence, I cannot perform the surgery. I could never justify the surgery to my colleagues."

I could not believe what I was hearing. What a roller coaster ride this was! It felt as though I had just crested a steep climb, prepared for the fall on the other side (the scheduling of brain surgery), but instead, the coaster took a sudden turn and whipped me around in another direction. My stomach flipped.

If I had any doubt that the fluid was CSF, the swing in events wouldn't have been so emotionally taxing. I would have welcomed hearing the words, "I cannot perform a craniotomy on you." Instead, I knew that the fluid was CSF, and I needed the leaks to be patched. Otherwise, I'd have to live with my intense headache and also risk further complications, which were life threatening. I never thought I'd be in a position to want a craniotomy. Maybe this was God's way of making sure I was ready.

I asked Dr. Cilluffo what I was supposed to do next. He didn't have an answer. I was frustrated. I could see he was frustrated. We both knew I had a leak, but because of liability and politics, he would not touch me.

Jerry and I walked out of his office. I was disappointed, and scared. What was going to happen next? Who would help me?

Jerry, being the analytical person that he is, said to me, "Wow, that is good news. You don't have to have surgery." He did not sense the effects this medical roller coaster was having on me. It hurt for him to say this, as it only reinforced how another aspect of my life was a roller coaster: my relationship with Jerry.

Upon arriving home, I immediately called Terry Whalen, Director of Munson's laboratory. I asked him what beta II transferin was. He explained it was something new they were using to test CSF, however, they did not perform the test at Munson. They sent the sample to the Mayo Clinic for testing. You can imagine what ran through my mind. I explained to him my test results, as well as how Dr. Cilluffo was so positive the fluid was CSF. I asked about the reliability of this test. Terry said he would be happy to call the Mayo Clinic laboratory to ask about the test and my specific results.

Terry called me back within ten minutes. He had talked with someone in the Mayo Clinic lab, who confirmed that although the test was new, it was more reliable than protein and glucose, because the only body fluid beta II transferin is found in is CSF. The lab technician offered to run the test again, and to report the results to Terry within three days.

Meanwhile, I tried to find out more about the beta II transferin test. I spoke with Dr. MacKenzie and asked if he had heard of this test. He had not. Norma Powers, Manager of Munson's Medical Education Department and Library did a literature search for me. She found some information on it. Again, her findings showed it was a brand new test; the most conclusive and reliable test for spinal fluid to date.

After learning this, I had mixed feelings. If this was the most reliable test, maybe my fluid was not CSF. (This would be wonderful.) On the other hand, I was not so sure that the Mayo Clinic was reliable in following test protocol. Since this was a new test, maybe they hadn't worked the bugs out yet. Their ratio of error could still be high. I did not want to get my hopes up prematurely.

Three days later, I received a call from Dr. MacKenzie. He said, "Karen, I just received another report from the Mayo Clinic. Your beta II transferin test was positive." My heart sunk. Here I go again. I had just fallen down the back side of the roller coaster and wasn't prepared for the peak waiting for me on the other side. It took me by complete surprise. It validated that this recovery process was not going to be typical or predictable. What could go wrong, would.

Dr. MacKenzie didn't know about my conversation with Terry, therefore he wondered why the test was done again. I explained that I had requested information from Terry. Dr. MacKenzie also had mixed feelings. I could sense his disappointment and uneasiness in having to tell me the results were positive. By this time, Dr. MacKenzie was riding the roller coaster with me. I could sense his devotion to helping me. We both knew what these results meant.

I called Dr. Cilluffo and told him to go ahead and schedule the surgery. There is nothing quite like "signing up for brain surgery." It was ten days before Christmas. Dr. Cilluffo would be on vacation until January 4, 1993. He scheduled my surgery for January 5.

I was able to half-heartedly enjoy Christmas. While it was difficult to keep my mind off of what was ahead of me, I also thought of it as a wonderful Christmas present. All I wanted for Christmas was to be headache-free.

To avoid the cold weather and snow, my parents usually move to Florida each October. This year they stayed in Michigan. Mom and Dad moved in with Jerry and I in mid-December. This made things a lot easier around the house. I was not in much of a mood for cooking and cleaning, and Mom always had endless energy for both of these tasks.

Part III

THE RUMBLE

Twelve

Number One

*Every experience in life, everything
with which we have come in contact in life,
is a chisel which has been cutting away
at our life statue, molding, modifying, shaping it.
We are part of all we have met.*

ORISON SWETT MARDEN

I T WAS A BRIGHT, sunny, and cold winter day. The snow was melting from the rooftops as people shoveled paths through the snow. After parking my car, I walked from the lot into the hospital. This time I wasn't entering as an employee, but as a patient; someone whose journey led to a very delicate and risky operation, a bifrontal craniotomy, brain surgery.

I couldn't help but consider the possibility that this Christmas was my last. As I made my way to the outpatient laboratory, Christmas music still played throughout many departments.

I needed to do an autologous blood donation. Although Dr. Cilluffo didn't think I would lose very much blood during surgery, it was a precaution.

Each of the preparatory steps I took made my impending brain surgery more real. It all seemed like a nightmare. I just needed to wake up.

During my last appointment with Dr. Cilluffo, we discussed the details of my surgery. This was my last opportunity to ask questions. He repeated the specifics of the surgery, how he'd make the incision from ear to ear and then cut my skull by drilling three holes. The holes were points for him to connect with his saw. Eventually, he would end up with a triangular-shaped piece of bone that he would remove. Dr. Cilluffo would then lift my brain up and backwards, away from the cribiform plate, the base of the skull. This would allow him to work under my brain and to make repairs. Then he would wire my skull back into place, using titanium plates. These would make the skull more secure, and prevent it from moving or sinking.

Dr. Cilluffo ended with a disclaimer, saying, "This is all I hope I will have to do. When I get in there, however, I might find surprises and need to do more. My biggest concern is to preserve your ability to smell. I think the leak is located very close to your olfactory nerve, and I might have to cut part of the nerve. Smell is very important in life. I want to make sure you are able to smell dirty diapers, when the time comes. But, I cannot guarantee that I can preserve this."

He went over the biggest risks involved with the surgery, namely meningitis and possible death. He assured me his mortality rate was very low. He said there was also a chance of blindness and permanent brain damage.

I surprised myself by not being as terribly anxious about the surgery as I thought I'd be. I had done everything in my power to investigate the options, and to learn about the damage and how it could be repaired. Theoretically, I had done my homework. Emotionally, I was doing my best. I was definitely nervous, but not deathly afraid.

I asked Dr. Cilluffo how long of a recovery he anticipated. He said I would be in the hospital approximately one week, and then be able to recover at home. I asked how long it would be until I could walk again. He felt confident I'd be back on my feet within two weeks of surgery, however, it depended on how well I came through the surgery. I was astonished. I anticipated at least six months of immobility.

I should have known better, considering my work in cardiac rehabilitation. After heart bypass surgery, it used to be patients were sent home to lie in bed for six months. Now, we get them up within a few days after surgery, and start them exercising to rehabilitate.

According to Dr. Cilluffo, I would only need rehabilitation if I suffered more brain damage from the surgery.

Dr. Cilluffo knew I had seen Dr. Scheiberger for a second opinion.

Therefore, he told me he would ask Dr. Scheiberger to assist him with my surgery. He said they normally helped each other out on the more difficult surgeries. I appreciated hearing this. It was comforting to know I would have two very experienced neurosurgeons working on me.

The surgery itself was expected to take approximately four hours. They would shave my head after I was put under anesthesia. I asked Dr. Cilluffo if he played music while performing surgery. He said yes. I thought it might help me if my favorite music was playing while I was under anesthesia, so I asked Dr. Cilluffo if he would play a tape of my music in the operating room. He looked surprised when I asked this.

"I always play my special music," he said. "I like instrumentals, especially piano players." I again asked if he would mind playing my tape. Finally, he conceded.

After leaving his office and thinking more about the music issue, I realized that, like myself, his music was very important to him. The more I thought about it, it was more important for him to like the music and to feel relaxed as he sliced into my head, than it was for me to subconsciously hear familiar tunes.

I returned to his office the next day (the day before surgery) and left a note on his desk.

> Dear Dr. Cilluffo,
>
> I have the utmost confidence in you as my surgeon and know you can help me. Thank you for your willingness to repair my CSF leak.
>
> I've thought about the music and want you to play your favorite selection. Do your best! I'll talk with you on the other side.
>
> Sincerely,
> Karen

I WAS SCHEDULED to check into the Same Day Admitting area at 6:00 a.m. on January 5, 1993. I was free to do as I pleased until the night before surgery. I managed to squeeze in a lot of last minute things. One was to order a single rose to be delivered to the offices of Cindy Monroe and Ronna Hoffmann, the morning of my surgery. I attached a note that read, "Thanks to you, the tide is coming back."

I was confident this was going to be another turning point; just like the one year anniversary of my accident and being able to drive again, after remaining seizure-free for six months. I was going to be "healed."

I wrote a note to Jerry, as well.

> *Dear Jerry,*
>
> *As I approach a craniotomy, I fear I will never see you again. I don't want to leave you behind. I don't want to say good-bye. My love for you is so deep. I would set you free, knowing my life may never be the same. Maybe the pain of losing me would be easier, maybe not. But the future is so uncertain, I could be blind, totally disabled, or comatose. I don't want you to hurt.*
>
> *But I need your support, without you I cannot do this. It's impossible. I need you by my side, holding my hand, seeing your smile, feeling your presence. You give me strength. You give me hope. You are truly remarkable.*
>
> *I find it difficult to even write words that can encompass the feelings I have for you. Words seem like objects, where as you are the essence of my being.*
>
> *All My Love,*
> *Karen*

In reality I was pleading for his support, hoping he would begin to understand my emotional needs.

On the day before surgery, I also visited Diane and Paul Fetter. They had been such wonderful friends and supported me throughout my recovery. It had been very hard for them to watch me go through the pain of my headaches, not to mention the frustrations of dealing with doctors. Diane surprised me by giving me a teddy bear she had made. It had a bandage on its head. This was a very special gift. I looked forward to having this bear with me in the hospital.

Although I did not consider myself to be a teddy bear collector, I was beginning to accumulate several. My first teddy came when I was first hospitalized with my seizures. My dear friend Jean Greene gave it to me. This was the bear I named "Seizure."

My mother suggested a name for the teddy Diane made, "Cilluffo." He too would be my greatest friend for awhile. Diane told me this was my good luck bear and if I needed to have any more surgeries, she would have to make me a bigger bear. I assured her there would not be a need for more bears. This was the only craniotomy I was going to have. I hadn't forgotten, however, a comment my mother had made about someone they knew who had a granddaughter who had seven craniotomies.

On the night before my surgery, I had a basketball game scheduled with my women's city league team. We played at the YMCA, which is normally a difficult court to play on, but on this night I could do no wrong. I played most of the game, and shot the lights out of the hoop. I sank every three-pointer I shot and scored 28 points. Mom and Dad came to the game (just like old times when they watched me play for Michigan State).

During the entire game there were times when my mind would wander to what was going to happen tomorrow. I kept thinking this could very easily be the last game I'd ever play. I might not be able to walk onto a court again, or have sight to see the basket or a ball. This was such a humbling feeling. We take so much for granted. With Mom and Dad there, and me playing so well, it was almost as though this was meant to be my last game. Or maybe it was God's way of saying, "See, even in the midst of a storm, you will shine and bring joy to others." I could still see the pride in my parents' eyes. It glistened through their smiles.

When the final buzzer blew, tears filled my eyes. Everyone knew what was scheduled for tomorrow. I received hugs from everyone. I was over-whelmed by the support from all the players on my team. This felt like the perfect grand finale to my physically active life-style; if it were to end this way. There was no place I would have rather been on the night before surgery.

There is a metaphor connected with my presence on the basketball court right up until the day of my craniotomy. I learned a lifetime of lessons playing basketball, all of which helped me prepare for and rehabili-tate from this life-threatening surgery. I have learned to enjoy challenges, but respect them to the highest degree.

Challenges are like climbing mountains. With a positive attitude, we view these challenges as tools to make us stronger. I was going into sur-gery with a very positive outlook, confident everything would go well and my headaches would diminish. I also felt positive, knowing if I ended up impaired in any way after surgery, I could make the most of my life, in whatever condition I remained. I was definitely having the typical pre-game/pre-surgery jitters, but I was still going into the game ready to win, not afraid to lose.

I needed to have the utmost confidence in my teammates. The outcome, for the most part, was in the hands of my surgeon and the nurses. Life is most certainly not an individual sport. I did my best to stay in the best physical condition possible, all the way up to the day of surgery, maximizing my potential to withstand the trauma.

After surgery, just like in-between halves of a game, there is a time to rest and a time to prepare for what comes next. I needed a balance of both to rebuild my body. Like training for competition, I used the same skills to build my strength. This included not only the physical skills but the emotional skills as well: desire, determination, and perseverance. These tools remained very valuable in my recovery.

I decided I wanted as few surprises as possible upon waking up after surgery. I figured there were two variables. The first was waking up and wondering what Dr. Cilluffo had done and what was my condition. The second was how I would look with my head shaved. It would be enough for me to handle the first variable, so I chose to eliminate the second. Therefore, I decided to shave my head the night before surgery. Then, I'd know what to expect and minimize the surprise.

After the basketball game I went to a friend's house, so they could help me. Since I knew it was a mandatory thing to do, I tried to make the most of it and have fun. I took the clippers (and a big deep breath) and made the first swipe down the middle of my head, from front to back. I just kept going, until I had nothing but stubble over my whole head. I handled this better than I thought I would. Knowing it would grow back, helped.

Late that night, I spoke with my brother, Lamar, and my sister, Kay, who both live in Atlanta, Georgia. It tore my heart to say good-bye to them. We were all so scared. It was twice as hard for them, being one thousand miles away from me. Tears flooded my eyes while I talked with each of them. I truly felt their pain, and thus it became my own. Two hearts beat as one, when the depth of love like ours penetrates life.

I know my fear was not as great as my family and friends. But I think it is pretentious to say, "I was not afraid to die." Even with the comfort of God's grace and mercy, and the promise of eternal life in heaven, there is

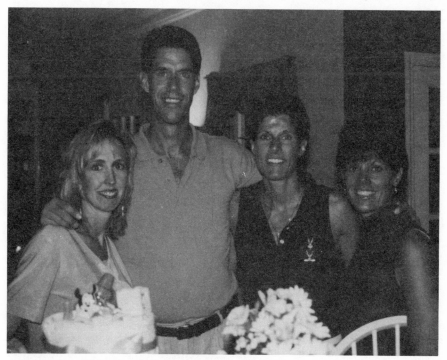

Sister-in-law, Teresa; brother, Lamar; author; sister, Kay.

fear. The fear is earthly fear. We certainly do not fear eternal life, but we may fear the moments, minutes, or hours before our death and the potential pain accompanying it.

We need to learn to die, just as we need to learn to live. It is a time of letting go and letting God. What we do in our lifetime certainly contributes to our feelings when we face death. Questions deluge our being. Have we fulfilled God's wishes? Did someone's life breathe easier because I lived? One can either be at peace or distraught at the time of death.

To welcome peace, we must remember who we are and have faith in the grace and mercy of our Lord, Jesus Christ. Serenity in our lives comes from the realization that God loves us and protects us.

After saying good-bye to Lamar and Kay, I prayed for strength and for God to watch over my family. I knew God would ease their worries, "Weeping may remain for a night, but rejoicing comes in the morning." (Psalm 30:5 NIV) While Lamar and Kay felt lost in the dark, God was their light. They needed a safe place. God was their refuge.

I DIDN'T SLEEP well. I laid awake most of the night, thinking about the surgery. I needed to be at the hospital the next morning at 6:00 a.m. Mom, Dad, and Jerry took me to the hospital, where we met Ronna, Paul, Diane, and Pastor Jim Helman. I wore a hat so I wouldn't look too strange, even though it really was not bothering me in the least to have a shaved head. That was the least of my worries.

Surprisingly, I was quite at peace with what was happening. My prayers were being answered. After I had changed into my lovely hospital attire, everyone took turns coming in to be with me. Jim came in and said a special prayer for me. Then we prayed the Lord's Prayer together. This was very special. He is such a wonderful pastor, and a great friend. I felt very comforted by his presence and later found out he was astounded by the level of peace he saw in me as I went into surgery. We all knew I was not going into surgery alone. God was with me the entire time.

I remembered the words to the song, *As You Go On Your Way.* "As you go on your way may Christ go with you. May He go before you to show you the way; May He go behind you to encourage you; Beside you to befriend you; Above you to watch over; Within you to give you peace." I felt completely surrounded by my Heavenly Father's protective arms.

I pictured God assisting the surgeons and nurses, and felt such solace, knowing He'd take care of me. I knew this had to be in His plans, and thus whatever happened, was for a reason. I had no control of anything at this point, so I did not attempt to take charge or convince myself I might have some dominion over my life.

I walked to the pre-surgical holding area with the nurse and had to say good-bye to everyone. This was the toughest part. I was at peace with myself, but I knew it was difficult for those around me to experience this peace. (This was another validation of my theory that it is harder to be the one waiting for a loved one in surgery than it is to have the surgery.) Not knowing in what capacity they will see me next was terribly frightening for all of us.

I was asked to lay on a gurney. Then the anesthesiologist came in to talk with me. He told me what he was going to do, that he would start my IV soon, and then he would give me something to help me relax.

Suddenly, six people were surrounding my gurney, doing six different things to me. One of them was an operating room nurse, Lois Laite-Zimmerman, who I had helped start an exercise program. She came to talk with me, asking if I had any questions, trying to help me relax. It felt so good to see a familiar face.

In the midst of our conversation, things started to fade away. The anesthesiologist must have given me his magic potion, because the lights went out mid-sentence.

It always seems like the very next second after you lose consciousness, everything is over and it's time to awake. This is the scariest time for me, waking up. The unknown, what Dr. Cilluffo did and my condition, are questions piercing every muscle within me, creating an enormous amount of stress.

I first recall hearing voices in the recovery room. Their conversation was about the snow outside. One voice was very familiar. My friend, Steve Hall, R.N. was again in recovery, as he had been for my previous sinus surgeries. I tried to open my eyes, but couldn't. I faded in and out, until finally, Steve noticed I was fighting to wake up. He came over to where I was laying and started talking with me. Once I managed to open my eyes, I saw his big smile. My eyes felt as though they had been glued shut by the Vaseline patches they covered them with before cutting into my skull. (The patches protect the eyes when the surgeons peel the scalp, forehead, and facial skin away from the bone.) Steve recognized I was having problems with the gunk still in my eyes and wiped them for me. We chatted for a while. He did most of the talking.

When they were ready to transport me to my room, Steve wheeled me out of recovery, towards the elevator. Mom, Dad, and the rest of my support crew came out of the waiting room to see me. They stood in the hall as I was escorted past them. I managed to give them the biggest smile I could summons, along with the thumbs up sign. I received a standing ovation.

I was anxious to hear how the surgery went and what Dr. Cilluffo had found. Of course, the jokes came first. "He did not find anything in your head Karen, not even a brain." Eventually, my parents and Jerry told me of the conversation they had with Dr. Cilluffo after surgery.

The surgery had lasted six hours. He found the leak near the cribiform plate, where he had suspected. It was very clear to him where I was leaking. He managed to save half of the olfactory nerve, which meant I should have part of my sense of smell. Everything went smoothly, but took longer than anticipated.

What a relief to hear he found the leak. I feared he wouldn't find it, or worse yet, I would experience more impairments as a result of the surgery. Thus far, everything seemed to be intact. They repeatedly did neurological tests to make sure I remained stable.

I slept most of the remainder of the day and the next. While there were several visitors throughout the first few days, I have very little recollection of my time with them. It was such a surprise to wake up to a room full of balloons, flowers, fruit, and cards. I was overwhelmed with the love, care, and support of my friends and family.

I have a very clear memory of one incident that occurred the day after surgery. A nurse came into my room and said she was going to get me up and walking. I wasn't sure I heard her correctly and asked her to repeat herself. I was right, she said, "Let's get you out of bed." I could not imagine how I was going to do this. I had not moved an inch since I was placed in bed. Even competitive, always active Karen wasn't sure she liked this suggestion. Fortunately, I hadn't temporarily lost my willingness to do what I was told. If she thought I could do this, I must be ready.

Sitting up required more effort than I ever imagined. Not even my most recent exercise workout took this much energy. I was sweating profusely. Half of my energy must have been expended on the emotional fear of moving. I was scared to move, thinking it would be extremely painful and might damage the work Dr. Cilluffo had done.

Consider how frightening it would be to move a broken arm that had just been set, then put it into perspective. I was moving the major operating system of my body, my broken head and damaged brain. Knowing the details of the surgery, didn't help. My friend Joy had filled me in on how they remove a large piece of the skull during surgery and lay it in saline solution, until they are done.

I was still in the process of moving to the side of the bed. I thought my headache was bad before surgery; it was nothing compared to what I felt now, though still not as bad as I anticipated. I could feel exactly where they had been working in my head. With two nurses, one on each side, I walked to the door of my room and back. I felt like this was a major accomplishment. Maybe, later in the day, I could go further. Oh yes, my competitiveness was still seeded in my brain.

Little by little I went further. Before long I was walking down the hallway, with assistance. The nurse pushed my IV pole and hung onto a belt wrapped around me. I held onto the pole with one hand and the railing with the other. I was not ready for a 10K race, but I was certainly making progress.

Postsurgical recovery was going smoothly, then without warning, I began to deteriorate. My neck got terribly stiff and sore, and I started running a fever. At 8:00 p.m. my nurse decided to call the Infectious Disease Specialist. She was concerned that I might have meningitis. Dr. Burke responded to the call and suggested a lumbar puncture to test my CSF.

My multiple experiences with myelograms made me very familiar with this procedure. Unfortunately, Dr. Burke was unable to get any fluid from his attempt at tapping my spine. He requested a CT scan, so I was quickly wheeled down to Radiology, for both a repeat lumbar puncture and a CT scan.

In Radiology, Dr. Williams attempted to tap my spine. By this time I was in and out of consciousness. I do not remember the CT scan or being taken back to my room. I woke up in my room. I was laying flat on my back and extremely uncomfortable. I desperately needed to urinate. I rang the call button for the nurse. I told her I needed to get up to use the rest room. She very sternly stated I was not to move from the flat position. I could not get out of bed to go to the rest room, instead she very generously offered me a bedpan.

I knew I was not going to be able to go in the bed pan, no matter how badly I had to go. I could barely use one while sitting up in bed. I could never figure out how anyone can go while laying down. There has to be a better design for bedpans.

Nurses must think people are immodest pee-ers. They stand next to the bed, waiting for the bedpan to be filled, like putting a cup under a soda fountain. I am not only a modest pee-er, I also have to request they run the water in the sink and give me a pan of water to play in with my fingers.

Even then, I still can't guarantee success. In this case, even cheating and propping myself up on my elbows did not work. I sat there for several minutes, mimicking with my voice the sound of urine hitting the toilet, trying to make myself relax. It was to no avail.

The nurse had to catheterize me, because by this time I was in pain. She apologized for not being able to get me up. She knew I was very uncomfortable, in many ways, but she could not do anything more than she had already done. I told her I was also very nauseated. So, she returned with a shot to help reduce my nausea.

The medication did not kick in soon enough. Before I could even press the call button or reach for the spit basin, I vomited all over myself, while still laying flat in bed. This was awful. I was helpless. I could not move, not because I was told not to, but because I still required assistance to move. I reached for the call button and closed my eyes to the mess surrounding me.

When the nurse walked in and saw what had happened, I thought for sure she was going to get me out of bed. How could she not? She needed to clean my whole bed. Instead, she requested another nurse's assistance and they changed my bed while I was in it. They gave me a new gown and helped me wash. As is usually the case, I felt better after vomiting and was able to fall asleep.

In the middle of the night, I awoke to the strangest thing. Dr. Scheiberger, the neurosurgeon on call, and a nurse who I did not recognize, were performing another lumbar puncture on me. When I opened my eyes, I was in the fetal position on my side, being held in this position by the nurse. Dr. Scheiberger was behind me. I looked at both of them, wondering what they were doing and why.

This is where the fun part, in a manner of speaking, began. My mind concluded I was in the accounting building across the street from the hospital. The nurse and doctor were on a scavenger hunt for hospital employees, and in one of the rooms they needed to get CSF for the hunt. This is where I came in. I was the volunteer from whom they were to take CSF.

I began moving and joking around with them, asking Dr. Scheiberger if he was finding all that he needed. He replied, "Please hold still, I am almost done. Yes, I was able to get the spinal fluid." I continued to converse with the nurse, who appeared heavily made-up, like someone working on a scavenger hunt for Halloween.

I said to her, "You aren't really doing a lumbar puncture are you? Why do you have to do your hunt on me?" The fact that Halloween had come and gone two months ago did not matter. My mind was not operating properly. I was hallucinating. I faded out of consciousness again.

The next morning I regained consciousness. I opened my eyes to Ronna shaking and shouting at me. She said I had been unconscious throughout the night and that no one could arouse me. When she walked over to my room from her office, she found a sign on the door of my room that read, "Do Not Enter: Isolation." Ronna panicked. She didn't know what happened through the night. She hustled to the nurse's station and asked a nurse if she could enter my room. The nurse was not willing to let her in, nor would she give Ronna information on my condition. Ronna then went to the Nurse Manager, who informed Ronna about my condition, explaining what had transpired during the night. She also allowed Ronna to go into my room to see me.

When Ronna first entered my room, I was still unconscious. She was unable to awaken me. She left in a panicked state, returning with the nurse. Ronna started to shake me, trying to arouse me. She kept saying my name over and over again. I regained consciousness in the midst of this.

When Ronna asked me how I was doing I answered very enthusiastically, "I am doing fine. But, why am I in the accounting building?" Ronna was quite taken by this response. I was not in the accounting building. I was still on East III, where I had always been. I continued telling her the story about Dr. Scheiberger doing the scavenger hunt and taking spinal fluid from me in the middle of the night.

Ronna knew what had really happened that night. She heard it directly from the nurse. She was floored by what I was saying, especially since I was dead serious. Ronna tried to convince me I was still on East III and that there had not been a scavenger hunt the night before. I would not believe her. I didn't even think I had undergone brain surgery.

While Ronna was trying to bring me back to reality, Dr. Burke walked in. By this time, I had tossed the sheets off of my legs and had one leg propped up and the other crossed over it. (Prior to this, I had not moved an inch, other than when the nurses got me out of bed for a walk.)

Dr. Burke must have read my chart before entering my room. His first question to me was, "Karen, where are you?"

I quickly replied, "I know you're going to tell me the right answer is East III, but I know I am in the accounting building." Ronna's eyes opened wide when she heard this, glancing at Dr. Burke to see his response. She explained to him how she was trying to talk sense into me.

Dr. Burke seemed quite concerned about my delirium, but didn't know what to do. He gave us the results of my spinal taps. They were mostly negative for meningitis, though all of them were not conclusive. He asked me if I remembered having the lumbar punctures. I could recall his unsuccessful attempt, getting sick on myself, and the scavenger hunt. That was all I could remember.

I could not figure out why all these people were trying to get me to believe I was in the hospital. I have always been very aware of my surroundings, so why would this be different? I would remain confident, until proven otherwise.

The nurses were still enforcing their mandatory flat position rule, so I stayed in this position until Dr. Cilluffo came in to check on me. He immediately demanded my head be raised. The CT scans had shown internal bleeding and increased swelling in my head. These symptoms were exasperated by me laying in a flat position.

I normally would know better than to allow anyone to lay me in a flat position after a craniotomy, but under the circumstances, my mind was not producing good decisions. The longer I was in a flat position, the more the swelling and bleeding increased, and my brain became less and less able to function adequately. It was causing me to hallucinate and lose consciousness. I didn't have meningitis.

It's amazing how the brain reacts to such trauma. It has its own built-in protection mechanism. Several hours after Dr. Cilluffo raised the head of my bed, I was beginning to make sense again. I was still not convinced I was on East III, or that I had had a craniotomy, but I had a hunch that what others were telling me might be true.

That night, the nurses requested Jerry spend the night in my room, otherwise they were going to have to put a Possey (pronounced posé) on me. I hadn't a clue what a Possey was, but I suspected it wasn't a flower. (It happens to be arm restraints to deter patients from going anywhere.) The reason for the Possey was because I kept insisting on getting out of bed by myself. Why wouldn't I think I could get out of bed on my own if I thought I didn't have surgery? I thought there was nothing wrong with me. Every time I made an attempt, someone in the room called out to me to stay in bed until a nurse came to help.

Jerry slept in a recliner in my room. Sure enough, in the middle of the night, I needed to go to the bathroom. I started to get up and Jerry quickly stopped me and called the nurse. I thought it was rather silly for this to be happening, still believing I was fine. They demanded I use the bedpan, despite my protests.

The next day, one of my nurses came in and wanted to take me for a walk. I was obviously eager to get moving and thus praised her for helping me get up from my bed.

The first thought that entered my mind when I stood up was, "If I have not had a craniotomy, what type of drug did they give me to make me have a headache like a craniotomy?" The pain was very intense. I moved slowly in the direction of the bathroom. Once I got to the mirror, I could not believe what I saw. My head was wrapped in a big bandage. My face was swollen and bruised. Yes, I did have a craniotomy. There was no way anyone could make me look like this, even for Halloween. The headache must be for real. I walked to the doorway and looked out into the hallway. It was not until I saw the hallway, and remembered it from before the pressure built up in my head, that I finally believed I was not in the accounting building.

Dr. Cilluffo came in and removed the bandage. He also pulled the drain that was draining blood from beneath my skull. This was an eerie feeling and sound. I could hear the fluid swishing inside my head, moving through the drain. When he pulled it out it sounded like a nail being pulled from a piece of wood. It creaked while sending a sharp pain through my head. He left the staples in for a few more days, which gave my mother time to count all seventy-eight of them. They completely crossed my head, ear to ear, just like he had described. I anticipated their removal to be painful, but it was no different than removing stitches. I hardly felt a thing. The skin in this area was still numb, as it is today.

I started to put the pieces back together again. Others told me the sequence of events and I began to describe my feelings throughout this period of time. My hallucinations were very vivid, though much of the past three days I had lost.

It was frightening to know I was so out of touch with the world. My brain was on the edge of completely shutting down, primarily due to an error in the physician's orders. Every physician who checked on me that night and the following day should have known to elevate my head.

During my entire admission for surgery, Dr. MacKenzie was on vacation. His expertise was greatly missed, as he is excellent at orchestrating the care given by several specialists. Throughout my recovery I've found that the biggest breakdown of patient care is when several specialists work on one patient. The lack of communication between them is significant. When the right hand fails to know what the left is doing, quality care is sacrificed. Dr. MacKenzie is excellent at seeing the whole picture, and thus, has been a critical part of my recovery.

While I remained in Munson following my surgery, I was overwhelmed with the love and support from my parents, friends, and co-workers. I was very touched by the generosity of a four year old boy, Jonathon, who didn't even know me. His mom, Liz Bailey, worked in the public relations department at Munson. She was always very supportive of my recovery. She stopped by my room to give me a teddy bear. It was not an ordinary teddy. It was her son's teddy. He had been in the hospital when he was two and three, and had this teddy with him to keep him company. When Liz told her son that a friend of hers was in the hospital, the boy insisted on giving his teddy bear to me. He wanted it to keep me company.

I was in tears when she gave this precious teddy bear to me. What an example of unconditional love!

Several months later, I bought her son a new teddy bear and wrapped it up with the old teddy bear. I was certain this child would be missing his teddy by now. Three days later, Liz came to me with the old teddy in hand and said, "Jonathon wants you to keep it. He gave it to you as a gift." My heart was warmed by such a gesture.

They kept me on a heavy duty antibiotic while in the hospital. Because all of the meningitis test results were not conclusive, I opted to go ahead with the entire ten day treatment as a precaution. Consequently, the home care nurse needed to teach me how to administer my own IV antibiotics so I could return home.

Although it was good to be home again, I was amazed at how very weak I was. Prior to my surgery, I was at a pretty good level of fitness, but it very quickly disappeared with such a dramatic shock to my body. Physicians have agreed that had I not been in such good shape going into the craniotomy, I wouldn't have recovered with such ease.

To regain my strength and stamina, there was still work to be done. Twice each day I infused a small bottle of antibiotics to make sure I wouldn't get meningitis. The home care nurse came every other day to check my heparin lock and make sure I was doing okay.

While Jerry was at work, Mom and Dad were able to assist me. During the first week after coming home, I mostly slept. When I was not sleeping I was laying on the couch or bed. I was most comfortable in this position. I could not be up for long periods of time. I began having major cramps in my buttocks each time I stood up, and this became quite uncomfortable. It took me at least a half dozen slow, painful steps before I could move with ease.

My sister, Kay, flew in from Atlanta to see me. What a wonderful feeling it was for both of us to be together again. After having fears of never seeing one another again on earth, it was a special reunion. We were able to laugh about my crew cut and permanent headband, as I kept singing the jingle Ch..Ch..Ch..Chia. After all I felt just like a chia pet must feel as the hair on my head began to grow. This was certain to bring a smile to all. Kay is so special to me, and our time was cherished. I cannot imagine what it would have felt like if the wheels were turned and it was her going through this surgery.

She had fun teasing me about my permanent headband, my scar. As kids, we wore headbands. I was always teased for wearing my headband in a goofy place across my forehead. At least now my permanent headband was in the right place. Actually in modern fashions, it looked like I was wearing a set of headphones to my Walkman.

By the second week, I was eager to see if I could exercise lightly. I knew my butt cramps would probably subside if they got more exercise. They were rejecting my sudden, sedentary life-style.

So with Dr. Cilluffo's permission, I first tried my stationary bike. I did surprisingly well. At first, it was hard to peddle with the cramping, but once I got peddling it seemed to relax the muscles. I started with just ten minutes at a time each day and gradually added five minutes every second or third day. I was up to thirty minutes of continuous peddling by the end of the third week of recovery.

Along with cycling, I had a burning desire to begin walking. I asked a friend of mine to take me to the mall to walk, because it was a cold, icy winter day outside. I figured if I could peddle a bike for ten minutes I could most certainly walk around the mall. The mall would be much safer for me. I did not need to risk falling on the ice and cracking my head open.

My first walk entailed one lap around the mall. I had really lost my strength and endurance. It felt wonderful to move.

I wore a hat to cover my head. It was not because of embarrassment, it was to protect others from being grossed out by seeing the huge scar on my head. It was still very visible. My hair was just stubble and the scar was quite ugly. Dr. Cilluffo had not done a very nice job of sewing my scalp together again. I ended up with an inch wide scar tissue headband. Hair follicles are not in scar tissue, and hair wouldn't grow in this area. It was going to take much longer hair than I was used to having in order to cover this bald stripe.

Recovery went very well. I lost a little more weight during this period, but once I started exercising, I was able to gain some weight.

It seems to work the opposite for me. The less active I am the more weight I lose. My normally muscular body atrophies. Then, when I am able to begin working out again, I gain a little back. My determination to continue exercising so soon after surgery would prove to be invaluable. I needed to build back my strength as soon as possible.

Thirteen

Devastation

Sweet are the uses of adversity.
WILLIAM SHAKESPEARE

I NEVER DOUBTED MY brain surgery would be a success or that it would take more than one surgery to repair my CSF leak. Sure, Mom had told me about someone who needed seven brain surgeries—no way would this happen to me.

Although Dr. Cilluffo had saved my sense of smell, he did change the effectiveness of it. What used to smell good, now smelled bad. For example, with food cooking on the stove, I no longer could smell the aroma of the food. Instead, I only smelled the burner of the stove. The same with toast in the toaster. It stunk. Of course, this hurt my appetite. I could still taste food, but it, too, was not the same. It almost would have been better if Dr. Cilluffo had cut the entire olfactory nerve.

One day I was drying myself off after taking a shower. Since my accident I had formed the habit of keeping my head up while I bent over to dry off my legs and feet—but this day, five weeks after surgery, with one more bend to dry my feet, fluid unexpectedly poured out of my nose—just as it did prior to my surgery. I was devastated. Was it really what I thought it was? Maybe it was only sinus fluid, like someone had once suggested.

I bent over again. Sure enough, more fluid flowed into my hand. This was not sinus fluid. I sat on the floor and cried. How could this happen? I did not know what to do. I called Jerry at work and told him what happened. His response was, "Really? I am sorry to hear this. I will be playing basketball after work tonight, so I will see you when I get home."I should have known better than to call him for emotional support.

I needed someone to share my grief. I needed a warm heart to cry with. I called Dr. MacKenzie. His response was similar to mine. He was devastated. He is such a devoted doctor. My pain was his pain, and he would do anything as a doctor and a friend to rid of this pain. He asked me to start collecting the fluid again, so we could have it tested. I did not relish the idea of doing this again, considering the roller coaster that Mayo Clinic lab put us on before.

It was easy to collect the fluid. I could produce it on call. Within a couple of days, Dr. Cilluffo met with me. He wanted to put a ventricular-peritoneal (VP) shunt in my brain. It was his belief my CSF pressure was too high. No matter what he'd do to repair the leak, it'd always start leaking again, because of the pressure. He used the example of patching a leaky basement. After one leak was stopped, the water would find a new place to seep through.

It was his belief the nerve receptors that told my body to absorb spinal fluid were damaged. My nervous system would always have an overabundance of spinal fluid, unless of course, I agreed to let him put another shunt in me; one that would run from the ventricle in my brain to my abdomen.

For some reason I was more afraid of having this surgery than my craniotomy. I have no doubt it was because I would be left with a foreign object in my brain—permanently. I wasn't sure I was willing to do this. I definitely needed more opinions.

I had already received Dr. Meyer's opinion regarding shunts in general. He was not in favor of them. Dr. MacKenzie convinced me to return to Dr. Scheiberger for more advice.

I knew something had to be done. I could not live with a CSF leak. The risks and the headache were too great. At this point, however, I would have preferred Dr. Cilluffo to go back into my head and repair what was still leaking, rather than have another shunt.

Jerry and I returned to Dr. Scheiberger. We were greeted by his words, "What are you trying to do, put me up against John?" He was only half joking. I told him about my recent surgery, subsequent reoccurrence of the leak, and what Dr. Cilluffo wanted to do next. I asked him what he would do in this situation.

He said he definitely would not use a VP shunt. He said I needed to find the best neurosurgeon to help me fix this problem, rather than waste my time with doctors in northern Michigan. He recommended that I see Dr. Julian Hoff, the Chief of Neurosurgeons at the University of Michigan in Ann Arbor. Dr. Scheiberger claimed Dr. Hoff was the best in the country, and that he could help me.

I wanted to remain in Traverse City for my care, so I asked him if he would consent to perform my surgery, if Dr. Hoff conferred with his recommendations. Dr. Scheiberger declined. "No," he said, "You need to get out of town. You are too well known in this area. No one is going to want to touch you, given the press that follows you."

While this was hard to hear, it was true. Practically everyone in the Traverse City area knew me. They were aware of my head injury and subsequent surgeries, as well as their failure. He was right. What physician would ever want to accept this load?

Dr. MacKenzie agreed with Dr. Scheiberger's advice. It was the third week in February. Dr. MacKenzie's office staff made an appointment for me to see Dr. Hoff at the end of June. This could not be possible. Had I misunderstood them? No, the first available appointment for new patients was June 23, 1993, four months away.

I spoke again with Dr. MacKenzie and asked if there was any way he could pull some strings to move the appointment up. I was learning to have more patience as time went on, but this was ridiculous. I was trying to take things one day at a time; but it is hard to do when even one day is too long.

As usual, the hardest part for me was not knowing what would happen next. If someone would have told me I was going to need another craniotomy, I would have rested a little easier than not knowing at all. Not knowing who, when, or what was going to be the next move was very stressful.

Dr. MacKenzie called Dr. Hoff personally and spoke with him about my case. Dr. Hoff agreed. I needed quicker attention than waiting until June. He told his secretary, Sandy, to squeeze me into his schedule ASAP.

My appointment was made for March 29, 1993. This was more reasonable.

The next hurdle was going to be getting my insurance, an HMO, to cover another referral to an out of plan physician. They had been willing to refer me to Mayo Clinic, but I thought I might be pressing my luck to try to get a referral and approval to yet another physician.

NorthMed HMO came through for me. They obviously recognized the seriousness of my condition and their need to send me elsewhere.

I drove down to Ann Arbor. (I felt a little like a traitor, given I am an alumni of Michigan State University.) I was well aware of the University's excellent reputation. Along with Mayo Clinic and Johns Hopkins Hospital, it was rated one of the best.

Dr. Hoff is a wonderful man. I was instantly impressed with his personality, thoroughness, and caring touch. Despite taking all of my records and films with me, he wanted to repeat all of the tests, including the myelogram, which he called a cisternagram. I told him how the test was performed and how it was not an effective method. He assured me they'd do it differently and felt confident they could locate the leak. I agreed to give it a try. I had nothing to lose.

The cisternagram was scheduled for the following week. I made reservations to stay in the Med Inn, a hotel connected to the hospital. Jerry and I went down the night before, since it was a five hour drive from Traverse City and I had to be there early in the morning. Staying at the Med Inn was most convenient. We got up, dressed, and walked down the hall to admitting.

The test went very well, but the results were the same as the previous two cisternagrams. By this time I could have performed the test myself. I was knowledgeable enough about the dyes they used and the angles scanned, that I could talk with the physicians who performed the tests very easily. While performing the test, they even asked me for suggestions.

I was admitted for an overnight stay at the hospital. This was their protocol after a lumbar puncture, but surprisingly, there were no restrictions. Unlike Munson Medical Center, I was allowed to get out of bed to use the rest room.

Dr. Hoff spoke with the Radiologist who performed the cisternagram and found the results to be inconclusive. He said from the looks of the CT scans I had a leak. "Your skull has been shattered," he said.

This time it did not surprise me to hear that there was more damage than previously diagnosed. I prayed, though, that this would be the last. There's not much worse than shattered.

He said he wanted to schedule surgery as soon as possible. It was scheduled for the following week, on April 16, 1993. Dr. Hoff said he was going to have to cut the entire olfactory nerve and lay a carpet of fascia down, over the leak. I would lose my sense of smell and taste. I told him it wouldn't be a great loss, since it was already impaired. Losing this sense was the least of my worries. Of any of the senses to lose I believed this was the least disabling.

I made reservations again for the Med Inn. This time, my parents joined us. Ronna also wanted to be with us, so she stayed there as well. Diane and Paul Fetter drove half way the day before, and stayed with family, then drove the rest of the way the morning of my surgery.

I had to go through a pre-op evaluation the day before surgery. Mom and Dad arrived that evening. By the time they arrived, I had already given myself my second buzzed haircut, hoping it would be my last.

All of us went down to the cafeteria in the hospital, for my last snack before fasting after midnight. I enjoyed my favorite frozen yogurt and chocolate chip cookies.

I didn't sleep well. Some might say the second bifrontal craniotomy should be easier, because I knew what to expect. This didn't seem to matter. For the first craniotomy it was fear of the unknown. For the second, it was fear of the known. I don't think either can be considered easy.

I had to be in admitting at 6:00 a.m. the next morning. My surgery was scheduled as Dr. Hoff's first surgery. I awoke at 3:00 a.m. and could not fall back to sleep.

I got out of bed and took my walkman into the bathroom. I thought I might get rid of some of my energy by dancing. I never got tired, and danced until 5:00 a.m., when everyone else started getting up to take their showers. At least the dancing filled my need to move my body, before my extended stay in bed following surgery.

We all gathered in the admitting waiting room. Diane presented me with a larger teddy bear, which she had promised. At the time of the promise, she did not know our worst fears would come true. She had said if I needed another craniotomy, she would need to make me a bigger bear. This bear I called Julian. It only seemed right since the first bear was Cilluffo.

We were all taken from one waiting room into another, where I was taken away from everyone except Jerry. I had to once again say my official good-byes. Jerry went with me to the pre-op area, where I had to change into my favorite designer hospital gown. Dr. Hoff came in to see me. He was shocked to see my head had already been shaved. I said I buzzed it in his honor. His nickname is "Buzz Hoff."

They gave me something to relax in my IV, and as always, it put me to sleep. Jerry said I continued to talk until they wheeled me out of this area, but I have not a clue what I said.

The surgery took six hours. Once again, another CSF leak was found. Dr. Hoff filled the right frontal sinus and laid a cadaver dural patch graft down over the area that was leaking. He used fibrin glue to seal the area. (This was glue made from my own blood.) He cut the olfactory nerve. My sense of smell and taste were gone forever. I came through the surgery with flying colors.

When I woke up I was already in the Neuro Intensive Care Unit (NICU). I was shivering. During delicate surgery of that length they have to lower the patient's body temperature, to reduce the level of bleeding. I always woke up very tense, and the cold only compounded this feeling. It was hard to relax when I was so cold. I kept saying to myself over and over again, "Karen, relax your shoulders, arms, legs, and feet. Relax." Eventually, after fading in and out of sleep, I managed to relax as well as could be expected.

I couldn't figure out what the noise was in my room. It sounded like a motor turning off and on. There was also something wrapped around my legs. I then realized that when I heard the motor run, whatever was wrapped around my legs filled with air. This was to keep my circulation flowing.

I had a horrendous headache. When the nurse came in, she said Dr. Hoff requested I be placed on a lumbar drain, which pumped CSF out of my spine to keep the pressure low. This reduced the stress on the area he had patched. Every now and then, an alarm went off on this pump and the nurse had to reset it.

While in the intensive care unit, a patient can only have visitors at certain time periods. My parents, Jerry, and everyone else took turns coming in to see me. Each brought a unique form of comfort to my recovery. I slept most of the day after surgery, but through the night I kept being awakened by the alarms from the monitors. It seemed that every time I was about to fall asleep, an alarm would go off.

First it was the heart rate monitor's alarm. The nurse had set the low end of the range at 50 beats per minute (bpm), but my heart rate was going lower than this. My normal resting heart rate is 42-56 bpm, so I imagined it was going even lower while I slept. I watched the numbers on the monitor for awhile. My heart rate was dropping as low as 40 bpm while I was awake.

I asked the nurse if she could reset the low end of the range, so that I could get some sleep. She reset it to 40 bpm.

I fell back to sleep. Suddenly, the alarm honked again. The nurse said she was watching the monitor while I slept. My heart rate was dropping as low as 36 bpm. She reset it once more to 30 bpm.

I thought I'd finally be able to get some sleep, but I was wrong. The next alarm to go off was the spinal fluid pump alarm. The nurse came in and tried to figure out what was wrong. The machine kept turning off. At this point my head pain reached a 15+ on a scale of 1-10, 10 being the worst pain. I had never felt pain as I felt on this night.

I asked the nurse if it were possible the machine had taken too much spinal fluid out of me. She replied, "They have it set at a level of 6, so it should not be taking too much out." I didn't sleep the rest of the night. Between the alarms and the pain, I couldn't.

The next morning the doctors came in to check on me. I told them about the machine turning off and on all night. They looked at the machine and immediately turned it off. They said I was right, it had drained too much CSF out. They reset the level to 8 and told the nurses to wait another two hours before turning it back on.

What a relief. Now I felt as though I had a chance to be comfortable. My head pain still persisted, but not nearly at the intensity it had been.

Jerry came in to see me that morning. He told me he was returning to Traverse City. This was supposed to be the man who was devoted to me and would care for me; and he was leaving me in the intensive care unit to go home. I did not have the strength or energy to question why. I guess at this point, the emptiness I felt deep inside left me at a loss for words.

I knew that Jerry and I had a lot of work to do to make our marriage work. I was trying to learn more about people, feelings, and relationships. I was reading everything I could get my hands on, and continuing counseling, with the hope of saving our marriage. I knew I could not do it alone, however, and Jerry was not doing anything to help us.

I tried to talk with him, but the most he would say was, "I do not know how to talk about feelings." I suggested books for him to read, not just about relationships, but about head injuries and survival. He showed no interest. He was more interested in his singular life, not his life with me.

Jerry could not accept the alterations in our life-style as a result of my head injury. He could not accept change at all, let alone a major change such as this. He wanted our life-style to go back to the way it was, not recognizing the fact it never could.

Even though Jerry was the one who left me in Ann Arbor, in reality, he was the one being left behind. I was moving forward in life, while he desperately tried to stay in the same place. It was sad to see someone I loved isolate himself as he did.

I GRADUALLY BECAME accustomed to the young residents and interns coming into my room. They usually filled my room at 6:00 a.m. every day, asking me questions about how I was feeling—before I even had a chance to open my eyes. Most often, the room was so full, there were tiny heads appearing in the doorway. I often felt like a monkey in a circus.

My case was a very unusual one, which made a perfect learning opportunity for residents. Thus, it was very common for more than one or two of the neurosurgical teams to be in my room at the same time. It was often difficult to rest, with so many residents and interns wanting to evaluate my condition. I will never forget the day eight residents and interns came into my room and asked me to tell them the whole story of my injury. I said, "Do you have a couple hours to spare?"

I proceeded by telling them, from beginning to end, the story of my injury, misdiagnosis, surgeries, and recoveries. It seemed like it took about two hours. Most of them stood with mouths open, seemingly in awe of this medical disaster.

It was not five minutes after they left when an intern returned to my bedside. "I was just here, when you told the history of your injury. Now, I need to write it in a report. Could you repeat it?" he asked.

I was shocked. "You have got to be kidding," I said. I remembered this intern. He was standing at the foot of my bed, and looked as though he had just crawled out of bed, yawning the entire time I was speaking to the group. Now, he was asking for a repeat of what I had said. I don't think so. I was polite, however, and repeated my story, summarizing much of it. He listened intently, holding his note pad in hand. Once again, he didn't write one thing down.

While on this neuro floor, I discovered that the head nurse, Etta, was a sister to one of my friends in Traverse City. Etta became my confidante at U of M whenever I was an inpatient. I always knew she'd find me and take time out of her busy schedule to talk.

After I was moved to the neuro floor, the nurses started to help me out of bed and to walk. I knew my biggest mission was to increase my stamina and to improve the motility of my bowels. I knew the importance of getting my bowels moving, so I that I wouldn't need to bear down, and thereby increase pressure within my head. Some people may think the pain of surgery is all one worries about, but there are many other factors that need attention.

I always took a few days to get my appetite back, but this time it took much longer. I had no sense of taste or smell. I couldn't smell the good or the bad. Everything tasted the same, like cardboard. All beverages tasted like water. This was somewhat difficult to adjust to, but fortunately I had never been a big food connoisseur.

At first, my lack of taste was frustrating, but eventually I placed more emphasis on texture. The first time I realized I was doing this was when I described how the bagels were at a new bagel shop in town to my friend Joy. I said, "They're good. They are hard on the outside and chewy on the inside, just how I like them."

She looked at me strangely and replied, "But how do they taste?" This was a good question. I couldn't answer.

On another occasion, someone asked me how the bread tasted. I replied favorably. Someone else asked, "Is it garlic bread?"

I quickly and confidently replied, "No it's not. It's just plain bread." It wasn't plain, it was garlic. I forgot there was a possibility it was garlic.

While I adjusted to eating without taste, I also began challenging myself to walk. I'd frequently ask Mom or Dad if they wanted to walk with me around the block. The corridors were arranged in a block formation and I worked hard to increase my distance with each trip out of my room.

Mom and Dad stayed in Ann Arbor until I was discharged. Before they drove me home, Dr. Hoff gave me very specific instructions on what to do and what not to do. He wanted me to begin walking for exercise right away, so I could regain my strength. He said to avoid things which increase pressure in my head, such as: blowing my nose, sneezing, coughing, and bearing down. He didn't want me lifting anything over ten pounds, and I was to get as much sleep as my body required.

I could handle this. I had done it before. I was looking forward to being home and closer to all of my friends again, though I was worried about my marriage. This seemed like an awfully large load to be carrying. I prayed our lives would smoothen out so Jerry and I would have a chance. I prayed God would lead me to do what was right in regard to focusing my energy in the right direction. All things pointed toward my health. Unless my health was restored, I wouldn't be able to work on my marriage.

Once again, I was overwhelmed by the support from my friends and family, both in Traverse City and across the country. I have saved every card I have received since my accident. I now have more than six shoe boxes full of cards and letters. Anytime I need a lift, I just dig into the boxes and start reading.

After returning to Traverse City, I continued with Dr. Hoff's prescription of walking. This time, I was able to walk outdoors. It was May, and the weather was just turning nice. Although I really appreciated hearing the birds sing and seeing the flowers bloom, there was something missing. I could not *smell* spring: the freshly cut grass, the flowers, and the moist air after a light rain. My sense of smell was completely gone.

I could only try to remember what these aromas were. I still had the habit of lifting things to my nose. Eventually it sunk in, I wasn't going to smell anything. It didn't matter how close something was to my nose.

One morning I put some bread in the toaster and walked into another room. Five minutes later, I walked back into the kitchen and saw smoke pouring out of the toaster. I didn't smell anything. I popped the toast up, sticking my head in the midst of the smoke. I still couldn't smell it. This was serious. I needed to make changes in how I did things. No more walking away from any kind of cooking. I had to rely totally on my sight. My house had smoke alarms, but I had to make sure, as everyone should, the batteries were always good.

Smoke is obviously not the only smell that is an alert to danger. One day, I was cleaning the shower, trying to remove the rust stains from the hard water. I was using a new, very strong cleaner. Suddenly, I couldn't breath. I ran to a window, stuck my head outside to get fresh air, and began breathing more easily. I went back and read the box, which I should have done in the first place. It said in big, bold, red letters, "Do not inhale fumes. Inhalation can severely damage lungs."

I was not sure how I was going to finish cleaning. I couldn't smell the fumes, and thus would not know when it was safe to return to cleaning the shower. The only measure I had was my breathing, which I guessed was beyond the safe level.

I needed to learn how to rely on my other senses. They say when you lose one of your senses, another one gets stronger. This is true, not only in the physical sense, but also in the emotional sense.

At this point in my life, I could have said, "My life stinks." In the face of losing my sense of smell, however, my life honestly didn't stink. To compensate for my losses, I experienced an increase in my sight, humor, and the most valuable component of wholeness: spirituality.

While I realize a sense of humor doesn't qualify as a physiological sense, it should. Laughter became a very important part of my healing. Learning to laugh at myself allowed me to focus attention outside of myself. When we share with others the joy of laughter, we free ourselves of the bondage of perfection. We accept our mortality and learn to play with life.

I still do funny things, like pop chewing gum into my mouth without taking the wrapper off. I have written checks to people while standing in front of them, not tear the check out, close my checkbook, and walk away. (One thing which has always puzzled me is why I still write 1989 on my checks, instead of the current year. Here it is almost eight years later, and I still do this. Maybe it is because my accident was in 1989. I haven't found anyone who can explain this.)

Occasionally, instead of saying good-bye, I say thank-you; or instead of please, I say hello. I continue to find personal items in the most peculiar places. I'm sure there's a logical reason for some things to end up where they do, but I haven't figured it out yet.

Within a few weeks after returning to Traverse City from Ann Arbor, I was shopping at a local supermarket. This was the second time I had been out in public since my head had been shaved for surgery. This time I did not care too much about what people thought when they saw my bald head and intense scar. I was standing in line at the check-out, minding my own business. I found very few people were bold enough to stare at me, except for the woman in front of me. She turned to me and said, "Wow, what happened to you? Did you get bit by a shark?" Traverse City is a vacation area, with lots of lakes nearby. Even Lake Michigan is very close, but we certainly do not have sharks in our fresh water.

I politely said to her, "No, I just had surgery," and managed to hold back my laughter until I reached my car.

The next day I stopped at my hair salon to talk with Mike about an area on my head that was refusing to grow hair. Except for a 3"x 3" spot that was shiny and bald, the rest of my head had stubble growing.

The receptionist asked if she could help me. I asked if Mike was available. She said he was in the rest room. I said I would wait. She walked to the door of the rest room and yelled through the door, "Mike, there's a guy here to see you."

This did not surprise me, but I wanted to make sure she knew who (or what) I was. So I said to her, "You can tell Mike, Karen is here to see him."

She was embarrassed, realizing what she had done. In the state of her panic she landed a great line, "Oh, are you here for a haircut?" I could not contain myself. Here I was, a woman with a shaved head, and this woman was asking if I needed a haircut.

Laughing at situations like this helps keep things in perspective. I began seeing with greater depth. My perspective and perception of life with a head injury changed. No longer did I see it as my enemy. I began embracing this valuable piece of me. It is a piece of me, by no means the whole. It is a part of me I need to use to serve the Lord, just like my faith and my smile. What happens to us is not as important as how we respond to it.

How I responded to the next series of events in my life would be crucial. It didn't seem like it was enough that I had a head injury, was misdiagnosed, lost my grandfather, and had two brain surgeries. What seemed like a minor injury at the time had turned into a major, life changing circumstance.

Each time something new struck me I felt as though this must be the grand finale to my tragedy. Then something more came about. I felt as though I had accepted each loss, and was ready to get on with bigger and better things; well, maybe not bigger. Once suffering is completely accepted, it lessens the pain, and allows one to move forward. No one ever said life would be easy. God said in the very beginning, after our fall into sin, life was going to be difficult. All of us carry burdens God never meant for us to carry.

It was May 1993. I had two craniotomies within three and a half months; yet, the challenges kept coming my way full force. The momentum was intensifying. Little did I know that the next two years would make the past year look like a fairy tale.

Fourteen

How Much More?

Consider it pure joy, my brothers,
whenever you face trials of many kinds,
because you know that the testing of your faith
develops perseverance. Perseverance must finish its work
so that you may be mature and complete,
not lacking anything.

JAMES 1:2-4 NIV

FROM THE MOMENT I arrived home from Ann Arbor, Jerry and I were at each other's throats. Feelings we both had kept repressed began to surface.

I was continuing therapy with Margo, who helped me tremendously. I could not, however, save our marriage by myself. Jerry was not willing to see Margo with me. He said if he couldn't talk with me, then he could never talk with anyone else.

It felt like I was paddling a two-person canoe upstream against a raging current, by myself. The saddest part was that Jerry seemed perfectly content with the way things were. He wouldn't acknowledge we had major problems. It hurt me deeply that he couldn't recognize my sadness and fear, even when I verbalized it very clearly to him. I kept trying to figure out what more I could do to help our relationship, while Margo kept saying to me, "You are doing all that you are capable of doing. You cannot do it all yourself."

Jerry must have finally recognized therapy was our only hope, because he suddenly changed his mind. He started to see Margo individually, as

196

well as jointly with me. At last, I felt some hope. He had decided to stick his paddle in the water. Whether he moved it or not would be another challenge.

Jerry began expressing his feelings, but in inappropriate ways. I began seeing sides of Jerry I had never seen before. His anger was evident. It was as if he had been a time bomb all along, just waiting for his fuse to be lit. Explosive behavior became commonplace. He had stuffed so much anger inside for too long.

Our marriage had been built around physical activities. Jerry and I didn't have an emotional or spiritual foundation. When I could no longer participate at the same athletic level, Jerry and I had nothing to share. I attempted to introduce an emotional and spiritual connection. Jerry remained focused on activity, resisting any kind of change in our life-style. We didn't need to give up our physical activities altogether, but the level at which they were performed and their status in our priorities did need to change. This didn't seem to matter to Jerry, as his fear of change and self-centeredness overruled. He didn't care about the "u" in "us." Rather than talk about how we were going to adjust to the change, we were pushed further and further apart.

Jerry didn't have the capacity to discuss the deeper side of what was happening in our marriage, and I didn't have the stamina to help him. I had my hands full with my emotional and physical therapy.

One of our fights occurred in the basement. The last thing I remember was Jerry pushing me out of the workshop. Next, I was waking up to my neighbors, Ron and Gloria Hodgins, telling me to relax and that Grand Traverse Emergency Medical Service was on their way. I was laying on the floor of the basement, feeling like a dish rag.

The paramedics arrived. Ron told them I had had a seizure and was post ictal. Gloria was taking my blood pressure and talking with me, trying to keep me calm. I believe she sensed my fear. She could see abrasions on my legs that could not have been caused by a seizure. They suspected more had happened than Jerry was telling them.

I was so thankful they were there when I regained consciousness. They had heard the 911 call on their band radio and came over immediately to see how they could help.

I was taken to Munson for CT scans, all of which came back negative for bleeding. The scans clearly showed, however, swelling and air in my head from my craniotomy. I was only three weeks post surgery, and still had a very distinct scar that had not fully healed from ear to ear. A few hours later they released me from the emergency room, and sent me home.

Occurrences similar to this happened a few more times before I finally admitted to myself something was wrong. I kept denying the fact it was happening to me. This was only something you hear about happening to other women in bad relationships. I was not in a bad relationship. At least, I did not want to believe I was. I trusted counseling would help Jerry and me get through these battles.

Jerry's anger was mounting. The last straw came on one of the nights he knocked me unconscious. I found out later from Margo that Jerry had called her, instead of 911. Margo asked where I was. Jerry said, "She's on the floor."

Margo replied, "Is she okay?"

Jerry said, "Hold on, let me roll her over."

Margo was panicked and urgently tried to persuade Jerry to call 911. He said, "No, maybe I'll just call our neighbors." He called Ron and Gloria, who rushed over to help me.

The first thing I remember was Gloria saying my name. I was laying on the floor in the hallway. They helped me to a chair. Wanting to make sure I was okay, they stayed with me for quite awhile. I had yet to see Jerry. I had no idea where he was. They said he was on the telephone, in another room.

I was so scared. Gloria had a wonderful sense of intuition. When they were about to leave, Gloria asked if I was going to be okay. I tried to say yes, but was not very convincing when I burst into tears. She held me as I cried. She sensed what was happening. She and Ron repeated several times to me, "Karen, you cannot keep living like this." They were wonderful. I am so thankful I had them as friends and neighbors.

After Ron and Gloria left, I was scared to death being in the house alone with Jerry. I grabbed the keys to my van and left. I could not stay there, alone, with him. I didn't trust him. This had far surpassed anything I should have tolerated. I drove to a parking lot of an apartment complex and laid in the back of the van, trying to sleep. I laid awake most of the night, only dozing off a few times.

My mind kept racing. What was I going to do? Jerry had to move out. We had discussed a separation with Margo, but we were not in agreement of who should move out. Jerry's insensitivity was obvious when he expected me to leave, in the midst of my recovery. I was not back to work yet and spent all day at home rehabilitating. I was hardly strong enough to move.

The next morning I went home, when I knew Jerry would be at work. Just walking into the house gave me an uneasy feeling. I had been living in a cyclone, sometimes in the eye of the storm, other times in the full force of high winds. Jerry called midday and said he would be moving out that afternoon. What a relief!

I asked Ronna to come over when I knew Jerry would be coming home from work. I was scared to be alone with him. Jerry and his father arrived to pack up his stuff. No words were spoken.

THAT EVENING, WHEN I bent over to pick up the paper, only five weeks after my second craniotomy, spinal fluid flowed out of my nose. "Not again," I cried, "Please God, not again."

I knew it was not sinus drainage. It was clear liquid, as it had always been. It was CSF. Enough of it flowed out to soak half of the paper. My tears soaked the rest.

I felt an urgent need for solitude. I got in my van and drove to my favorite thinking, contemplating, figure-out-life spot. It is tucked away deep in the woods, overlooking a beautiful lake. The only living creatures to come near this spot are usually wildlife.

Once I arrived, I took a deep breath and let out all the feelings that were overflowing my cup. "How much more God?" I yelled. "How much more?" I let my emotions fill the air and break the silence. With arms raised to the heavens, I shouted, "No-o-o-o-o-o-o! Please let it stop." "No-o-o-o-o-o-o! Please let it stop." The echo repeated back to me off the opposite shore, "No-o-o-o-o-o-o! Please let it stop."

I was feeling as though everything that could go wrong in my life was going wrong. It had only been eight months since the leak was detected, and I had been hit with almost every possible tragedy under the sun. My marriage was breaking up. As far as leaking again, bad luck would have it that I would leak after the first craniotomy. It seemed more like an unknown plan of God's rather than bad luck that I leaked again after my second craniotomy. I know God doesn't want me to encounter pain, but He must have wanted to use me for more than I previously anticipated.

I always felt comforted when I was at "my spot." I felt closer to God. It just seemed easier to release everything I had within the depths of my being. It might not help solve problems, but it did help me be more at peace. The solace of this area was a wonderful expression of the peace God grants us.

As I returned home that evening, I saw five rainbows. This day had been my lowest so far, and God had showed me that he cared. I believe these rainbows were specifically meant for me (and every other suffering soul within sight of them).

The first rainbow was a full half-circle. The second one, adjacent to it, was a full half-circle. The third rainbow came completely down to the ground and was transparent. I could see the trees behind it, through its colors. I saw the beginning of the rainbow and could hold onto hope of someday seeing the end. The fourth rainbow was amidst the clouds, over the water, and radiated technicolor ever so brightly. The final rainbow was the least expected. In the dark of the night, I looked up at the full moon. There, around the moon, was a ring of colors. One full circle, no ends at all. It was a rainbow around the moon. I got the message. There is no end to hope. God grants us hope, even during our darkest days and nights.

God is not going to give me the score of my game of life until I reach His finish line, because God is not done with me yet. This doesn't stop Him from showering me with hope. He loves to do that, just as someday He will love to welcome me into His kingdom.

The day before this all happened I had seen Dr. Hoff for my postoperative checkup. We had celebrated his success at stopping the leak. We were confident I was heading in a very positive direction. When I called him to give him the most recent update, that I was leaking again, he was devastated. As he searched for words, I could hear the disappointment in his voice. Almost in a shameful way, he asked if I would come down to see him again, so he could have another shot at it. In a note he wrote to Dr. MacKenzie this same day he said, "We start all over again."

Jerry and I continued to see Margo jointly, as well as individually. We had several conversations about our future. It always boiled down to Jerry saying how much he looked forward to our lives returning to the way they used to be. No matter what I or anyone else said, he truly believed he was going to return to the past. Personally, I could not wait until a better tomorrow.

I prayed for daily guidance. I seriously needed God's help in deciding for my future. This was not a decision I wanted to make, but I had always relied heavily on my own thoughts rather than God's. Prayer took on a new meaning for me at this time in my life as I began having more frequent conversations with my Heavenly Father.

I knew I could never trust Jerry again. If I were to stay with him, I'd live in fear. I thought I knew him as a person, a friend, and more importantly, as a husband. Evidently there was a hidden side to him. In the heart of adversity, change, and emotional upheaval, he could no longer conceal his dark side. I firmly believed this side didn't have to be so dark and filled with emotional extremes, if Jerry would learn to express himself in a more appropriate way. I was heartbroken by his resistance to learn.

I felt as though I had failed. It was hardly like losing a game or a race. This was a promise I had made to God, "...until death do us part." Yet, unless Jerry could keep his promise, "...in sickness and in health...", I could not keep mine. I was devastated by his broken promise.

This didn't take away the feelings of shame, guilt, and defeat. I was full of guilt that I wasn't able to live up to my promise to God. I had never given up on anything before, and now, even though I was not the one who was walking away, I was accepting the defeat of my marriage.

In the midst of all my problems, I began to lose confidence. I lost confidence in myself, but even more devastating, I also began to lose confidence in God. I dwelled on the fact I was disappointing Him in a major way. Rather than continue to let God be in control, I tried to take control back into my own hands.

Oswald Chambers says it very nicely in his book, *My Utmost for His Highest*. "Sometimes we wish He would make us be obedient, and at other times we wish He would leave us alone. Whenever God's will is in complete control, He removes all pressure. And when we deliberately choose to obey Him, He will reach to the remotest star and to the ends of the earth to assist us with all of His mighty power."

It is unfortunate that we have to make choices of whether to take control on our own or let God stay in control. It is less fortunate that we too often choose to take control.

When I turned to find strength within myself instead of God, I did not find any. This was a heart shattering period of my life. I was not capable of standing on my own at any time in my life, let alone at a time such as this. I was in the midst of insurmountable pain from my head injury. I didn't think life could get any worse. It did. I was on the brink of losing my marriage, I needed another craniotomy, and I was overloaded with endless uncertainties. Consequently, I almost gave up.

G IVING UP IS the most painful of all human experiences. In the midst of my seemingly hopeless storm, I wouldn't have seen a rainbow if it were resting on my fingertips. All I saw was the doom and gloom of living the rest of my life alone and in pain. Whether I was going to remain married to Jerry or not, I saw myself emotionally alone. I saw no end to my emotional or physical pain.

I focused on the damage to my head, recognizing it was far more extreme than I ever realized. I began to wonder how much more damage there was than what had already been diagnosed.

It was getting harder and harder for me to continue working. I was working more than I should have been, but I didn't know where else to channel my stress energy, and I was extremely afraid of losing my job. My headache was averaging a ten on a ten-point scale, with ten being the worst possible headache. It felt as though someone had blown holes through my eye sockets. I couldn't imagine what I'd do if the pain ever got worse. I didn't know what to do with the pain as it was. Nothing relieved it, not even Percodan, a strong narcotic.

I could no longer concentrate. My headache was a major distraction and I couldn't bury my head deep enough to protect it from environmental conditions.

It was looking more and more like I was going to have to live with the endless pain, even though this seemed impossible. I have a very high tolerance for pain, but it was wearing me down. I no longer had the energy to fight it, as I once did. I was physically and emotionally drained.

I was losing confidence in my surgeons. Thus far, neither one was able to help me. Even Dr. Hoff, who was supposed to be one of the best neurosurgeons in the country, had been unsuccessful.

I had to manage my own care continuously. While I realize the patient is ultimately responsible for the care they receive, it is a full-time job to ensure everything is done properly and in a timely manner. I was expending precious energy by doing this, and had no one to help me. I was constantly having to call physicians and ask them to call one another. It seemed as though I was always waiting for a physician to call me, never knowing when the phone would ring. I finally got smart and enrolled in call waiting, so I didn't have to be afraid of missing a doctor's call while using the phone.

If I wanted to get things done within a reasonable time frame, I always had to be available at the drop of a hat. I was very fortunate my job allowed for this. I often spent several hours in doctor's offices or hospitals during the day, then ended up working until all hours of the night. Nervous energy often kept me up, working at my computer until four or five in the morning. I'd get a ton of work done in a very efficient way, but was exhausted the following day.

My life seemed so shaken and scattered. I didn't see an end to the madness. I didn't see an end to my headache. I only saw an end to my marriage.

I felt a great deal of pressure from my parents, who were against the breakup of my marriage. I knew no matter what was happening between Jerry and I, they'd have difficulty understanding. They had only seen one side of Jerry, the kindhearted one. They never believed he was capable of doing anything to hurt me. Consequently, they blamed me for the breakup of the marriage.

Jerry did everything he could to keep himself in a positive light with them, lying to them and telling them I was the one exhibiting violent behavior. Like many aspects of my injury, I chose not to share with my parents the details. I believed it would have been too hard for them to worry about this, on top of everything else. It made it more difficult for me, because I sacrificed the support I'm sure they would have given me had they known the truth.

Jerry and my parents had been going behind my back to talk with my doctors and therapists about me. They didn't think I knew what they were doing, but I did. This was Jerry's attempt to protect himself. As for my parents and their actions, they were merely desperate for information and didn't know how to help me. They wanted to know the long-term prognosis of my condition. As I look back on it now, if I would have shared the truth with them there would not have been a need for them to go behind my back. Instead, in my defensive mode, I accused them of deceiving me and not trusting me. This only made matters worse.

As everything came to a peak, my life seemed worthless. Rather than reach out to God, my therapists, or my friends, I carried the entire load. It felt as though God had abandoned me, when the reality was I had abandoned God. I was scared to let anyone see my weakness, my doubt. People constantly complimented me on my strength, and told me what an inspiration I was to them. How could I disappoint them by revealing how much I was struggling? I was embarrassed. I did not feel worthy of the praise. I was trying to remain strong, but it had been four years since my accident. There was never a break in challenges, never a time to rest. The pain kept intensifying, like a blazing fire.

I thought, "I have done everything possible to work through my emotions, grow spiritually, overcome depression, let go of control, reach acceptance, and embrace change. Why am I still overwhelmed with pain? I've experienced more pain in the last four years than most people experience in a lifetime. God, I've learned from this. How much more is there to learn? Hasn't this been enough?"

If I would have heard God's answer, I believe He probably said, "Yes Karen, *you've* experienced it all. Now you have to learn to experience it with Me." But my ears were closed. I was only thinking of myself, and how much pain I was having to endure. I felt very alone.

Too embarrassed to ask for help, I gave up. I lost my will to live, and contemplated ending my life. I am ashamed that I failed to remember the one who loves me most, the one who would never leave my side, the one who was carrying me through these trials, my Heavenly Father.

It was as if I was climbing Mt. Everest and focusing on the peak of the mountain, rather than each small step along the way. To anyone looking only at the mammoth amount of work ahead, this climb would seem impossible.

I hesitated to end my life each time something happened that caused my emotional strength to vacillate, like seeing five rainbows. There were periods of despair, when everything seemed hopeless. Yet, there were also uplifting times, when I was very positive and confident that things would work out for the best. It was truly a roller coaster of emotions. The hardest part was when I felt I was riding the coaster alone, feeling the need to scream, but not a sound would come out.

It was two weeks after Jerry moved out, the middle of June 1993. I went out into the garage, where my van was parked. I put my dog, Akita, outside, so she would remain safe, and closed the garage door. I started the engine of the van and left it running, while I laid down in the back. I was tired. I would fall asleep and never wake up.

I laid there, thinking about what I was doing and questioned whether it was right or wrong. I started to do what is natural for me when I'm in the midst of uncertainty and fear, I began to pray. When I began talking to God, I suddenly realized there was someone else in my life. Although I felt like I had been abandoned by everyone, I had not considered God. He had not abandoned me. In fact, I was, at this very minute, abandoning Him. I was giving up and not trusting Him to take care of me. I was trying to take control away from Him. I worked real hard to fight back the tears, trying not to be overcome with guilt.

Unexpectedly, I heard Akita cry from outside the garage. Again, I recognized there was someone else in this world who loved me unconditionally and who needed me, Akita. This convinced me. What I was doing was not right. It wasn't fair. It's not my place to determine when my race is over. It doesn't work this way in any competition, and it doesn't work this way in life.

I moved to the front of the van and turned off the engine. My lungs had already inhaled a significant amount of carbon monoxide. I had started to cough. I was extremely light-headed. I laid back down until I regained some strength. I opened the garage door and Akita jumped into my arms. We both had tears in our eyes. She truly loved me, as did many other people in this world. She licked the tears from my face and I held her close to my heart.

God used Akita to give me two very important messages. "I need you," and "I love you." I heard them loud and clear, and was ashamed I had doubted God's promise. I prayed for forgiveness and promised never again to try to take my life, which He so generously had given me. I had tried to take control into my own hands, and was as close to destroying God's work as I could ever be. I vowed to give complete control over to God from this point onward, no matter what the circumstances. No matter how dark my life looked, how disastrous the storm appeared, or how much pain I encountered, I would persevere with the help of God. My outlook would remain positive, and I would radiate this understanding to everyone surrounding me.

This positive person is truly who I am. I have never been one to focus on the negative or to be pessimistic. I had temporarily conceded to temptation, and lost my true self and my faith in God. I am not a quitter, but without focus on the promise of God's love, I was lost.

I'm in awe of God's willingness to forgive. I was literally kicking Him in the face that day, and He still loved me and forgave me. I was on the verge of giving up. I know it was only because of God's grace that I did not quit. His loving, merciful heart said, "No, Karen, I'm not done with you yet. I will not let you do this. I will not let you go,"

To ACCEPT I was on the edge of giving up was to acknowledge the underlying weakness in my competitive nature. I know at any given time I might feel as though I am in the midst of a hopeless storm, however, I've also learned nothing can be hopeless enough to warrant loss of life. Rainbows will always shine over me.

I failed to remember God is not going to give me more than I can handle. He was surrounding me with countless friends and family to support and love me. He also promised me He has the game plan. What is happening to me is not without purpose. I just need to trust in Him and not try to understand why things are the way they are. Nor should I ever try to take my life into my own hands.

Life is a never-ending course of combating our sinful nature and our desires to live according to what we want to do or how we think it should be. We are continuously tempted to take control. In the competitive world we're taught to be winners, and in the corporate world we're taught to be leaders. But what about God's world? I believe we should be followers. God has already given us the victory, and He is now leading us to the awards ceremony. In the mean time, however, He's teaching us that it's His way of helping us mature. If we throw our hands up in defeat, we abandon this process, and miss out on life's most valuable lessons.

Life is just like kayaking down a river. There are a variety of potentially dangerous circumstances we might encounter. To become skilled in maneuvering through obstacles and safely handling the current, we can only learn by experience. There is no way to simulate what actually occurs on the river. There is no way to practice, other than to be right out there, doing it. This is a frightening thought.

As spectators observe kayakers moving with the current, they may think they are watching highly-skilled people. They are not. Kayakers develop their skills with the help of the potentially destructive force of the river. They learn while they play. With each rock or overhanging branch, they develop more proficiency to maneuver safely. As the current gets faster and the white water rumbles, breaking the silence of nature, the kayaker acquires the ability to capitalize on the power of the water.

In the midst of this learning, if the kayaker suddenly decides they are too tired to continue or they do not want to be challenged by these obstacles anymore, their position can be fatal. What once was teaching them and developing greater skills and strength, now is likely to destroy them.

Just like kayaking, in life we learn as we go along. There is no way to practice beforehand. The challenges we face are our teachers. Each experience provides us with a new set of skills for the future. If we throw up our hands and refuse to paddle, the challenges we face have the potential to be destructive.

When I made the decision to end my life, I was throwing my paddle into the river and saying, "I cannot do this any longer." I was tired. I couldn't see any progress, and I couldn't remember anyone telling me how I could practice this game called life. I knew there were going to be challenges. I knew I could learn the skills necessary to maneuver safely around the obstacles. I failed to recognize, however, the intense emotion and physical challenges I would experience while riding the white water. I never considered how difficult it might be for my family and me to remain by one another's side, as all of us were challenged to maneuver down the river independently. Each of us were faced with different obstacles and various forces along the way. One cannot be without loneliness, fear, doubt, anger, and hopelessness when fighting the force of the current. They are there to guide us.

Prior to giving up, I was learning how to move forward with great fear and apprehension. I was only beginning to trust God's intentions, but was not yet ready to buy stock in them. I was learning to accept the flow of the river, but at times still turned around and tried to paddle upstream. At these times, my doubts surpassed my level of confidence and trust. I lost sight of the learning process, feeling as though we might as well tally up the score of the game. I was confident I had lost.

This was one of the biggest lessons I have ever learned. This segment of my life is one of the wildest rivers I have traveled. Along the way, I gained countless skills and became proficient in many others. It's a hard way to learn. Fortunately, God got my attention.

My readiness to give up happened for a reason. It might have been so I could withstand the next several years of recovery without questioning if I could go the distance. Now I knew I could do anything God wanted me to. I would float forward with a richer sense of peace.

ONCE JERRY MOVED out of the house, it only took a few days before I knew it would be impossible to get back together with him. It took another six weeks before I was ready to file for divorce.

I worked with Margo on my feelings and my decision. She supported me wholeheartedly. She encouraged me to take care of myself, to not put myself in a vulnerable position. She wanted what was best for me, while at the same time she was unable to tell me what to do. She maintained her professionalism, guiding me toward making my own decision.

Margo was a key player on my recovery team. A whole new world was opened to me when I started working with Margo. I had been so focused on the physical world around me, I never learned to understand the emotional side of life. Margo helped me see inside myself and nurture a part of me I previously never knew existed.

I prayed for God's guidance. I was assured my life would be better without Jerry. I knew divorce was not okay in the eyes of God. I could try to justify it all I wanted, but it still did not make it right. God never intended for us to separate from one another. It is *our* inability to live according to His will that brings divisions to relationships, marriages, families, churches, and many other aspects of life.

I had to move forward in my life and take care of myself. The distance between Jerry and I had only increased over the years. I could accept I would never return to the past, because what I was uncovering was even better. Jerry could not accept this, nor could he see a value in my true self.

Just as it is said, "Life is like an onion. We peel one layer off at a time, and sometimes we cry." I was peeling several layers off throughout my recovery and getting closer and closer to the most flavorful part, my soul. Every experience, good and bad, happy and sad, was the source of my growth. They've provided me with a wealth of knowledge and valuable tools I will use during the balance of my life. I will use my mistakes to the betterment of my being and my successes to enhance my hope.

I made an appointment to see Patrick Wilson, P.C. to discuss my divorce. Pat had been a friend since I moved to Traverse City, nine years prior. He offered to handle my case, encouraging me not to worry about anything. I was comforted by the fact he was genuinely concerned and eager to relieve me of as much stress in my life as possible.

Within three days, Pat had the papers prepared and ready for me to sign. I cannot compare signing divorce papers to anything. What else terminates a promise to God and a commitment of love to a man for the rest of their life? I can think of only one other thing close to this, death. It was as though I was signing papers to terminate life, not my life, not Jerry's life, but our life. Along with this, came the same grieving process.

Denial had already passed. I had been through the stage of refusing to believe this was happening to me. I experienced depression, which remained with me at varying degrees, throughout the divorce process. I encountered anger, inside and out, sometimes letting it get the best of me. Eventually, I moved onto acceptance and hope for a happier life.

My decision to divorce Jerry was validated by several incidents that occurred after he had moved out of the house. One evening, I was invited to Paul and Diane's for dinner. We talked until 11:00 p.m. and finally Diane asked me if I was afraid to go home. I thought about it for a brief moment and realized, yes, I was fearful of going home to an empty house.

I suspected Jerry was following me, and thought maybe he was trying to get in the house when I was not home. I was afraid I would come home one night and find him there, waiting for me. My distrust of him was evident.

Paul suggested that Diane ride home with me and stay with me. Diane replied, "I don't want to be alone in that house with her either, no way. You take her home Paul." Paul agreed to take me home. He wouldn't let me go alone.

We drove my van. As we drove into the entrance of the subdivision, Jerry's van drove through the subdivision, past the entrance in front of us, with its lights out. I said, "There's Jerry with his lights out." Paul, stunned by what I said, asked if I said what he thought I said. I confirmed my statement and told him where Jerry was headed. We stopped my van and turned off the lights, waiting to see where Jerry was going and what he would do. I couldn't believe what was happening. My intuition told me Jerry was following me, but I never thought we'd actually catch him.

Jerry turned around and began to head back towards us. He made the mistake of stepping on the brake. I saw the brake lights come on in-between the houses. Jerry was moving towards us very slowly, with the van's lights off. As he moved closer to us and my house, Paul decided to confront him. Paul drove towards Jerry, shining our headlights on him. "What are you doing here, Jerry?" he asked. "I'm driving through the neighborhood because I was passing by," Jerry replied.

I wanted to say, "And you thought you'd turn your lights off so you could see better in the dark, right?" but I restrained myself. There was enough evidence to prove his guilt.

After this happened, it was very hard for me to feel safe. I had the locks changed, but that didn't stop Jerry from breaking in. He had duplicate keys made without telling me—though he made the mistake of bragging to my neighbors that he had the keys. I had the locks changed a second time.

This type of stress was the last thing I needed while continuing my medical care at the University of Michigan Medical Center. It was difficult to control my anger towards Jerry, knowing very well he knew my physical condition. It reinforced my belief that he never really cared.

Fifteen

Somewhere Out There

Even if you're on the right track,
you'll get run over if you just sit there.

WILL ROGERS

I N THE MIDST OF divorce I needed to proceed with my medical care. My health was a very valuable commodity, no matter what happened between Jerry and me. I needed to continue my efforts to improve my health.

I was overwhelmed by the magnitude of tragedy and loss in my life. Although it would have been very easy for me to give up, I held onto hope as tightly as I could. My faith carried me through these difficult times. God's love embraced and carried me through the impossible moments. Looking back, these challenges are a reminder of God's unfailing love.

I clung to God's promises. These trials would ultimately increase my endurance and strength to face other matters. The hard part was seeing this perspective when I was surrounded by trials. My feelings are illustrated in a poem I wrote during this period of my recovery.

SOMEWHERE...
Somewhere out there,
      Beneath a brand new day;
Life will begin again,
      More will go my way.
Does life wait while I live,
      Or do I travel my destined path;

New paths of exploration,
>> Paved with love, smiles and a laugh.

Somehow I'll keep moving,
>> Without an end or destination;
Be it answers to my prayers,
>> And the power of determination.

Earth's destiny undefined,
>> Forever changing in every way;
Once a goal, once a time,
>> Then a road traveled each day.

Each day marking a new beginning,
>> New challenges, new feelings, new friends;
Sunset is only an intermission,
>> A transition of what life sends.

The beauty of a sunset,
>> One chapter coming to a close;
Dawn turning to daylight,
>> Like a blossom of a rose.

As time passes by us,
>> We sprout, bloom, and grow;
With the fresh morning rain,
>> Giving us the power to go.

Some may call each rain a storm,
>> Some see only clouds so dark;
Others focus on the rainbow,
>> The promise God will do His part.

Never allowing the storm to last,
>> Always making the rain cease;
The hope of new beginnings,
>> Minutes, days, and weeks.

The rainbow is a reminder,
>> For me everything will be fine;
Given to me at opportune times,
>> When I most need a sign.

When the storm seems relentless,
　　　Battering me, tearing me down;
When feeling ever so helpless,
　　　Hopeless and spun all around.

Then I look to the heavens,
　　　And there amidst the gray sky;
Shines a rainbow just for me,
　　　Not needing to ask why.

For this summer is filled with rainbows,
　　　More hopes than one each day;
Multiples seen in the distance,
　　　Some closer, not just far away.

Never would I have thought I'd see,
　　　The end of a rainbow touch the earth;
Yet there between the trees and I,
　　　Brilliant colors, not an end but birth.

The birth of new hope,
　　　Close enough to touch;
Hardly out of reach,
　　　As long as my focus is as such...

That when I'm up above it,
　　　Seeming to see the perfect line;
It's a very different view,
　　　Yet when in it, it's not so fine

Rainbows circling the moon,
　　　Hope even in the dark of night;
A rainbow without an end,
　　　A symbol of eternal hope and light.

A light of beauty beaming bright,
　　　A ring of everlasting hope;
Reflecting down from up above,
　　　Giving me strength to cope.

Counting five in one day,
　　　I needed more signs this time;

As my doubts and fears intensify,
        Questioning abilities of mine.

It seems insurmountable,
        These obstacles towering above;
Yet I know I have the tools,
        I know I have the love...

Of friends watching over me,
        Climbing the same trail;
Someone to hold onto,
        Never without fail.

Someone always beside me,
        Never a moment alone;
Be it hand in hand,
        Or even via the phone.

I'm letting down my guard,
        Showing what's behind;
The strong willed face, the permanent smile,
        Showing feelings of every kind.

Here lies two ends so opposite,
        Once again they stand apart;
Feeling good, letting my doors open,
        But scared to build more than the start...

Of the closest friendships,
        I've yet known;
Where love is felt,
        Where love is shown.

Where tears flow,
        Like giant raindrops;
Flooding our hearts,
        Filling our pots.

As I'm high upon these mountains,
        I'm frightened by the view;
While beautiful and wondrous,
        It is overwhelming too.

How can I have such feelings,
    All at the same time;
At two ends of the spectrum,
    Very difficult to define.

I look out over the valley,
    And see the easiest way;
Then I end up miles from nowhere,
    So what do I learn from this day?

From the deepest valleys I walk,
    Through the storms I come;
Doubts and fears with each step,
    Wanting to just run.

Wanting to be on the high road,
    It feels like the way to see;
The beauty of life beneath me,
    The beauty of life in me.

Yet, looking up from below,
    The beauty can be seen;
It's easier to view this perspective,
    If on others I lean.

For it's common to lose one's balance,
    Being overwhelmed while looking up;
But it's okay to hold on,
    To others when things get tough.

Wandering through the valley,
    At the foot of the mountains so high;
Ready to begin my ascent,
    Having no idea why...

I was placed at the foot,
    Of the biggest mountain range;
Many miles to travel,
    By foot, by rope, by brain.

Please find it, please fix it,
    Give me back a life;

> Please heal me, please give me,
> A feeling it'll be all right.
>
> I know You have an ultimate plan,
> One I may never know the look;
> Just give me strength to have the faith,
> Your plan is by the book.
>
> May Your presence continue to guide me,
> Throughout my life, every part;
> May You light my path ever brighter,
> To remain ever close in heart.   (Written: July 1993)

Throughout the summer of 1993, I made several more trips to the University of Michigan Medical Center. I was still leaking spinal fluid and Dr. Hoff was trying desperately to find the location of the leak. He wanted to avoid going back into my head at all costs.

We made several attempts to find the leak with a radionuclide isotope labeling study. This test involves the placement of pledgets (a strip of gauze attached to string) into each of my eight sinuses by an otynlaryngologist. A lumbar puncture was performed, and then radionuclide isotopes were injected into my CSF. I was scanned every hour for six hours, and then twenty-four hours later. The hope was to see the radioisotope move into the area of the CSF leak.

The first time I had this test, I was shocked when I saw the pledgets. I wondered how in the world they were going to fit into my sinuses. Fortunately, the doctors numbed my nasal passages beforehand; amazingly enough with cocaine. The amount of cocaine used was minimal, but very effective for reducing the discomfort.

When all of the pledgets had been placed in my sinuses, I thought my head must be hollow. How in the world was there enough room for the equivalent of eight cotton balls up my nose? Nevertheless, they were up there and attached to a lifeline string. (Was this to prevent them from getting lost in my nose?)

After running the first scan, I was allowed to walk around the hospital, until it was time for the next scan. The unique part of this, was the fact that the strings from the pledgets were hanging from my nostrils. Fortunately, having been through so much already, I was no longer modest about my appearance. The radiology tech simply taped the strings to my face in the form of a handlebar mustache, and off I went to walk the hallways. It became very common for people to see me walking with strings hanging out my nose.

After one scan, they sent me to the parking garage, so I could run up and down the steps. This activity would increase my spinal fluid pressure, and thereby increase the opportunity for the doctors to find the leak. The only problem was that the cocaine numbed more than my sinuses.

The first time I got up from the table, after receiving the cocaine, I felt a little queasy. While I walked down the hallway, I felt as though I had a little buzz going, which was totally unexpected. Diane Fetter, who accompanied me every time I went to Ann Arbor, kept an eye on me. I was really fine, though we had a good laugh over my new experience with "cocaine."

The results of the radionuclide isotope study were inconclusive. This didn't surprise any of us. I had yet to have a positive test, despite two neurosurgeons being able to clearly see my leak when they operated on my brain. Therefore, Dr. Hoff decided to check to see if my lumbar shunt was working. It had been in me for eight months.

X-rays showed the shunt had completely pulled out of my spine and was not functioning. Dr. Hoff guessed the shunt had pulled out of my spine soon after it was placed. When I told him how sick I was immediately after the surgery and how extreme my headache became, he acknowledged this was a result of the shunt detaching. Dr. Hoff felt it best to replace the entire shunt, since there was still a need to keep the spinal fluid pressure low, to reduce the chance of a continued leak. Once again, there was only a small chance this would work, but one we were both willing to try.

Diane and I drove to Ann Arbor, the day before surgery, for my pre-op tests. We stayed with some friends of hers in the Ann Arbor area that night, and I was admitted to the hospital the following morning. Upon walking into the admitting department, the woman at the desk said, "Hi, Karen. Here we go again, huh?" This was impressive. It made me feel comfortable and cared for, while at the same time reinforcing the fact I had been there too many times.

The surgery went very well. It only took an hour and a half to remove the old shunt and install a new one. I was told this shunt had a valve on it, which would control the amount of fluid flowing through it.

From the recovery room, I was taken to a semi-private room on the neuro floor. I was getting to know most of the nurses on this floor, including Etta.

I was quite uncomfortable after this surgery. The incisions were located in two places, my abdomen, where the shunt dumps fluid into the body, and in my back. This made sneezing, coughing, and laughing difficult. I remained in bed, with full privileges to use the bedpan. Boy, was I thrilled.

I slept most of the day. Eventually, I really had to use the bedpan. I called for the nurse, who was happy to assist me. Unfortunately, no matter what tricks we tried, I could not go. She had to catheterize me to relieve my bladder.

Throughout the day my back became more and more uncomfortable, even though I had not moved from a thirty-degree angle in bed. The resident doctor came in to check on me and asked to look at my incisions. When I bent forward in bed for the first time, he was quite surprised to see a large amount of swelling at the site of my incision. He quickly left to find Dr. Hoff, not giving me a chance to ask him what this meant.

After he left, I reached my hand around to my back and felt a lump the size of a baseball. This, of course, increased both my worry and my pain. Dr. Hoff came in shortly. He immediately wanted to see my back. When he saw it, he said he probably needed to take me back into surgery. It was a blood clot, and had the potential to do some damage.

This ignited fear, as I remembered my father's back surgery three years prior to this. He also had a blood clot that pinched his spinal cord and left him paralyzed from the waist down. They rushed him back into surgery to dissolve the clot. Afterwards, he regained movement in his legs.

Within another ten minutes, several other doctors came in to look at my back. By this time, the swelling had grown to the size of a grapefruit. The doctors consulted with Dr. Hoff. They convinced him to wait, to observe the clot, and to see if it would dissolve on its own. The nurses began drawing circles on my back with a pen to track the growth of the swelling.

Meanwhile, I continued to eat and drink, but still could not urinate without being catheterized. After eating dinner, I suddenly felt extremely full. I'm not one to over-eat, so it was strange to have such a full feeling. Shortly thereafter, I became very uncomfortable. I had pain in my thoracic cavity, and no one knew why. Was it related to the clot?

On this evening, Dr. Hoff's son, who was a resident, took care of me. He ordered x-rays of my abdomen, to determine the cause of my pain. (This was a very long night for me.) At midnight, they finally took me down to Radiology, where I laid on the stretcher in the hallway for over an hour. Diane stayed at the hospital with me, extremely worried about my condition, not knowing if I would require more surgery.

Once they read the x-rays, they could see that my bowel had stopped working. This was the cause of my discomfort. The clot pressed up against the nerves going to both my bladder and bowel. Neither of them were functioning. The doctors decided to hold off on further surgery, because the blood clot had stabilized. They anticipated it would dissipate on its own.

Before giving me medication to help me sleep, they gave me a suppository to get things moving in my bowels. I woke up the next morning to a roomful of interns asking me how I was feeling. On this day, I could again see heads bobbing in the doorway, trying to hear the conversation. Of course, the million dollar question was, "Have you had a bowel movement yet?"

"Negative," I replied.

This prompted their recommendation for alternative methods of relieving the pressure inside my bowel, none of which I was looking forward to. I could see this was going to be a very humbling day.

I was still very uncomfortable and becoming irritated by the increasing amount of noise from my roommate's visitors. She was waiting to go to surgery, and had eight family members and friends packed in our room, with the television blaring. This was not a pleasant environment for someone with a headache and an obstructed bowel. I complained to the nurse, and asked her if she could suggest they wait in the lounge and turn the volume down on the television. This helped for awhile.

The nurse then began trying to get my system running again. The size of the clot had reduced, so they figured if they could get my bowels working, everything would be fine. Their first attempt was with enema. I don't normally care what type of medical procedure is done on me, but this was the most humiliating of any I'd had. It did not work.

Next, they tried a big bag enema, with no success. This was followed by me drinking magnesium citrate, a liquid similar to acid. I counted my blessings that I couldn't taste it. (Not having a sense of taste or smell did have its advantages.) The magnesium citrate was supposed to dissolve the obstruction from the top down, since we hadn't had success from the bottom up. The nurse was most confident this would do the trick. It failed.

They tried everything short of dynamite, which at this point I probably would have agreed to. By late morning, Etta came in to check on me. She had heard of my predicament. A mischievous grin came over her. I asked what she was thinking. She said, "The doctors have ordered an M&M, if all the other attempts fail."

"What in the world is an M&M?" I asked.

With a frisky look in her eyes, she explained, "It is warmed whole milk and molasses."

I knew I better ask more questions. "Do I drink it?"

She replied, "Oh no. It goes in the other end. It is an enema." The expression on my face must have been a dead give away as to how I felt about this. She laughed and said, "It works every time. I will call down to dietary to have them put it together."

I could not believe this was happening to me. I thought once I experienced a craniotomy I had experienced it all. I jokingly said to Diane, "I wonder how this will show up on my bill?"

It wasn't long before the nurse came in to tell me they were waiting for the M&M, and would use it as soon as it arrived. This nurse seemed quite unfriendly that day. Even though she was not familiar with me, usually I can warm people up by talking with them. She was difficult.

Before long, she reappeared in my room carrying a huge bag of brown fluid with a tube on the end. This bag was so big she had to hold it above her head to carry it. It must have been eight inches in diameter and three feet long. This is not an exaggeration. She hung it on an IV pole and pulled the curtain. She said, "Please lay on your side so we can get started."

I said, "Wait a minute. We're going to do this in my bed?"

"Affirmative."

"No way. How will I ever get to the bathroom? I'm not even in the bed closest to the bathroom." She assured me she'd get me there in time and then followed it with a quick comment.

"That's one way to get rid of her visitors." I looked up at her, and she had a big smile plastered on her face. I was seeing another side to her that I liked.

As I laid there she kept saying, "Relax." I could feel the stuff moving inside me. She continued to express her wit and humor by saying, "Tis better to give than to receive." Laughing was not an option at this point, though it was hard to contain myself.

After she had inserted the tube into my rectum, she blew up a little balloon that helped keep everything inside. I still had the feeling I was going to explode any second. I couldn't believe the entire tube was going in me. Once the bag was empty, she detached the tube from the bag, leaving the tube inside me. She said, "Relax for fifteen minutes. I will come back to help you to the bathroom."

I shook my head saying, "I can't keep this inside me for fifteen minutes."

She said, "Call me if you need me," and walked out the door. As soon as she stepped one foot out the door, I hit my buzzer. She returned and asked what I wanted.

I pleaded with her to help me to the bathroom. She said, "It works better the longer you can keep it inside you. Just hold it for ten minutes. Buzz me if you need anything."

As soon as she stepped out of the room the phone rang. I debated whether to answer it or not. I did. It was Dr. MacKenzie, wanting to know how I was doing. Boy did I have a long story to tell him with only seconds to spare. Without appearing rude, I told him, "I really need to talk with you, but it will have to be at another time. I am confident you will understand when I tell you what is happening at the moment."

As soon as I hung up I buzzed for the nurse again. She returned a few minutes later and asked my roommate's visitors to leave the room. She pushed back the curtain and helped me to the edge of the bed. I was scared to death to move, feeling as though I was going to explode. The M&M felt like dynamite. This would not be a pretty sight.

As it was, it was quite a sight to see me walk across the room, knees pinched together as close as possible, bare butt hanging out of my hospital gown, and a funny looking tail (the tube) hanging out of my butt, as I tried to move as quickly and smoothly as possible.

The nurse and I could not contain our laughter. We were having fun. I threw all humility out the window. After she deflated the balloon and removed the tube, I sat down on the toilet. She said once again, "Try to keep holding it inside you as long as possible. I'll go get some towels."

"Towels? Towels? There is a need for towels?" Oh no, I thought to myself. This is going to be messy. What is going to happen? I was trying desperately to hold it in, more relieved now that I was in position to at least have a safe accident.

As the nurse was walking back into the bathroom, I lost control. My bowels started to move at an increasing rate. Just as the nurse said, "Have you had any big ch..u..n..k..s.....?" I exploded. It felt as though I had blown the bottom out of the toilet. She smiled and nodded her head, "Yes, I guess that answers my question."

What a relief. It had worked. I felt as though all of my insides came out of me within five seconds. The M&M did its job. I immediately took a shower and cleaned up, then returned to bed for more rest.

The shift changed shortly after this major constipation relief. The first thing my next nurse said when she walked in my room was, "I hear there was an explosion in this room earlier." Word travels fast. Anyone who knew me and came into my room that day, made wisecracks at my expense.

Later that afternoon, I decided to put some real clothes on, instead of the hospital gown, so I pulled the curtain. I began putting my underwear on, when suddenly I saw feet with scrubs walk up to the curtain and say, "Ms. Wells, are you here?"

I said, "Yes, you can pull the curtain back. I'm just putting on my underwear." Instead they sat down in the chair next to the curtain, and began asking me how I was feeling. I gave a simple answer, "Much better, now that I exploded. But really, you can pull the curtain back."

I reached from my bed to pull it back myself. Much to my surprise, there wasn't just one resident in the room, there was an entire roomful of residents listening to our conversation. I was embarrassed, and they all had smiles on their faces, knowing I had no idea they were there.

This M&M story has been a fun one to share. It has drawn a lot of laughter, along with many other stories of my humbling experiences.

A LTHOUGH THE SHUNT was supposed to reduce my spinal fluid pressure, Dr. Hoff also prescribed Diamox, a medication commonly used by mountain climbers to reduce altitude sickness. Diamox is a diuretic that helps decrease spinal fluid pressure by reducing the rate of its production. Spinal fluid is produced at a rate of approximately two pints per day. We only need about one cup of spinal fluid at any given time. Typically, bodies absorb the overflow and eliminate it through the urinary system. Since our entire nervous system floats in spinal fluid, it is a very essential fluid. The miraculous part is that we manufacture more fluid than we actually need, to ensure the nervous system is protected.

I had been leaking spinal fluid for four years, and unbeknownst to anyone, my brain was experiencing additional permanent damage as a result. Due to the extremely low pressure caused by the leak, my ventricles (the cavities inside our brains), were shrinking from a lack of fluid circulating through them.

Despite the shunt lowering my pressure even further, and the effects of the Diamox, my leak persisted. So did my headache. In fact, the headache became worse. I could tell the pressure was too low by doing a very simple test. I could lie flat on my back and increase the volume of spinal fluid to my head, reducing my pain. I called Dr. Hoff, who was always very prompt at returning my phone calls, regardless of where he was.

After discussing the changes in my symptoms since the new shunt was inserted, both on the phone and during a routine checkup, Dr. Hoff decided to clamp it off that very same day. Soon after he evaluated my status, we walked down to the procedure room together. Dr. Hoff was always eager to ease my pain, taking time as though I was his daughter. This is very unique, especially for a surgeon of his caliber.

Throughout my recovery, I found that the surgeons who worked at a lower skill level were the ones whose egos stood in the way of their patient care. These surgeons wouldn't give me the time of day, whereas, the two most highly-skilled neurosurgeons in the world gave me all the time I needed.

Dr. Hoff and his assistant prepped my abdomen, where the shunt was attached and dumping spinal fluid into my peritoneal cavity. Dr. Hoff numbed the area with a local anesthetic before making his incision. He made a very tiny cut, and began digging around for the shunt. Although he could palpate it from outside my body, Dr. Hoff had some difficulty getting his instrument to connect with it inside. I squirmed a few times, but for the most part was very comfortable. In fact, while he was digging around in my abdomen, trying to bring the shunt to the incision, Dr. Hoff began bragging to his assistant about my level of competitive success. He explained that I had played basketball for Michigan State University and then became a champion triathlete. It was interesting to hear Dr. Hoff bragging about me, when he was one of the top neurosurgeons in the world. But this was typical of his personality. He cared more about his patients than about his own accomplishments. Then Dr. Hoff asked me if I had ever competed in the Ironman Triathlon in Hawaii.

I replied, "No, but it's always been a goal of mine. Do you think someday I'll still be able to do it?"

He responded confidently, "Certainly, you will get there."

"Will you be a part of my medical support staff when I do?" I asked.

"Most certainly," he said, "I'd be proud to be there with you. You can count on it," he said with a huge smile.

This is a good example of my rapport with Dr. Hoff. This gave me great comfort, even in the midst of pain and frustration. I am so thankful I had such a fine doctor, one who was both very skilled and extraordinarily personable. I continued to be surrounded by angels.

Between Dr. Hoff and Dr. MacKenzie, I knew I was in good hands. They are two of my four most-loved doctors. They embody the finest in health care professionals.

Once Dr. Hoff completed this minor surgery, I hopped off the table and adjusted to the pressure change very quickly. He sent me on my way, saying there was no reason for me to stay in the area. I could go home to Traverse City, as long as I called him the next day to report my progress.

Diane and I got back on the highway and put the van on autopilot. We were becoming quite familiar with this trip.

I felt fine, except for one minor detail. The local anesthetic to my abdomen must have affected my bladder. I had a great urgency to urinate, but when we stopped at the rest area, I could not relieve myself. I became increasingly uncomfortable, and as we traveled further north, there were fewer and fewer rest areas. It was the longest trip from Ann Arbor to Traverse City I'd ever experienced. I went to bed as soon as I arrived home, hoping whatever was wrong would correct itself by morning. It did. I have a new appreciation of our urinary system.

Diane was such a blessing. I do not know what I would have done without her. She was there for me whenever I needed her. During this time, our friendship moved to a new level. We spent a great deal of time on the road, driving to and from Ann Arbor. You would think we'd run out of things to talk about, but this was hardly the case. Our friendship was very valuable and therapeutic for both of us.

My friendship with both Diane and Paul was strong. We were like the three musketeers. They helped carry me through one of the most difficult times in my life. I was in the midst of my nasty divorce, distanced from my parents, and fighting to tolerate constant pain and fatigue from my headache.

They say when tragedy strikes, you suddenly find out who your true friends are. I ended up finding out how deep seeded all my friendships were. I am moved by the depth of these relationships. Everyone surrounded me with a blanket of love and tenderness; everyone except my husband. After seven years, our marriage would end in divorce, at a time when I needed a companion the most. But what was lost in my marriage was made up in friendships, both long-standing ones and new ones made during my recovery. Whether these friends were geographically close to me or not, they still remained ever close in mind and heart. Each and every one of them supported me in a unique way, which complemented the others. I truly believe God had a hand in this. It was as though He orchestrated the whole performance, and everyone harmonized their support in a most beautiful way.

My parents were trying desperately to stay with the orchestra, but they didn't know what song to play. When they played a duet, choreographing beautiful music, it was as though I pushed the mute button, not knowing how to receive their support.

It was during this time the movie "Free Willy" came out. I don't think I've cried as hard at any other movie than I did at this one. The timing was right. My life coincided with the message of setting Willy free from captivity and returning him to his family. I yearned to be held in the arms of my mother and father. I was feeling held captive by my injury. Whenever I heard the words of the song "Will You Be There," I cried. I felt it was written for me. The words were very fitting for all my friendships, but especially my relationship with my parents.

> Hold me, like the river Jordan, and I will then say to thee you are my friend. Carry me like you are my brother, love me like a mother, will you be there? When weary tell me will you hold me, when wrong, will you mold me, when lost will you find me? But they told me, a man should be faithful, and walk when not able, and fight till the end, but I'm only human. Everyone's taking control of me, seems that the world's got a role for me, I'm so confused, will you show to me, you'll be there for me, and care enough to bear me. In our darkest hour, in my deepest despair, will you still care? Will you be there? In my trials and my tribulations through our doubts and frustrations, in my violence, in my turbulence, through my fear and my confessions in my anguish and my sorrow, in the promise of another tomorrow, I'll never let you part for you're always in my heart.
>
> by Michael Jackson

I was being faithful to what I had been taught through competition, fighting to the end, while trying to walk when not able, and screaming beneath my coat of armor, "I'm only human." I kept repeating these words over and over again, using them to help me accept my weaknesses and desires to give up. I gave myself permission to feel this way.

I wrote a poem that speaks of my friendships with those who have stuck with me through my recovery. I consider each family member and friend, an angel sent by God to watch over me. I cherish these connections.

MY ROCKS

The waves keep rolling in,
  With a thunderous roar;
Collapsing over my head,
  Not one, but two and more.

The force is relentless,
  The power hard to overcome;
With great intensity it keeps coming,
  Making me want to just run.

I can see them off in the distance,
  Predicting the size almost;
Yet they seem to keep building strength,
  As they near my coast.

I stand with feet firmly planted,
  Confident I can hold my own;
Ready to withstand the blow,
  Prepared for the danger zone.

One wave strikes,
  Knocking me unsteady;
The second wave hits,
  Not when I'm ready.

The third crashes down,
  But I still hold my ground;
Number four weakens me,
  And turns me completely around.

The fifth is a shock,
  Even though I saw it coming;
The sixth has hit me before,
  But I've always kept running.

Seven is on its way,
  Yet I have a moment to see;
These rocks shining beside me,
  They're there to rescue me.

The back water washes over us,

Swirling the sand making us shine;
Never leaving us completely covered,
Holding life's beauty for us to find.

These friends, these rocks, see me weakening,
Trying to persevere;
They recognize the difficulty,
They detect my enormous fear.

As the waves rumble over us,
They reach out their gentle hands;
Giving me a base to hold onto,
Sharing their love as plentiful as sand.

Their abilities are wondrous,
As if to calm each wave;
Listening, caring, and sharing,
A unique path we pave.

The gift of their friendship is priceless,
They are so faithful and true;
They give me hope and strength,
I just wish they only knew...

How much it really means,
To have them next to me;
As the waves test my spirit,
My capacity to be...

True to myself in every way,
Holding onto what means the most;
Giving one to another,
Even when waves rip the coast.

To describe their friendship would limit,
What seems limitless and deep;
For if I dig the sand around them,
Their depth would only keep...

Me digging for a lifetime,
They're here for the duration;
Not a ripple, crest or tidal wave,

Could falter this relation.

With their help I persevere,
    Not knowing what's still in store;
Knowing they'll always be there,
    Not once, but twice, and more.

We laugh, we cry, we feel the pain,
    While the water rushes over our feet;
We don't give in, we don't give up,
    Each challenge we're here to meet.

Lord, thank-you for these rocks,
    They're gifts I know, from You;
Please let the waves make us strong,
    We can endure, with You too.   (Written: August 1993)

Each wave has a significant meaning. The first one signifies my accident, while the second one was the death of my grandfather. The third is my first craniotomy, and the fourth is when I realized the surgery did not fix the leak and I needed another craniotomy. The fifth was my divorce. The sixth was finding out I was leaking spinal fluid after my second craniotomy, and the seventh meant I was headed for more surgery.

I surely felt as though my friends were the backbone, or in this case the rocks, of my recovery. They were the surest earthly things I had to hold onto. And, hold onto, I most certainly did. Each friend played a very unique role in my recovery. While some assisted me by doing things around my house, others were available to listen and to talk about my feelings. Some, like Diane and Paul, also traveled great distances with me, as I began seeking medical care further away from Traverse City. The everlasting care and concern from these friends has been a wonderful gift from God. It is miraculous!

The most intense feeling, however, was that God was my surest rock. Just as the song goes, "...and He walks with me and He talks with Me, and He tells me I'll never be alone," I felt His presence. I knew with God and the angels with whom He surrounded me, I'd never be alone. God was constantly directing and protecting all of us. "Who shall separate us from the love of Christ? Shall trouble or hardship or persecution...? No, in all these things we are more than conquerors through Him who loved us." (Romans 8:35 & 37 NIV)

These friendships are miracles that dwell within our hearts. It's interesting to think of how they happen. They can only be an act of God. How else would it be possible for so many people to have such deep connections that keep growing stronger? Just when I think a friendship is as close as it could ever become, it gets even stronger.

Sixteen

Dreaded Words

Hear my cry , O God; listen to my prayer.
From the ends of the earth I call to you,
I call as my heart grows faint;
lead me to the rock that is higher than I.

Psalm 61:1-2

O NCE DR. HOFF CLAMPED off the shunt he was at a loss about what to do next to fix my leak. He kept saying to me, "I don't want to go into your head again, without knowing where the leaks are. But, I also don't want anyone blindly packing your sinuses, with the hope of stopping the leaks. This is not the answer. We have to find the location of your leaks first." I appreciated his caution.

On the other hand, my patience was shrinking. It had been four years since my accident and no one had solved the puzzle. I was beginning to wonder if there would ever be a solution, or if my case could not be solved. My biggest fear was that one day, after exhausting all options, a doctor would say to me, "Karen, we have done all that we can do," despite my condition still being critical.

I had to ask myself, "Can I live with the pain I am experiencing every minute of every day? What will my life-style be like? Will I still be content and at peace living life at a much slower pace, with less competition, and possibly less success? Will I still be able to perform my job and maintain my career? Will I still be able to help people (this gives me my greatest

232

satisfaction)?" These thoughts raced through my mind daily, and I didn't have answers to any of them. It was terrifying.

I would most certainly try to live with the pain and to carry on with an active life-style, knowing there would be some trade-off. I focused on the positive sides of the trade-off, such as: slower might be better and the biggest competitor I had was myself. The greatest threat to my success in life would be my pride. Once I got over the hurdle of feeling like a victim and recognized I was a survivor, I began attaining greater levels of success.

I will continue to find success on whatever path God leads me. Maybe my scars from healed wounds will be profitable to God and to other people. I believe that there is a reason for everything. Life is God's plan.

Throughout my recovery, I have needed to welcome and accept new phases of my life. I have not chosen these changes, but my faith tells me it is best that they were chosen for me.

The most difficult thing to accept, and to believe that God has chosen for me, is my pain. To this day it puzzles me. The only reasoning I hold onto is maybe there are still many more parts of life to learn. God needs more time with me. In order to learn the lesson well, maybe I need to continue experiencing pain.

My pain has a way of slowing me down. Without it, my lessons might be forgotten. Until I am completely sold on this new way of living and comfortable with being just Karen Wells—not Karen the cyclist or Karen the competitor or Karen the let's do everything I can in one day—maybe I need the pain as a reminder. God has uncovered me from all the glitz, showmanship, and rapid speed. Why would He risk my ego taking back the reigns and ruining His design?

I moved closer and closer to complete acceptance of this, recognizing I was probably getting closer to the day when I'd be told, "We have done everything. You must now live with the pain." Yet I was still not willing to give up hope on a solution. I wrestled daily with whether God wanted acceptance from me, or did He want hope and perseverance. I continued to choose hope and perseverance, wanting to use acceptance as a backup plan. I knew that even within acceptance there was hope and perseverance. Hope for peace, and perseverance to go the distance, despite the pain.

D R. HOFF AND I discussed our next strategy to find my leak. Not only was it a matter of relieving my pain, but also eliminating the critical risk of meningitis. Everyday that I lived with the leak, I lived with a very high risk of death. An infection of this nature could kill me.

He recommended I see Greg Wolfe, M.D., an Otynlaryngologist at the University of Michigan. He wanted Dr. Wolfe to use a flexible scope to locate my leaks.

I was getting very run down from the weekly ten-hour round-trip drives to Ann Arbor. But, if Dr. Wolfe could locate my leaks, I was willing to make the drive again.

I met with Dr. Wolfe. For the eleventh time, I told my entire story to a physician. My story began with the day of my accident and included details of everything that had occurred over four years. The longer it took to repair the damage to my skull, the longer my story became. It was becoming increasingly more difficult to make it a condensed version. I learned, however, from telling my story over and over again to every resident and intern who entered my room while I was in the hospital.

After listening to my story, looking at my scans, and examining me, Dr. Wolfe recommended surgery to pack my left ethmoid sinus. While he had no proof this was the area where I was leaking, he suspected this would help stop the leak. His plan was to go in and blindly pack the whole sinus cavity, patching the leak from beneath the skull.

I immediately began asking questions. "How do you know it is in the left ethmoid sinus? Aren't you going to use your flexible scope to try to find it first?"

Dr. Wolfe quickly became very defensive. His change in temperament was frightening. How could I ever trust someone like this to perform surgery on me? It was as if he was intimidated by my wealth of clinical knowledge on my injury and medical care. I was beginning to believe all Otynlaryngologists were rude and arrogant, especially since my experience with the physician at Mayo Clinic had been very similar.

I was very apprehensive about the decision for more surgery, especially considering Dr. Hoff's convictions of not wanting anyone to blindly pack my sinuses.

I left Dr. Wolfe's office feeling like I had been stolen away from Dr. Hoff. Dr. Wolfe did not seem to care what Dr. Hoff's opinions were. He went ahead and scheduled surgery, without consulting Dr. Hoff.

I couldn't travel all the way back to Traverse City without speaking with Dr. Hoff first. I knew if I could talk with him, my worries would lessen. Either he would agree with the scheduled surgery, giving me more confidence, or he would advise me not to have the surgery. In any case, I knew talking with him would help. I was worried I might not be able to reach Dr. Hoff before he left the hospital, as it was already late afternoon. I called his clinic, to see if I could speak with him. I had seen him earlier in the day, and knew he had been there.

The woman I spoke with was only performing her job by being very protective of Dr. Hoff's time. She said that unless I had an appointment, I couldn't see him. I explained I had seen Dr. Hoff that morning and pleaded with her to just give Dr. Hoff a message and let him make the decision if he wanted to see me or not. She agreed, and said she would need to call me back. I was on a pay phone two floors below her, so I said I'd come up to the office and wait for a reply. When I arrived, Dr. Hoff's nurse came out to the waiting room and said, "If you can wait around until 5:00 p.m., Dr. Hoff could see you after his last patient leaves.

What a gift this was. I knew he'd come through for me. Dr. Hoff had no idea what I needed to see him about, yet he trusted it was urgent enough to warrant his extra time in the clinic. I was constantly amazed at how devoted Dr. Hoff was in helping me. I patiently waited for Dr. Hoff to finish seeing his other patients. Eventually, he came into the examining room to talk with me.

He seemed very concerned about my meeting with Dr. Wolfe. After telling him what happened, he quickly said, "No, I said I don't want any-one blindly packing and I don't want you going through with the sched-uled surgery." He asked if Dr. Wolfe used his flexible scope. I replied by telling him how defensive Dr. Wolfe got when I started asking questions. Dr. Hoff seemed quite disturbed over this, and disappointed that our hopes had been shattered.

He wasn't willing to stop here, however. He wanted me to have another opinion and gave me the name of an otynlaryngologist in the Detroit area, who was a highly respected physician. He knew this physician used the flexible scope.

The following week, Diane and I drove to Detroit to see Dr. Eugene Rontal, M.D. only to receive yet another conflicting opinion. He believed I was leaking from the right sphenoid sinus, and he also wanted to pack this area blindly. He was very thorough with his examination. His technician tested my hearing, which was followed by a thorough examination by Dr. Rontal. But once again, the flexible scope was not used. I was beginning to wonder if there was such an instrument, or if Dr. Hoff had heard of the eight-inch steel rod and fallen victim to jokes of its incredible flexibility. Given my feeling of horror every time these physicians brought out their rigid, steel scopes, this flexible scope seemed quite inviting.

I asked Dr. Rontal about the flexible scope. He said, "I wouldn't waste my time using it because my suspicions are usually right." I didn't feel comfortable with suspicions. He then said, "I will prove to you it is leaking there. I will put a glucose strip at the entry to the right sphenoid sinus." (Glucose strips, which differentiate CSF from sinus fluid, are used because CSF has glucose in it) When he pulled the strip out of my nose, sure enough, it was positive. He was convinced of his theory.

I returned to Traverse City extremely disappointed because no one had used the flexible scope. I called Dr. Hoff immediately. I was mystified by the contradicting opinions; so was Dr. Hoff. I think he began to question himself at this point, wondering if he was doing the right thing and probably thinking I might be questioning his decisions. So, he referred me to another physician in the Detroit area, S.M. Farhat, M.D., a neurosurgeon who he respected a great deal.

I saw Dr. Farhat, out of respect for Dr. Hoff's opinion. I had not lost confidence in Dr. Hoff. I felt he was doing all he could to help. I was impatient with his indecisiveness of going back into my head to repair the leaks, but I had not lost confidence in him. In fact, I respected him for caring enough to hold back on performing another craniotomy until he knew for sure where he was going. On one hand, I wished he would just go ahead and do another craniotomy; on the other hand, I was glad he was being conservative, given the risks involved.

Dr. Farhat agreed with Dr. Hoff's decision not to perform more surgery until the leak was located. He also agreed that my sinuses should not be packed blindly, which left us with very few options.

After talking it over with Dr. Hoff and Dr. MacKenzie, it was suggested I return to Mayo Clinic to see Dr. McCaffrey. They both spoke with Dr. McCaffrey to see if he could possibly use the flexible scope to locate my leaks. Dr. McCaffrey was more than happy to see me again, if, of course, I didn't have a cold.

I didn't have a burning desire to see Dr. McCaffrey again. Yet, it seemed like my only hope of finally having someone use the mysterious flexible scope. I took the first available appointment, which was two weeks away, in the middle of November 1993. I worked very hard to have an open mind. I had to look beyond the previous insensitivity of Dr. McCaffrey and remember his expertise.

The one year anniversary of my grandfather's death came before I left for Rochester. It had been a difficult year for me, and I was still grieving. Because of my own physical complications, I felt as though I never had time to grieve his death. There had been so much attention focused on me for the past year, I never allowed myself to grieve this loss.

I knew the best way for me to process some of these feelings was to write about them. In addition, I had also started to paint as a way to uncap hidden emotions. (I began therapeutic painting shortly after Margo asked me to draw pictures for therapy.) I don't pretend to be good at painting, but I recognize its therapeutic benefits.

Therefore, I first painted oak leaves, reminding me of the days I spent with Grandpa raking leaves at the cabin. I framed this piece and have it hanging on my wall. Then I wrote a poem called "Missing You."

Missing You

One year has passed,
    Yet your presence has not;
As you live on in my heart,
    Your love I've not forgot.

I treasure the times,
    You talked, laughed, and told;

Stories of your life,
> The memories you'd unfold.

I did not know you first,
> Even after twenty-two years;
Then our bond grew strong,
> Which made for many tears.

Ever since your soul departed,
> I hold on to my memory so clear;
Of your smile, your voice, your words,
> Spoken from afar and near.

Thoughts, ideas, and wisdom,
> Not even expressed aloud;
Were powerful, bright, and true,
> For which I am very proud.

You shared with me your heart,
> Giving this precious gift of you;
Being my dear Grandfather,
> And a beloved friend too.

Even right until the end,
> You were giving yourself to me;
Never once did I feel an emptiness,
> I trusted you'd always be...

There with me in every way,
> Showing how much you care;
Lying in pain, ready to die,
> You even asked how Karen did fair.

I thank God for the time we shared,
> In your last few weeks of life;
The opportunity to tell you my feelings,
> As I sat peacefully on your right...

I said "I love you Grandpa,
> With all my heart and soul;
You're in good hands now forever more,
> God will play His role."

You held my hand so tight,
>I knew you were in pain;
I prayed for God to take you Home,
>Knowing for me He'd do the same.

Oh how I cried outside your room,
>Not knowing how to say to you;
All in a moments time,
>The lifetime of love I have for you.

I longed for just one more time,
>Not wanting to turn my back to you;
I held your hand and touched your head,
>I said quietly, "I'll see you soon."

I couldn't bring myself to say good-bye,
>It was the hardest thing I've ever done;
I just wanted to hold you tight,
>And stop the movement of the sun.

As if I thought you'd never die,
>Not prepared for your life to pass;
You're a man I thought had hung the moon,
>I wanted every minute to last.

I really knew as I turned away,
>This was the very last time;
I knew I had said everything I could,
>Also giving you the heart of mine.

My last days with you on earth,
>I wouldn't trade for a pot of gold;
One last chance to show my love to you,
>Even though you'd already been told.

I knew it would be my last chance,
>To laugh, to touch your heart;
To hold your hand with such wonder,
>Not wanting you to depart.

I felt my heart tear open inside,
>It hurt for I really knew;

There wasn't going to be a miracle here,
  Grandpa was preparing to leave too.

I awoke at 7 am,
  November 7th of '92;
Fell back for 16 more,
  Then recognized I really knew.

Awakening in a pool of tears,
  This would be Grandpa's final day;
He wanted me to know,
  Prepared if there was a way.

So I relayed a message through Mom,
  Even though in silence he lay;
"I'm strong because you're strong",
  He then responded in his usual way.

I'm strong because you are strong,
  He knew just what this meant;
I had told him years before,
  These words were heaven sent.

I trusted the Lord to give me strength,
  To bare his death with song;
The Lord's My Shepherd, I Shall Not Want,
  He knew these words for long.

I dedicated this day to you Grandpa,
  Accompanying your every step;
Not wanting to be left behind,
  I prayed, looked at photos, wept.

Recalling our fun with lemon drops,
  I never thought I'd see;
Your grin and comment break the ice,
  "We didn't do so well did we?"

When I turned and walked away again,
  I felt more peace inside;
I knew you were more comfortable,
  Back by Grandma's side.

For a Grandfather's life is never lost,
  You're with me in my heart;
The memories I have are your gifts,
  Never to depart.

To tell a joke or see your grin,
  Just as the flowers grow;
I plant a tree as you live on,
  In my heart and soul.

Magical memories bring you close,
  Each day the sun rises;
As I smile and say thank-you Lord,
  For my Grandfather, yes he is mine.

Thank-you Grandpa,
  For giving me so much;
For sharing your life with me,
  And teaching me how to love.

I carry you with me,
  As I travel through life's way;
Holding your strength and courage,
  To assist me through each day.

I'm proud to be your granddaughter,
  Still believing you hung the moon;
We'll be together again,
  I'll see you again soon.   (Written: November 7, 1993)

After completing this poem, I found greater peace with my grandfather's death.

Prior to leaving for Mayo Clinic I made the necessary reservations, making sure all accommodations were satisfactory. My parents had already left Michigan, to spend the winter in Florida. Once again the Fetters came through for me. They offered to drive me to Rochester, Minnesota. In order to decrease the stress of our trip, I arranged for us to only go as far as Milwaukee the first day, where we would stay with my dear friend, Mary Prange. It was a welcomed bonus to the trip.

MARY HAS BEEN my friend ever since I was a student in her fifth grade class. She has been a tremendous influence on my spiritual life. Her faith is unwavering, and her understanding of how faith connects with everyday trials is extensive. I can always count on having wonderful conversations with Mary about faith, hope, and joy. She is a living example of how one should walk with God. She is a spiritual hero of mine.

Mary has taught me a lot about faith and God's promises. She has seen firsthand the lessons she has taught being put into practice. I remember very clearly a phone conversation I had with Mary the night before my first sinus surgery, two months after my accident. With a horrified tone in her voice, she said, "Karen, are they going to cut into your brain?" It felt good to relieve her of her fear, by telling her they'd be going through my nose and mouth. Then, when the time came for me to have brain surgery, I had to break the news gently. I wanted to reassure Mary I was in good hands, God's hands. I could tell she was scared of what this surgery might do to me.

I had not seen Mary since before my first two craniotomies. It was a marvelous reunion. I know from seeing friends going through this recovery process with me, it was always a big relief for them to actually *see* me after each surgery. Until then, they could not believe I was okay. I know I would feel the same if the tables were turned.

It was difficult for Mary to go through my recovery process. It has forced her to acknowledge the vulnerability of her own life. Most of us walk with this fear daily, but it is brought closer to reality when someone dear to us lives with a tragedy we fear.

It was from a foundation of spiritual faith—a foundation that Mary helped my parents build within me—that I was able to view my accident not so much as a tragedy but as a blessing in disguise. It is a blessed tragedy. Mary saw very clearly how I reacted to my head injury. She has listened to me speak of the many blessings it has brought into my life. What Mary once gave me has been returned to her tenfold. It is a comfort to her to hear me speak of this as a blessing, and to see me live my life in such a way, giving her strength and courage, as it does many others.

During a visit with Mary, two years after my accident, I was talking with her and Elaine Timm, a good friend of Mary's. Elaine began asking

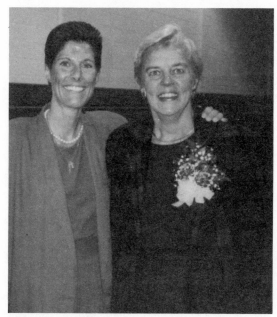

Author and her spiritual mentor, Mary Prange.

many questions about my injury and its circumstances. It was the first time Mary heard me talk about the damage to my brain. As I spoke, Mary listened intently. She was very quiet, asking few questions. I have no doubt Mary was shocked by what she heard. She wanted desperately to believe I was perfectly okay, just as I appeared on the outside. It hurt her to know I was struggling, while at the same time she recognized this could very easily be her someday. Her reply was, "I cannot imagine going through this myself. How do you stay so strong?"

It was finally my turn to witness to her. I said, "It is my faith, Mary. I know God has a plan for me, and this must be a part of it. Trust me, God grants me peace beyond any human understanding." I went on to quote the Bible verse, "For my thoughts are not your thoughts, neither are your ways My ways,' declares the Lord. 'As the heavens are higher than the earth, so are My ways higher than your ways, and My thoughts than your thoughts." (Isaiah 55:8-9 NIV)

Mary knows I would never have chosen this way of life, but then my ways are not His ways. She is not the only one who has said to me, "I do not believe I could ever be as strong as you are Karen, if I were faced with this tragedy." I am of the opinion she would be as strong, just like any of my other friends who doubt their strength. One never knows until it happens, but with faith, we know we have been given all the tools.

Every morning before she goes to school to teach other children how to walk with God, Mary puts a lightning bolt necklace on. She wears it, remembering me and how quickly life can change. It reminds Mary of her own mortality, and the impact she has on children. Her finest remembrance, however, is of the strength and courage God gives to each of us as we walk with Him.

T HE FETTERS AND I arrived in Rochester the next day. My appointment was for the following day, so we had some time to wander around and get settled. Diane and Paul made the trip as fun and lighthearted as possible, knowing I was a bit anxious. They were overwhelmed by the clinic, as I had been a year ago. I registered at the front desk of the clinic a half hour before my appointment. Then we went to the fifth floor, to join everyone else in the auditorium-sized waiting room.

By the time I was finally taken into the examining room, I was quite nervous. I did not know what to expect from Dr. McCaffrey. I didn't have a cold this time, but it hadn't taken me a year to rid myself of it, either. I'd need to explain what had happened since our first meeting.

Dr. McCaffrey seemed very pleasant and examined me with my favorite eight-inch instrument. I asked, "Can you use a flexible scope to find my leaks?" At last I received a definitive answer (and description) of this infamous flexible scope.

He said, "It is used during surgery to find leaks. I need to inject dye, fluorescein, into your CSF and look for it with the flexible scope through your nose and mouth, with the use of a black light. When I find the leaks, I patch them from beneath your skull."

I questioned the effectiveness of patching them on the side of the skull that would be most likely to give way to the pressure of the CSF. He expressed confidence in his ability to secure the patches so they wouldn't leak again. One thing is for sure, Dr. McCaffery didn't lack confidence (as he did personality).

He continued, "If I'm not able to see the fluorescein leaking through your skull during surgery, I'll leave pledgets in your sinuses for at least six hours after surgery. They would collect the CSF, and then I'd be able to determine where the leaks are."

I began to get excited about the potential for this to be over soon. If he could repair my leaks, it might mean no more headaches, no more weekly trips to doctors, and finally a return to a decent life-style.

The surgery was scheduled for two days later at St. Mary's Hospital. Between now and then I had to go through some tests and a pre-operation exam. The rest of the time was spent relaxing, reading, shopping, and trying to keep my mind off having another surgery. That is, until I received a phone call from Bryant, a man who was house-sitting for me.

I was still in the midst of a nasty divorce. My primary reason for having Bryant stay at the house was to prevent Jerry from breaking-in. Bryant was calling to inform me that he had come home from work that day, only to find Jerry trying to get into the house. Jerry had already made it through the small garage door, and was working on the house door. He obviously knew from stalking me that I was out of town. Even though Jerry had moved all of his things out of the house, he had a hidden agenda in attempting to break-in.

This was the type of stress I didn't need going into surgery, and it was a clear demonstration of Jerry's uncaring, unloving, and insensitive personality. I was angered to hear of the episode, but glad I was seeing Jerry's true colors after all these years.

Fortunately, I managed to put this aside. Instead, I began preparing emotionally for my surgery. I was not nearly as nervous about this surgery as I had been for the others. Going through my nose and mouth seemed less invasive than going through the top of my head, even though he was still going into my head.

The surgery lasted two hours. When I returned to my room, Diane and Paul were there, waiting for me. Dr. McCaffrey came in to see me shortly after the nurses settled me in bed. He told me he hadn't found any leaks and, therefore, did nothing to patch them. I was devastated. My hopes had been way too high. He then proceeded to remove the gauze pads from my nose, even though it was less than two hours after surgery. I questioned why he was doing this. He said, "There is no reason to keep them in any longer. I did not see any leaks." Then, he left my room.

Diane, Paul, and I could not believe what was happening. We didn't understand why he was not following through with his plan. The nurses came in to check on me. I asked them why he removed the pledgets. They weren't certain why, but insisted on having me keep a piece of gauze taped under my nose to catch any drips.

Within six hours after my surgery, fluid leaked from my nose. I rang the call bell for my nurse. She came promptly. I told her about the fluid. She told me to keep soaking it up with the gauze and that she'd call down for the black light in the operating room. The fluorescein appears clear to the naked eye, but under a black light turns a different color.

The black light arrived within twenty minutes. We immediately put the soaked gauze pads under the light, to see if it looked a different color. The gauze pads turned green. My heart fluttered. I could not believe what I was seeing. Even though I knew I was leaking CSF, each time I was faced with evidence as clear as this, it felt as though someone had hit me in the chest. It was real.

I asked the nurse what color the fluorescein normally turns under a black light, hoping she would say orange. She said, "I think green. I will put this in your chart."

I was discharged the next day and told to return to the clinic to see Dr. McCaffrey in two days. By this time, my parents were on their way from Florida. They decided to drive up to Minnesota to be with me, which boosted my spirits. They arrived the evening I was discharged. It was so good to see them and to have them with me. I felt as though I was being bombarded by loads of stress, and having them with me always gave me a sense of security.

When my parents heard about Jerry's attempts to break into my house, they were struck with awe. Until this point they hadn't believed me when I told them details of what he'd done. It was becoming more real to them.

After being discharged from St. Mary's, we returned to the motel so I could rest. The headache I was experiencing was excruciating. I could not lift my head above my shoulders for more than fifteen seconds at a time, before the pain was intolerable. It reminded me of the pain I had experienced after my first shunt surgery. As long a I laid flat, I was fine.

That night the pain was so intense my parents and the Fetters took me into the emergency room. Our biggest fear was meningitis. I had all of the symptoms, and knew I couldn't afford to wait until my appointment with Dr. McCaffrey. We spent half the night in the emergency room. It took them forever to get me into the CT scanner and also to get the results back from the lumbar puncture. My parents took turns coming in to be with me, since there was limited space in the exam room. The resident physician finally returned. She said the fluid tests came back negative for meningitis. She sent me back to the hotel with a pain killer and said it was important to keep an eye on my symptoms, and to make sure I told my surgeon when I saw him.

I returned to the clinic for my appointment, hoping Dr. McCaffrey had checked the nurses' reports and read the account of the fluorescein under the black light. Paul and Diane went into the exam room with me, as they had before. But, when Dr. McCaffrey came in, he asked me to go to another room. Paul and Diane stayed and I followed him to a different exam room. Dr. McCaffrey had me on a table, where he proceeded to look up my nose. This was very unusual. During my previous appointments, he examined me from the special chair in his exam room, where Paul and Diane were waiting.

While Dr. McCaffrey was reading over my chart, I told him about my trip to the emergency room and how excruciating the pain was. I also asked him what color fluorescein shows up as under a black light.

"Green."

I asked if he had checked the nurses' charts at St. Mary's, the day after my surgery.

He said, "No."

"We collected fluid after the surgery and it showed up green under the black light," I said.

"Where did you get the black light?" he asked defensively.

"The nurses got it from the operating room. It was the only one in the hospital."

Without even turning to look at me, he harshly said, "You do not have a leak. You may think you have a leak, and you may want to have a leak, but you do not have a leak."

I was furious. I had never in my life had so much anger towards a person. How could he say something like this? No wonder he wanted me in another room, away from witnesses of his behavior.

I could not think of how to reply. I simply said, "I cannot believe you have been so negligent and can even make a statement such as this." I walked out of the exam room, got Paul and Diane, picked up my stack of MRI and CT scan films and left.

I had given him a second chance after he was rude to me during my first visit to Mayo Clinic, but this time I knew I would never return.

I called Dr. MacKenzie from the motel. I was very upset and knew he'd put things in perspective. I don't know what I'd do without him. He was always there for me.

Dr. MacKenzie returned my call within ten minutes. After hearing what happened, he said, "Karen, just come home. We can help you more here. It does not sound like this physician is very interested in helping us find the leak. You and I both know you are leaking CSF, so let's talk about our next move when you get back to Traverse City."

We packed our bags and left for home that afternoon. My parents decided to go to Traverse City before heading back to Florida, so they could spend Thanksgiving with me.

ONCE I WAS back in Traverse City, Dr. MacKenzie called Dr. Hoff at U. of M. to get his thoughts on what we should do next. Dr. Hoff said he wanted to try at least one more cisternagram and also to test the fluid again for beta II transferin.

Before having the cisternagram, I met with Dr. Hoff to discuss his plan of action. For most people, it would be a shock to have a renowned neurosurgeon ask them for suggestions. It was no surprise to me, however, when Dr. Hoff said, "Karen, if you were to design a test to find your leak, what would you do?" What a compliment. He respected my opinion and expertise.

His ego was definitely not standing in the way of showing his need for help. It never did. This, along with his display of confidence in me, increased my respect for him tenfold.

Oddly enough, I was ready for the question. Throughout my recovery I learned by reading, asking questions, and doing everything possible to stay with the clinical thinking of my doctors. I knew practically all aspects of every test, surgery, and procedure performed on me.

I told Dr. Hoff that because of the position of my body when fluid came from my nose, and the amount flowing, it was my belief fluid leaked throughout the day into my sinuses. When I bent over, gravity pulled the fluid through the open passage out my nose. I recommended the cisternagram be performed in a way that allowed the spinal fluid and radio-isotopes to leak for a minimum of twelve hours. During this time, my body should remain in a position so that my head was lower than my pelvis. Meanwhile, CT scans should be performed frequently, while I remained in this position.

Dr. Hoff agreed with my recommendations and arranged for another cisternagram the following week. Much to our dissatisfaction, the test was again inconclusive.

I took more fluid, which I had collected from my nose, with me to the hospital. It was sent off for analysis. Dr. Hoff told me he'd call me with the results. Within a week he called me and said, "The beta II transferin test came back negative. So I think we better stop. If we cannot prove it is CSF, I cannot justify doing anything more to you."

I reminded him how the other beta II transferin tests had first come back negative and then came back positive when retested. He said he did not think the likelihood of that happening again was very great.

There was a pause in our conversation. There was something more to say, but he hesitated. My heart leaped into my throat. I didn't know what more to say or ask.

Then he said it, "Karen, I have done all I can for you. I'm sorry."

He said the words I had dreaded for more than a year. The horror of hearing those words had haunted a small part of my psyche ever since I began leaking after my first craniotomy. It was then that I realized there was no certainty in any type of surgery. Until then, it had never entered my mind that surgery of this high scale could fail.

Once reality sunk in, my mind shifted to, "What if there isn't a way to fix this?"

As Dr. Hoff surrendered, my heart broke. All hope diminished. With great feelings of despair, I sank to my knees.

As I tried to get the words thank you out of my mouth, my voice quivered. I knew he had tried everything he possibly could, and that he was just as heartbroken as me. To have one of the best admit defeat made it even more difficult.

After I hung up the phone, I cried. "Where do I go from here? Is this the end? Must I live with this pain? Help me God, please help me."

Seventeen

New Hope

*The privilege of a lifetime
is being who you are.*

JOSEPH CAMPBELL

I STILL HAD A tremendous amount of respect for Dr. Hoff. The impact
of his words hurt badly, as hopes of relieving my pain were shattered.
Suddenly my future looked very grim. I had been on heavy duty
narcotics to relieve my pain since the day of my accident, four and a half
years ago. Would I need narcotics forever? Questions flashed through my
head like lightning bolts. I had no answers.

My pain hadn't diminished since my injury. If anything it had increased in severity, or my tolerance and strength to withstand it had lessened. It truly wore me down. I had to manage my own care, despite
battling the pain. In addition to this, I continued to work.

I was forever thankful of my employer's willingness to accommodate
my needs by allowing me to work from home and to work restricted hours.
I know my dedication to my job was evident. Also, the Americans with
Disabilities Act (ADA) was a critical factor. Under this law, it was Munson's
obligation to accommodate my needs. Looking back on it now, my desire
to keep working may have been at the expense of my health.

There was always pressure on me to maintain my job, my income, and
more importantly, my health care benefits. Therefore, I kept working as
much as I could, knowing if I didn't, Munson Medical Center could pull
the rug out from under me. I was always the first one to praise Munson

when someone asked how I was able to maintain my job. I did this, despite never receiving praise from Munson about the exceptional work I performed with a head injury. I was devoted to my career, and I channeled all of my excess stress into work energy. My pride kept me working, even when my body and head said quit.

As I thought about the prospect of living with pain, my thoughts turned towards my career. How could I maintain my career if my pain persisted? I was already struggling with the pain, and I could sense my stamina wasn't what it once was.

I prayed for guidance. Should I keep searching for a doctor who could help me or should I accept the prognosis from Dr. Hoff? Was this really the end of the puzzle, even though it wasn't complete? Was I only one step away from finding a solution? If I stopped searching, I would never know. Or, maybe a solution didn't exist. I always believed that giving up was always giving up too soon. The answer could be around the next corner. I prayed, "God, You have given me signs before, when I have needed them. Please give me a sign, some direction, as to which way to go."

Within a week, a door to my future opened when I was talking with Carrie Mayes. She told me about a friend of a friend who had a child with a brain tumor. The parents took this child around the country, trying to find a doctor who was willing to help. Every doctor they spoke with told them there was no hope for their child. The tumor was inoperable. Somehow, they were connected with a neurosurgeon by the name of Ben Carson, M.D. at Johns Hopkins Hospital. He is the chief pediatric neurosurgeon for this most prestigious medical institution.

Dr. Carson not only told them he could help their child, he performed surgery to remove the tumor, and the child is now a healthy adult.

Carrie said, "I will get Dr. Carson's phone number for you. Even though he is a pediatric neurosurgeon, maybe there's an adult neurosurgeon at Johns Hopkins who can help you." Hope filled my heart. Maybe this is the answer to my prayers. Carrie continued, "Dr. Carson has even written several books. You could probably pick one up at the bookstore in town."

The next day I stopped at Horizon Books, to see if they had any books written by Dr. Carson. Not knowing the titles of his books, I asked an employee if she could locate them on the store's computer. She found several authors by the name of Ben Carson and read the list to me. It didn't show which of the authors were doctors, so I had to go by title only. I took a guess when I chose *Gifted Hands*. This sounded like it might be talking about the hands of a surgeon. I placed an order and received it five days later.

Carrie called the day after I bought *Gifted Hands*. She had the phone number to Dr. Carson's office. She asked if I had looked for his book. I told her I found it but had only skimmed through it quickly, to see what type of book it was. I had looked at the photos in the book, to see if there were any other doctors shown. In one picture, the Chief of Neurosurgery at Johns Hopkins, Don Long M.D., was included. I tried to find a place in the book where Dr. Carson talked about Dr. Long. I came to a page where he spoke of Dr. Long as his mentor. He spoke very highly of Dr. Long's personality, expertise, and especially his willingness to help people.

I called Dr. MacKenzie to ask if he had ever heard of Dr. Long. He said, "No, but I'd be happy to call him and see if he's interested in your case."

I was excited, but had to remain cautiously optimistic. I could hardly wait to hear back from Dr. MacKenzie. Would he be able to get through to Dr. Long, and if so what would Dr. Long say? A few days later Dr. MacKenzie called and said he had spoken with Dr. Long. "I talked with Dr. Long for about an hour. I told him about the difficulty of your case, summarizing the whole picture, the tests, surgeries, and failures. He said, 'I think I can help her. Send her out to Baltimore. I will arrange for a time to meet with her, a time for her to meet with Michael Holliday, M.D., an otynlaryngologist, and I'll also go ahead and block off time for tests and surgery as well. This will save on the expense of Karen having to fly back if we decide to do surgery.' Then he told me about another patient of his who has a similar problem. Everything sounds very promising."

After getting off the phone with Dr. MacKenzie I looked to the heavens and prayed, "Thank you God. Thank you for giving me another chance. You are truly amazing!" My prayers had been answered. It wasn't time to sit back and accept a life-style full of pain. It was also very reassuring to know I was not the only one with a persistent CSF leak. Dr. Long said he had another case like mine. I may be unusual, but I'm not the only one with problems, by any means. I was relieved to hear that Dr. Long was willing to help me, and seemed confident that he could. My flame of hope still burned.

D R. LONG SCHEDULED my appointment for July 6, 1994, three months away. He wanted to schedule enough time for testing, surgery, and follow-up care, without me having to travel back and forth to Baltimore, Maryland. He is a world renowned surgeon, and travels extensively to other countries. He was scheduled to be in China just before I would arrive at Johns Hopkins.

While this seemed like an eternity away, I was actually very fortunate to be able to see him this soon. Considering it was now four and a half years since my accident, three more months wasn't going to make a difference. The only risk was meningitis and living with extreme pain.

I WAS CONCERNED about how my parents would react when they found out I was going to Johns Hopkins. I always felt they were critical of my decisions, thinking I had poor judgment and was not capable of making wise choices. A trip to Hopkins would be costly for me, which was always a concern of theirs. Because none of us were communicating the way we should, we never knew exactly what the other was feeling.

They were coming to visit one afternoon, so I decided to leave Dr. Carson's book, *Gifted Hands*, on the counter top, where they'd easily see it. I prayed one of them would pick it up, and that it would stimulate a conversation about Hopkins. They didn't yet know I was planning to go to Hopkins for treatment. I thought if I told them the story of how I found out about Dr. Long, they would think it was a farfetched idea of mine. However, if they knew of Dr. MacKenzie's conversation with Dr. Long, and read Dr. Carson's book, they might support me.

I spent a great deal of energy trying to protect my parents from riding the roller coaster with me. Thus, I never told them Dr. Hoff had said there was nothing more that could be done. There were many situations like this, throughout my recovery, when I thought it best they didn't know all of the details. The conflicting beta II transferin test is another example.

The emotional highs and lows were hard enough for me to handle, let alone someone who has even less knowledge of the medical care system. I really think because I worked in the medical care system my emotions were probably multiplied due to a greater depth of knowledge. In most cases, ignorance would have been bliss. This was my reasoning for filtering the information I gave my parents.

I knew if Mom read Dr. Carson's book, she'd be sold on the idea of me going to Hopkins. She'd be most impressed with his strong faith in God, his exceptional skills, and the credit he gives to his mother for his success. It worked. Mom picked up the book and asked what it was about, leading me into the story of how I became connected to Dr. Long. Before leaving my house she had read the introduction and a few chapters, finding it difficult to put down. She asked to take the book home with her, for which I was very happy. My plan was working.

Mom read the book. Within two days she called to tell me how much she was impressed with Dr. Carson. She was very eager to tell me about the chapter in which Dr. Carson talked of his mentor, Don Long, M.D. I could tell she was excited. It felt as though I had their approval. Mom went out and bought a book of her own and started telling all her friends about it. She loaned her copy to several others, while many friends bought a copy. I'm certain Mom has been one of Dr. Carson's best marketers.

It was such a relief to have my parents' support. It also reaffirmed that my decision was good.

MEANWHILE, DR. MACKENZIE worked hard to ease my pain. He recommended that I see the local Pain Clinic specialist, get advice on the relief of my pain, and begin biofeedback training with psychologist Vince Cornellier, Ph.D. I agreed it would be worth it to try both.

I scheduled an appointment at the Pain Clinic, but couldn't see Dr. Nelson for another four weeks. I told Dr. MacKenzie my dilemma. He said he'd try to get it moved up, but in the mean time he'd recommend I try using a medication which comes in the form of a patch. A Fentynal patch is a class two narcotic used to control chronic pain. Unlike the Percocet I was taking, it helps to keep a therapeutic dose in your system at a more constant rate. I only needed to replace the patch every 12 hours.

Dr. MacKenzie knew I didn't like taking medication, and thus, it was hard for me to take the Percocet every four hours. Instead, I waited until the pain became extremely bad, then I took it. By that time it was too late. The patch took care of this problem. Taking the dose soon enough was no longer in my hands. It was nice not having to remember to take pills.

The drug worked immediately. My headache disappeared. Along with it, however, came sedation. All I wanted to do was sleep. When I laid down during the day, I'd have intentions of sleeping for one or two hours, but wake up four or five hours later. I managed to get used to it after awhile, but I still slept more than usual.

Eventually, my body adapted to the dosage and my headache started to break through. Dr. MacKenzie advised me to use two patches. After doing so, I noticed my hands falling dead asleep in the middle of the night. I'd wake up and couldn't move them. As time passed, my arms did the same. They'd ache terribly when I'd try to get them to come back to life. I'd kneel on my bed and swing my arms by using the force of my shoulders, trying to increase their circulation. I was in tears while doing so, the ache was so bad.

I called Dr. MacKenzie and told him about my problem. He asked me to come to his office that afternoon and he'd do an EMG on my hands. He suspected carpal tunnel syndrome. Sure enough, the EMG confirmed his suspicions. I told him I didn't believe this was the real problem. I was doing nothing repetitive to cause this condition. I suspected the Fentynal Patch as the culprit. He disagreed, but was willing to change the prescription and suggested I buy wrist braces to wear at night to stop the nerves from being pinched.

He changed my prescription to MS Contin, which is in the morphine family. I didn't like the idea of taking morphine, even if the Fentynal was just as strong. I considered morphine to be an abusive drug. I tried it anyway, but quickly stopped because it was very nauseating.

Even though I didn't have the ability to smell or taste any longer, everything I ate tasted like the vapor of the medication. Some medications were stronger than others, and some were more tolerable than others. The MS Contin was very bitter, and thus, all food tasted nasty. This was another reason I stopped taking it.

I bought one wrist brace to try at night. It worked. Every night I wore it I didn't have a problem with numbness. This still didn't seem right to me. Why would I have carpal tunnel syndrome, if not due to the new medication I was taking? I began to debate whether I should stop taking the Fentynal patch as well.

In the midst of trying these medications to control my pain, I began meeting with Vince Cornellier, Ph.D. He was the fourth psychologist to whom I was referred. While it may seem strange that I worked with four psychologists, I found each of their styles and strengths to be very different. I was appreciative of the opportunity to work with all of them. Each one contributed a significant amount to my recovery, helping me to uncover Karen Wells beneath a lot of extraneous debris. This shows how far I came in just accepting the role of a psychologist in my recovery. At the time when my accident occurred, I thought psychologists worked only with the mentally ill.

I found my conversations with Vince about biofeedback very fascinating, given my background in exercise physiology. It was very easy for me to grasp the concepts and to apply them. My personal athletic experiences blended well with the techniques I used in biofeedback for muscle relaxation and pain reduction.

We focused on the extremes of muscle contraction versus muscle relaxation, attempting to increase blood flow and warm each muscle group, enhancing this ability to relax. I became acutely aware of my constant tendency to hold the muscles in my head and face very tight. I was apparently attempting to brace myself from the pain of my headache. Releasing this tension helped reduce the ache and fatigue of these muscles, but left me with headache pain just the same.

Many of my biofeedback sessions turned into dynamic discussions rather than active progressive relaxation. Vince and I seemed to communicate well, and I found our conversations very helpful. He had a nice perspective on the mechanics of my life, and recognized the pieces that needed to be addressed.

It didn't take long for him to see inside me and identify my operating system, the over-achieving, competitive, hard-driving, never say die person. I could talk a good line about my ability to relax. I knew all the right things to say, given my knowledge of human kinesiology, but the software (my personality) loaded on my hard drive (my body) was not about to allow me to implement these techniques. It was quite easy to see from our conversations that I had a very difficult time letting anything go. Letting muscle tension go was just a tip of the iceberg. As Vince would say, "You are attempting to hold the world and control which way it spins."

He was right. I didn't admit it at the time but I know now Vince was right on target. My sessions with Vince were most productive. When I went into his office, I knew we would accomplish something very specific. He made me work, challenging my thinking and testing my disposition. I felt as though I had made some major breakthroughs in my persona while working with Vince.

I improved my ability to let go of things I could not control. I have learned how to implement the last phrase of "The Serenity Prayer." "...and the wisdom to know the difference." I can better judge the difference between what I do have control over and that which I do not, and act accordingly.

Dr. MacKenzie's suggestion to try biofeedback might not have worked in the way he had intended it, but it did ultimately help me tremendously. It did not relieve my pain, but it relieved my instinctual need to control everything around me, which took a huge load off my back. Until it was lifted, I never realized what it was doing to me. Once I said no more of this, I am not going to play other people's game, it was like emptying a huge load of rocks at God's feet and saying, "I cannot do it alone anymore. Please help." But then going one step further and saying, "God, I never had control in the first place, thanks for helping."

The recognition of the need for help is the hardest part. The rest comes easier, as you feel the reduction of stress and then wonder why you fell into the trap of carrying rocks in the first place.

Rocks come in many different shapes, sizes, and temperaments. Many individuals carry them in the form of career stress, family pressures, a need for perfection, anger, pride, unwillingness to forgive, and countless other burdens in disguise. During this time, I came across a poem that helped me let go of many different shapes and sizes.

Letting Go

To "let go" does not mean to stop caring
it means, I can't do it for someone else.
To "let go" is not to cut myself off
it's the realization, I can't control another.
To "let go" is to not enable
but to allow learning from natural consequences.
To "let go" is to admit powerlessness
which means the outcome is not in my hands.
To "let go" is not to try to change or blame another
it's to make the most of myself.
To "let go" is not to "care for"
but to "care about".
To "let go" is not to "fix"
but to be supportive.
To "let go" is not to judge
but to allow another to be a human being.
To "let go" is to not be in the middle
arranging all the outcomes,
but to allow others to affect their destinies.
To "let go" is not to be protective
it's to permit another to face reality.
To "let go" is not to deny but to accept.
To "let go" is not to nag, scold or argue,
but instead to search out my own
shortcomings and correct them.
To "let go" is not to adjust everything to my desires,
but to take each day as it comes,
and cherish myself in it.
To "let go" is not to criticize and regulate anybody,
but to try to become what I dream I can be.
To "let go" is to not regret the past
but to grow and live for the future.
To "let go" is to fear less and love more.   Author Unknown

I had a difficult time admitting powerlessness in many aspects of my life. Letting go of this piece alone opened many doors. I allowed myself to take a breath of fresh air. Once I did, I recognized I had been suffocating under the rocks for too long. I was ready to sit back and watch others suffocate, while they operated on the same system. It's so much easier to see the madness of this operating system from the outside. I felt sorry for those still living their lives like this, seeing the tremendous stress it created. I wonder when they, too, will let go.

While working with Vince and trying Dr. MacKenzie's prescriptions, I waited for my appointment at the Pain Clinic. I finally met with Dr. Nelson and repeated my story to him. He asked what medications I was currently taking and how they affected me. He then began rattling off a number of medications that he recommended I begin taking to relieve the pain.

He suggested I begin with MS Contin, Ritalin, and Calan. I told him I had already tried the MS Contin and would not take it again. As he talked about these medications and their interactions to control my pain, I couldn't help but think of the side effects that might come along with them.

I left his clinic with a handful of prescriptions. There was no way I was about to take all of these drugs. I didn't even take aspirin before my head injury, and now he was suggesting a cocktail of drugs. No way!

I called Dr. MacKenzie and told him what Dr. Nelson recommended. He agreed with me. He did not want me taking a mixture of drugs either. He knew how sensitive I was to medications. He advised me to continue taking the double Fentynal patches.

I was becoming increasingly more frustrated with my increased dependence on these medications, and also scared I'd reach the point of being dangerously dependent. The more I thought about the visible effects the drug was already having on my body, the more I was convinced I needed to get off the Fentynal Patch.

I thought I could quit cold turkey, but learned very quickly that going off this drug was not going to be easy. It wasn't just a matter of the painful headache introducing itself back into my system. I was freezing cold one minute and blazing hot the next. I felt awful. I laid in my water bed, after having cranked its thermostat up ten degrees, with a sheet, a blanket, two comforters, and two afghans on top of me. I was still freezing cold. This was mixed with periods of hot flashes. I'd throw off all the covers, and still be sweating.

Several friends stopped by my house after learning what I was doing and what I was going through. My dear friend Dosie Kermode brought me food, flowers, and a children's book, *The Lord Is My Shepherd* (having no idea how special Psalm 23 was to me). I had obviously not been out of the house that day and opening the windows didn't even cross my mind. I was in my cold stage when Dosie arrived. She was quite surprised, as was I, to see that it was 82 degrees inside my house. I was covered with so many blankets, I couldn't move beneath them, and I was still freezing.

I was going through all the classic symptoms of detoxification. At times I had to get out of bed, even if I felt lousy, because I was spooked. It felt like something was after me, a feeling of suffocation.

I finally called Dr. MacKenzie to see if there was anything he or I could do to make me go through this easier. The first thing he suggested was putting a Fentynal Patch back on. He said, "It has been the only drug to give you relief from your pain."

I replied, "No, I am not going to continue using these patches. The negative impact this drug is having on me is now outweighing the positive. I don't like the side effects. I'll try to deal with the pain for another six weeks. Then I will be at Johns Hopkins, where maybe Dr. Long will be able to finally repair my leak."

He told me to at least take two tablets of Percocet every four hours, so my body would get some of the analgesics it was craving. He said this would lessen the withdrawal effects. I took two immediately, praying it would help me feel better.

I acquired a new appreciation for the difficulty abusers go through to come clean. I was sure my de-tox days were not even close to what theirs are really like. I give them a great deal of credit for this accomplishment. It would have been extremely easy to do exactly what Dr. MacKenzie suggested, and put the patch back on. I thought of it well before he made the suggestion and had to work very hard to persuade myself not to fall prey to the drug.

I had to keep my long-term goal in sight and block out all need for instant gratification. This was difficult, especially since my long-term goal not only meant freedom from side effects, it also meant the return of pain. My goal was bittersweet, but I knew it was something I needed to do.

I was able to persevere through the worst of it. Once I reached the crest of this mountain, the other side didn't look much easier, as my pain returned immediately. It took two weeks before I felt as though the Fentynal was completely out of my system. I was glad to be off the drug.

After two days of not using the Fentynal patch, I slept without the brace on my wrist. The numbness in my hands, wrists, and arms was gone. There was definitely a connection. I was pleased with this response. Similar to when taking the Depokote, I knew my symptoms were a direct result of the medication. Sometimes we know more about our own bodies than a physician or textbook.

I JOINED A Small Group Ministry group from my church to fill my spiritual cup. I was never involved in a group such as this before. Beyond attending a Christian Day School, I never studied the Bible. It took one meeting for me to decide this was an important tool for my life. It not only helped me learn more about the Bible, it also developed into an essential support system. These friends became my Traverse City family. Weekly we studied, laughed, cried, shared, and prayed, walking away filled with inner peace and the Holy Spirit.

This stimulated my interest to study God's Word more on my own, reading the Bible as well as other Christian literature. Likewise, it took me to a new level of prayer. My prayers specifically pleaded with God to give Dr. Long the answer to my pain. I was confident there was a doctor, somewhere, who could help me. The missing piece of the puzzle existed, it was just a matter of finding it. I remained cautiously optimistic, knowing there was also a chance I'd never find it. Previous experience taught me that even exceptionally talented neurosurgeons can be challenged beyond their capabilities.

A S TIME DREW closer to my departure for Johns Hopkins, I began making arrangements. I asked my parents to go with me, and it was decided it was best for Mom to travel with me and Dad to stay home. It was difficult for Dad to travel with his chronic back problems, and this way he could take care of my dog, Akita, and mow my lawn. Mom would be my travel companion, medical support person, mother, and friend.

I made flight and hotel reservations for our expected stay in Baltimore. I was impressed by the travel agency that helped me with these accommodations. It is located right at Johns Hopkins Hospital. Since most patients travel from all over the world to Hopkins, the hotels work very closely with the hospital to be accommodating.

Everything seemed to be falling into place. It took nine months from the time I filed for divorce and the final judgement to be made, but now it was behind me and I was ready for a fresh start. I made sure things were in place at work for me to be gone about three weeks. My only concern was a change in the reporting structure of our department and my new director not having any knowledge of my department or my job. Fortunately, it was summer and our slow period. Unfortunately, I wasn't aware of hidden agendas.

The weekend prior to leaving for Baltimore I went to my parent's home, both to relax and also to leave Akita with Dad. Akita had some behavioral problems and was very vicious towards men particularly. I was a little nervous about my dad taking care of her, even though Akita had never been aggressive towards either of my parents.

Akita was also having health problems, which more than likely aggravated the situation. She had countless cysts growing beneath her skin. They had to be removed over and over again. People say dogs often look like their masters; we most certainly did. After multiple surgeries, both of us sported a bald look with scars.

Before leaving, I tried to show Dad how to protect himself and not put himself in a vulnerable position, but it made no difference. Akita turned on Dad when he attempted to let her out of the house. She did not break his skin, but bruised him badly.

I decided I couldn't risk having Dad take care of her, and I could no longer risk keeping her. I would never forgive myself if she hurt someone. Although I loved Akita dearly—she was a special friend—I had to ask the veterinarian to send her to puppy heaven. This was one of the most difficult decisions I had ever made, but I knew it was the right decision.

The hardest part for me was not only losing a very dear friend, but also the thought of taking the life of the one who had saved mine. If it wasn't for Akita's cry, I don't think I would be alive today.

Now it was time to say good-bye to Dad. Leaving him behind wasn't easy, knowing the chances of me having another craniotomy were very high. We both knew it would be difficult for him to stay home, but given his own health, it was for the best. Dad doesn't shed tears very often, but we were all overcome by emotion.

It's hard enough for me to hold back tears when I say good-bye, but when I saw tears in my father's eyes I was overwhelmed. He's a very loving, caring father, and also very quiet, keeping his feelings to himself. I knew he was feeling the pain of saying good-bye to me like at no other time before. There were too many unknowns. The only certainty was that this was going to be my last hope of receiving help.

Many bad things seemed to be happening to me. I was beginning to think I would never enjoy life again. I was devastated by the multitude of losses I was experiencing. I knew God was using these things to make me stronger, but I thought by this time I was strong enough.

Everything happened so quickly, I had little time to mourn the loss of Akita. Fortunately, I didn't experience the bulk of my grief until I returned home. It felt as though I had left Akita with Dad. In reality, I couldn't allow myself to experience the grief of her loss. I had to concentrate on my health.

Just when I thought God gave me more than he and I could handle, He showed me His plan to handle my grief. His plan for me to leave home, as if Akita was still with us, worked beautifully. My tears flowed freely as Mom and I left for the airport, after going to the veterinarian. But, once we arrived in Baltimore, my focus changed. I felt a new sense of peace. It felt as though I had just stepped off the roller coaster and was getting on the "It's a Small World" ride, sitting between my mother and my Heavenly Father. I wasn't alone. It was a peace beyond my human understanding.

Part IV

THE
REFRESHING RAIN

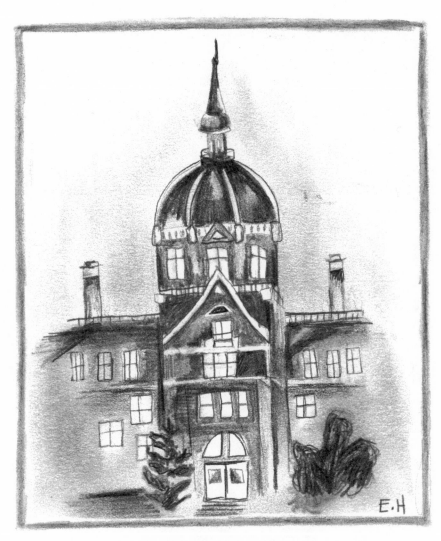

Johns Hopkins Hospital
Illustrated by Emily Helman

Eighteen

Peace Beyond Understanding

Sometimes the Lord calms the storm;
sometimes He lets the storm rage
and calms His child.
GOD'S LITTLE INSTRUCTION BOOK

UCH TO MY AMAZEMENT, this was Mom's first trip of this nature: flying into an unfamiliar city, renting a car, and finding a specified destination. She was quite nervous about the trip and our reason for going. My mind was focused on the uncertainty of what would happen at Johns Hopkins Hospital. This made our adventures through Baltimore amusing, as both our minds were working overtime, in different directions.

We checked into the Tremont Plaza in downtown Baltimore, and then went exploring. The Tremont Plaza was within walking distance of the Inner Harbor, where most of the city's activity takes place. It was fun to explore with Mom, this being our first time traveling alone together. I was excited. She's a fun person to be with, always ready for adventure and exploration.

Every family vacation left us with a heartwarming, lifelong memory of something Mom said or did. My favorite was in Florida, when I was a teenager. We were going to spend the day at the beach, and Mom, making sure she was in fashion, asked my sister and me if she looked *beachy*. You can imagine what was going through our minds! Mom always supplies good one-liners.

We shared many laughs in Baltimore, as well. It was rather funny the day I was waiting for the traffic to begin moving, after a red light had turned green several minutes ago. Mom very discreetly said, "Karen, I think you better pull out from behind this car if you want to go anywhere. It's parked."

The day I turned down a one-way street the wrong way, Mom remained very calm on the outside, while her arteries probably reached stroke level on the inside. I proceeded to keep driving until I reached the next available turn, while casually saying, "Oop's, sorry Mom."

We spent most of our time down at the Inner Harbor, walking around and watching people. We took in some of the attractions, but were most fascinated with the sea lions in a pool outside the aquarium. It was fun to watch their interactions with one another. We weren't quite sure who was watching who. Whenever we were near the harbor we'd go say hi to them.

All of this helped relax our anticipation of going to the most prestigious hospital in the world, Johns Hopkins Medical Institutions. Looking around the hotel lobby, it was easy to see we were not the only travelers from afar to visit Johns Hopkins. We came to know many others, as we shared stories, both of our treatments at Hopkins and our expeditions around the city. Suffering seems to have a way of drawing those within it together. This is one reason I believe all who suffer will never suffer alone, if they allow others into their lives.

My anticipation of meeting Dr. Long was building. It felt similar to my anticipation of meeting God someday. What should I say? What questions should I ask? Will he really accept me and want to help me? What if he says he can't help me? There were a million things racing through my mind.

As Mom and I wandered around Johns Hopkins, trying to become familiar with its enormous layout, I was in awe. I never dreamed I'd be in need of coming to a place like this. I felt very fortunate to be among those receiving the best in quality health care. Johns Hopkins Hospital had been selected numerous times as the number one hospital in the United States. It was such a blessing to be here. This was not an opportunity that just happened by accident. I was standing in Johns Hopkins Hospital because God put me here. I didn't know what else He had in store, but I was there, about to meet a very warm-hearted, caring, and patient physician. There would be no greater opportunity than this.

There was something very different about this trip, compared to all the others. I felt an overwhelming sense of peace. I had ridden the medical roller coaster long enough to finally be able to turn everything over to God. I no longer felt a need to manage my own care. I had a stronger sense of security and confidence, not merely with Johns Hopkins Hospital and Dr. Long, but with God. Until this point, I had expended a great deal of energy making sure everything was done correctly and in a timely fashion. I had to be my own advocate and was fortunate to be functioning well enough mentally to do so. I held the reigns very tight, not giving up control. I wanted to know everything there was to know and everything there was to do. I wanted to make suggestions, even with the little that I knew. The bottom line was, I didn't trust.

I had reason not to trust the medical care professionals helping me. They were only human, and several had proved worthy of my distrust. But, I had no reason for not trusting God. My journey, thus far, was one of give and take. I'd give the front seat of my tandem bike to God, only to take it back again. I wasn't content to just keep pedaling.

This time it was different. I not only accepted I didn't have control now, I also completely accepted I never had control in the first place. I turned every worry and fear over to God, Dr. Long, and his assistants. It was not only time to let God and others take over, but I also had used up every last bit of energy. I no longer had the energy to manage my care. Fatigue was getting the best of me. I needed to rely on others to do everything, and to trust it would be done as well as if I had orchestrated it myself. Even better yet, now I recognized God was conducting, and I knew each instrument of my care would be played by its finest musician.

This was going to be different, since I was so far away from my friends in Traverse City. It would have been very difficult to have had my first craniotomy this far from home. However, since I was anticipating my third, it wasn't so bad.

It truly astonished me how much energy my friends put forth in supporting me over so many years. Many friends sacrificed countless hours of their time to talk with me, hold me, and have fun with me; anything to keep me positive. They took on my pain as if it were their own. I don't know how they gave me the support they did. The only answer I have is they are true friends.

They entered the storm voluntarily, never once turning their backs on me. They carried me when I was weak, and cheered me when I was strong. They were God's tools to keep me going, as God rotated and recharged them to maintain their own strength. It seemed as though different groups of friends took segmented times to provide support, before passing the baton onto the next group. God must have been filling out the relay schedule each year, because I never went without support.

My first appointment at Hopkins was with Dr. Holliday. With his big, full mustache, Dr. Holliday reminded me of Albert Einstein. I was already prepared for the "inflexible scope." I knew it was painful, but if this surgeon could do anything to help me, I didn't care how far he reached with his scope. Not only was Dr. Holliday a very nice physician, I was also impressed with his steady hands. As he pushed the scope further into my nose, he didn't so much as touch the lining of my nasal passage. It was painless.

Dr. Holliday renewed my confidence in the specialty of otynlaryngology. He was very patient and understanding, and I felt very comfortable talking with him. His professionalism and personality places him in the top four of my all-time favorite physicians.

He didn't give much hope of being able to fix my leak through my mouth and sinuses. Given the extent of my skull fractures and volume of leaking, it was Dr. Holliday's recommendation we try to locate the leak with another cisternagram, which he called a RISA Study. He also referred me for more hearing tests (the results were negative for hearing loss). He said he'd be in touch with Dr. Long to discuss a plan of treatment.

The following day I met with Dr. Long. He walked into the exam room with a big smile and introduced himself. With a very deep, confident voice, he started the medical history routine. It was getting harder to summarize five years of history for these doctors, and thus I was beginning to see God's humor. Since I dislike history so much, He was making me a part of it.

I felt at ease with Dr. Long. Like Dr. Hoff, he didn't have an ego problem. This supported my theory, that if someone's good enough, they don't have to flaunt it. Their skill speaks for itself. Dr. Long was the best, yet he had two feet on the ground at all times. I knew right away he was going to treat me as he'd treat his own daughter.

During this initial meeting with Dr. Long I asked very few questions. I knew the routine. I was at peace with myself and my caregivers. Without holding firmly onto God's hand, I would have never been able to walk into a strange doctor's office, in a strange hospital, in a far away city, and say, "Please do whatever it takes to make me well again." I was finally handing God all the pieces, whereas before I handed over only a few broken ones. I had faith.

This was the biggest turning point in my entire recovery. I saw the miraculous things God did to get me through two brain surgeries within four months. Nevertheless, nothing was as incredible as how I came to be connected with the best neurosurgeon in the world.

God had a plan, and I was watching it unfold before me. It was time to let go. Trusting God should be like trusting gravity. If only our faith could be so strong. God's plan works. Ours doesn't. We don't need to add anything to His plan; we only need to receive it. It's difficult to avoid the temptation of substituting our own plan for His. There is no need to waste energy on figuring out His plan; it will happen as we allow it. If we try to add more to His plan or manipulate it, it's not help, it's interference. Our job is to align our heart and mind with the Holy Spirit and allow His plan to take place.

Dr. Long also scheduled tests for me, an MRI, CT scans with contrast, a blood workup and the RISA study Dr. Holliday suggested. Although this would be my seventh RISA study, I hoped Hopkins' methods of performing the test would be superior.

Surgery was already scheduled for July 15, 1994, giving us ten days to complete the tests. Surgery was contingent on what the tests revealed, but Dr. Long explained how he'd perform the surgery anyway. He'd go in through the same incision as the previous two craniotomies. After locating the leak, he'd suture the dura and use some of the lining within my skull to seal the area of the leak. I was ready, it was just a matter of going through the tests first.

In between appointments, Mom and I took in the sites of Baltimore and Washington, D.C. I also continued exercising, to maintain my strength.

The goal of my physical training had changed drastically since my injury. It was now part of my surgery preparation. I knew the importance of being strong and healthy. It had proved to be vital in my previous two brain surgeries, which were performed within a short period of time. Therefore, I wanted to do everything I could to maximize my ability to withstand another surgery and to recover quickly.

On the day of my RISA study, Mom and I walked through the clinic, while we waited for my next scan. We were both looking at people in white coats, hoping we'd see Dr. Carson. Finally, while standing near an elevator, I discreetly said to Mom, "There he is." We both stood in awe, as we watched Dr. Carson talk with his colleagues, completely unaware of us watching him or the impact he had on our lives.

Everything went well with the RISA study. The radiologist commented on the amount of fluid leaking from my nose, but he wanted to take more time to study the scans before telling me the results. Unlike either of the previous two hospital's protocols for post-study recovery, I was released to go back to the hotel immediately afterwards. I walked out the door without assistance. This seemed odd, since Munson required twelve hours at one angle and another twelve at another, and U. of M. required an overnight stay in the hospital with my head elevated. I began to wonder who was right, though I had the most faith in Hopkins, considering their level of expertise.

The night before my scheduled craniotomy, Dr. Long called our hotel room to say he still hadn't received my study results. He was confident he'd speak with the radiologist prior to surgery, so everything remained on schedule.

The next morning, I woke up early enough to go to the hotel's gym to ride the stationary bike. I wanted to ride for thirty minutes before showering and getting ready to leave for the hospital. In my mind this was the perfect way to warm-up for surgery.

We arrived at the hospital and found the Same Day Surgery department with little difficulty. The nurses were extremely nice while prepping me for surgery. Dr. Victor Perry, a neurosurgical resident, came to talk with me, seeking to answer any questions I had before going into the operating room (OR). He reviewed the procedure, wanting me to feel as comfortable as possible. He was such a nice doctor that he put me at ease very quickly.

A pastor from a Lutheran church in Baltimore was also with us this morning. The Sunday before surgery, my mother and I attended Atonement Lutheran Church. We met the pastor and many of the members. The pastor offered to come visit me while in the hospital, for which I was very grateful. I was shocked, however, when he walked into the Same Day Surgery room at 6:00 a.m. to say a prayer with my mother and me before I went into surgery. It was a big relief to know someone would be with Mom during my surgery. I was worried about her having to be alone.

Fifteen minutes before they were to take me to the OR, Dr. Long came to speak with me. He just talked with the radiologist who performed my RISA study. Dr. Long said, "Our results of the RISA study are also inconclusive, so I don't know where the leaks are. If I were to perform surgery I'd have to explore first, trying to find them. At this point, I want to leave the decision up to you. I believe I can find the leaks, but I cannot guarantee it. Do you still want to go through with this surgery?"

This was a loaded question. I knew I was leaking fluid. My last beta II transferin test had been positive, despite all of the cisternagrams being inconclusive. I had traveled all this way for Dr. Long to help me. He was the best. If I returned home without surgery and continued to leak, I'd never know if he could have helped. I had no choice but to go ahead with the surgery.

The lack of evidence didn't diminish Dr. Long's confidence. He also knew I had no choice, given the risks. I told him, "Go ahead with the surgery. I need your help. Do your best."

I'm not sure if this was faith or desperation. I was scared, but I had faith in a man who, prior to seeing him in surgery, I had met only once. I had faith in the OR staff. I met the resident anesthesiologist five minutes before surgery, but never met the attending anesthesiologist who put me under. How could I have this kind of faith in people I didn't know? It was my faith in God.

Because of my faith, I could entrust my body in the hands of these individuals. Without God, there would have been too many doubts. God provides us with a promise, "Never will I leave you; never will I forsake you." (Hebrews 13:5 NIV) I find it fascinating that I have more faith in God than I do any machine or human on this earth, and yet God remains sight unseen. Or does He? Doesn't He reveal Himself to us in many ways? He has to me.

God revealed Himself when He answered each and every prayer. He revealed Himself with messages of rainbows, smiles from friends, and incidents that happened not because of coincidence. They are Godincidences. These were only a few of the ways God made His presence known to me. The more I recognized His work, the stronger my faith grew.

My faith grew stronger as my body became weaker. Just because the previous surgeries failed to work didn't give me reason to lose trust. It seemed as if God was using each surgery to build my faith. God used people, circumstances, places, and things to help me learn and grow.

For the third time, I said good-bye to Mom before going into surgery, knowing she had the hardest role. Only this time she had to wait and worry without my father. I was confident Mom's faith was strong enough for her to feel God's presence with her as she waited. She knew God was with me, too. I still couldn't imagine myself in her shoes. I know I'll never know how she felt each time they'd take me from her, but I can speculate. My guess is it feels just as painful as someone taking a newborn baby from a mother's arms and saying to her, "Your baby may or may not come back to you."

Throughout my recovery, I felt the presence of angels. These angels were humans who connected with me in a special way, just when I needed them most. Prior to being taken to the OR, Keith, the head nurse in charge of the OR came to talk with me. Like many others, he was very kind and showed great compassion. He assured me he'd be with me for the duration of my surgery, making sure everything went smoothly.

As they wheeled me into the OR, my thoughts were focused on God walking next to me and His presence within me. I visualized Dr. Long and his assistants working on my head, while God handed them their tools.

Before going into the OR, they wheeled me to a holding area. Keith stood by my side, talking, trying his best to keep me relaxed. I could hear conversations inside the OR. Unlike both of my previous craniotomies, I wasn't sedated before arriving in the OR. I was aware of everything. It wasn't until after they wheeled me into the OR and hooked me up to the monitors, that they finally put me to sleep. Until then, I carried on conversations, as if it was another typical day in the OR for all of us.

Seven hours later, Dr. Long came out of surgery with a smile on his face. He told my mother he found the leak. He was very pleased we had decided to go ahead with the surgery, despite a lack of evidence. He said he found the leak very easily and was able to repair the area. He anticipated I'd feel much better without a constant headache. He again marveled at the fact I hadn't contracted bacterial meningitis since my leak began five years ago.

I woke up in the Neuro Intensive Care Unit (NICU), extremely cold. I was nervous about hearing the results of my surgery. I kept telling myself to relax, and tried to use the biofeedback skills Vince had taught me. These skills helped relax and warm my whole body.

This transition of consciousness was always difficult for me. My low body fat percentage (lack of insulation), combined with my low heart rate, increased my sensitivity to the cold. Lowering my body temperature during such delicate surgery helped reduce bleeding, but created great discomfort upon waking.

One of the medical students who had observed Dr. Long during my first appointment, came in the NICU to check on me. He asked a few basic questions for the routine neurological check. "What is your name? Where are you? What day is it?" He asked me how many fingers he had up. When I replied four, he quickly asked me to repeat the test. Obviously I was incorrect. My repeat performance was not any better, prompting his departure to tell Dr. Perry, the resident on call in the NICU.

I realized I had failed his test, so I started to practice seeing better by looking at the clocks on the wall. (There was only one clock.) I was terrified at the thought of any nerve damage.

Over the next several hours, nurses and doctors came to check my vitals and neuro functioning. Dr. Long came to tell me the good news of his success in finding my leak, and his ability to repair it. He was as excited as a little boy at Christmas. He shared with me the details of the leak's

location. It was difficult to retain this information, given my level of consciousness. Later, it helped to read his operative report:

> Under general anesthesia, the patient was prepared and draped in
> the usual fashion. The old skin incision was incised and the thinned
> portions of it removed. The skin flap was turned down with some
> difficulty because of scarring, but this was not a major issue. I took
> the periosteum with the flap in order to dissect it free later. The bone
> had healed nicely and had to be recut with a saw. It was then el-
> evated without injuring the dura beneath. I then elevated the dura
> subfrontally bilaterally, going over the cribiform plate, and exposing
> all the way back to the planum. The defect was found immediately. It
> was in the right side in the ethmoid sinus far lateral and was a clear-
> cut fistula. I repaired the dura with a single suture and then created
> a flap of pericranium to cover the whole floor of the frontal fossa,
> including the defect. It measured about 6 x 6cms. When I had dis-
> sected it free, I swung down this living graft, put it over the floor of
> the frontal fossa, and then allowed the frontal lobes of the brain to
> return to normal position to hold it in place. The bone flap was then
> put in place with plates and screws and the wound closed with a
> subgalial drain.

What most startled me when I read this was, "The defect was found
immediately." This must have meant it was very obvious and easy to see.
Why hadn't the RISA studies, cisternagrams, and myelograms shown the
location of the leak? Most noteworthy was that Dr. McCaffrey (at Mayo
Clinic) told me I didn't have a leak. At least Dr. Hoff was willing to admit
he didn't know what to do next. I'm sure if he would have gone into my
head again, he would have found the leak, too.

All day, I faded in and out, sleeping most of the time. There were
numerous machines hooked-up to me, as is the case after a craniotomy.
They were monitoring my heart rhythm and rate, respiration, oxygen satu-
ration, and blood pressure. I was on oxygen and had an arterial line fed
into my heart that monitored my blood pressure. This arterial line astonished me, since it went into an artery at my wrist and ended all the way up
into my aorta. There was a drain in my head, a tube penetrating through

a hole in my skull, emptying excess blood and fluid from within my skull. This reduced the intracranial pressure.

My first night in NICU was quite similar to my first night in NICU at U. of M. My heart rate dropped below 45 beats per minute and the nurses came flying into my room at the call of my monitor. I encouraged them to set the alarm at a very low level so I could get some sleep. In addition to alarms waking me, another patient was moved into my room, accompanied by many family members. She had just had emergency surgery because of an aneurysm in her brain. My first reaction was, "Wow, that's serious stuff. She had brain surgery." Then I remembered, that's what I had just been through. It was very easy to forget the seriousness of my own injury.

I felt more alert this time, somewhat aware of what was happening around me. For each of my previous brain surgeries I only remembered small fragments of time during the first three to four days post surgery. You would think I'd be kept very heavily sedated after such a traumatic surgery, but this was hardly the case. In fact, after brain surgery it was important for me to receive nothing more than Tylenol for pain. This would allow the nurses and physicians to accurately evaluate my level of consciousness and neuro functioning. Given the critical nature of this type of surgery, pain was the least of anyone's worries, including mine.

Like my caregivers, I focused my attention more on my capacities than on my extreme pain. I laid on my back with my head elevated, doing as much self-evaluation as possible. I practiced doing simple things, like looking at the clock to check my vision. Double vision was the only complication with my eyesight, and each time it presented itself, it corrected over time.

Another area of great concern to me was my ability to move my extremities. I constantly checked for movement and feeling in my hands, arms, legs, and feet. Fear of paralysis haunted me. I was fortunate not to have any major complications.

I was also anxious about my ability to speak understandably and fluently. Having gone through speech therapy immediately following my accident, I already knew the frustration of these difficulties. I was very proud of the progress I made (and fearful I'd lose it). After each surgery, I noticed my speech was noticeably delayed and word finding more difficult, though probably more noticeable to me than anyone else.

I became a pro at performing the neuro function tests. Every nurse, physician, and student who came to my bedside took me through this evaluation. It consisted of actions such as holding both arms up in the air, palms up, eyes closed, as if holding a pizza pan. Following the evaluator's finger from side to side and up and down was another test. They'd ask me to touch my finger to my nose and then to their moving finger. Something so simple as smiling was part of the test, to make sure the trigeminal nerves controlling facial muscles were intact. Everything had a purpose, and while it often seemed redundant, I appreciated the close observation.

As I laid in NICU, alone except for the monitors, my mind traveled to all sorts of areas. Most amazing to me is that I never felt the need to get out of bed. Even though I wasn't physically able to do so, I am surprised that I did not at least have the urge. My body was used to activity, but since my brain needed all of my energy, my body succumbed to those needs. It was entirely okay for my inner drive to just be still.

As I laid in bed, surrounded only by monitors, God's presence was within me. I drew strength from this inner peace, allowing my brain to heal, as all of my energy was channeled in that direction.

I didn't look at it as control having been taken from me, nor was it me giving control to anyone. After all, I never fully had control in the first place. Instead, I viewed this peace as a life force. I had the power and control to channel my energy in the direction needed. I could choose to direct it towards worries, defense mechanisms, or anger. On the other hand, I could choose to direct it towards positive energy, relaxation, increased circulation, and brain inactivity. All of which would promote my healing.

Simply allowing my brain to do what came naturally helped my entire body heal. Our bodies are designed to heal themselves. Our bodies send platelets to the exact area where we are cut, to stop the bleeding. When our skin is broken or removed, our bodies replace it with new skin. This feat cannot be accomplished by the most technologically-advanced automobile or computer. Our brains are our nucleus. Each of us is one of

God's miracles, and it is primarily external forces that hinder our bodies' optimal capacity to heal. Stress is one of these forces. Being at peace physically, emotionally, and spiritually optimizes our ability to heal.

This was my third craniotomy. Finally, I was truly at peace during my post-surgery recovery. My muscles did tense, as if to brace myself against and to resist the inevitable pain. But then I visualized increased blood flow to these areas, which gave me a feeling of warmth; leading to relaxation. As muscles relaxed, as a part of my body's natural pain killer, my pain subsided. It required continuous monitoring and effort to maintain an effective level of relaxation, but it was worth taking an active role in my recovery.

T HE MORNING FOLLOWING surgery came none too soon. It was a long, sleepless night. I was happy when they told me I'd be moved to a room on the regular neuro floor, Meyer 8. This was an indication I was doing okay. (I didn't know it, but Meyer 8 was about to bring me a wealth of experiences I would cherish for a lifetime.)

I was placed in a private room. My first nurse, who became a good friend, was Jennifer Accenelli, R.N. Her expertise was remarkable, but what was even more noteworthy was her ability to connect with patients on a personal level. Not only did she attend to a patient's physical needs, but also to their emotional needs. I was fortunate to be cared for spiritually by Jennifer.

The first four days after surgery were quite challenging. I felt very nauseous, either from the pain or leftover effects from the anesthesia. The depth and duration of sedation during brain surgery was significant. This, combined with my sensitivity to medications, made me feel lousy. I ran a low grade fever, raising suspicions of meningitis and fear of infection. As a precaution, Amoxicillin was prescribed for five days following surgery. It was administered every six hours through my IV, even during the night.

One day, as the Amoxicillin was infusing, I had a book of Max Lucado's, *When God Whispers Your Name*, next to me. Jennifer came in to detach the empty Amoxicillin bottle. We started talking. She asked me what the book was about. Whenever I don't know a person well enough to know their level of spirituality, I am very careful with my choice of words. I gave her a brief description of what I had read so far, and stated a little of how I felt about it. She got excited about my willingness to share with her my faith and began telling me of her own walk with God. She told me about the spiritual and inspirational books she had recently read.

From this point on, Jennifer felt free to speak with me about God, using her faith to complement her nursing skills. This friendship was a wonderful gift from God. At this critical time in my recovery, I needed a sister in Christ to be my friend. I needed to feel the closeness of a friendship, especially while I was so distant from my longtime friends. I needed a soul mate, someone who would share the Holy Spirit with me freely, not out of obligation, but purely from the soul. Jennifer was another one of my angels.

When I started to get depressed, Jennifer made a neat suggestion. She asked, "Have you ever written letters to God?" I must have looked puzzled, because before I could reply, she began explaining what she meant. "Try writing prayers down on paper, as if you are writing a letter to God. It really helps me talk to God. It's the same thing as praying, only you write it down. Have you ever seen the book *Children's Letters To God*? I'll have to bring it in for you to read. It's really neat."

Prayers are real. They are not phantom thoughts or words. They are conversations with God, and they can be in the form of a letter. That night, before going to bed, I pulled out some paper and wrote my first letter to God. At first I was a little apprehensive, feeling that this was too formal. Like writing a letter to a very important person, it's always difficult to come up with the right words. I didn't know what to say. Then, after I realized it was no different than a spoken prayer, I managed to write a couple of pages quite easily. I recognized that God never intended our communication with Him to be formal. The neatest part for me was realizing I didn't have to mail this letter. God was actually reading it as I wrote it, quicker than even the fastest fax machine. Part of my first letter went like this:

Dear God,

Thank you for sustaining my life during surgery, guiding and instructing the surgeons and helping me come through it as I have. I struggle each day with the pain and frustration, but you always seem to get me through it. Thank you. I'm scared to death that I'm leaking still and pray for You to not let this happen. Please let this part of my life pass, so I can continue on another journey, whatever and wherever You may take me. But Thy will be done. Thank you for letting me be at peace with what is happening. Sometimes it seems impossible but I'm working on it.

Today was a difficult day. Beginning with the sweats and feeling lousy. I never thought they'd get me out of bed, but I did.

I look forward to tomorrow, not knowing what you'll send me.

Love, Karen

This placed a whole new perspective on prayer. My spoken prayers meant more to me, because I could visualize how God was receiving each and every word.

In essence, ten years ago I wrote a letter to God but called it a poem. I wrote it following the death of my mother's best friend, Maxine Marshall. It was at a time in my life when I really wondered what God's agenda was, while recognizing that I was the one needing to adjust. God's plans weren't going to change.

Mrs. Marshall's death was one of the most tragic things to happen to my mother, and yet Mom's feelings remain a mystery. I know it was her strong faith that carried her while she watched her friend die. The words in this letter describe what I felt at the time. I assumed they paralleled my mother's feelings.

"Lord Give Me Strength to be Happy"

Dear Lord,

I need a friend, but I always ask for two.

I need food to eat, but I ask for a feast.

I need a roof over my head, but I ask for a mansion.

I need a car, but I ask for a limousine.

I need the sun, but I ask for blue sky.

I need the rain, but only at night.

I need the snow, but make it powder.

Lord, I am forever blessed with your gracious gifts,

yet I am never content.

I ask for one thing, but always want another.

I ask for You to take a friend from her suffering,
yet when it is done, I cry.
I ask for strength, but really want answers.
I ask for more faith, but really want proof.
Lord, instead of being happy with the blessings I receive,
I merely say thank-you and pray for more.
Lord, please accept my humble apology and thanks,
but Lord, may I ask for yet one more gift?
please help me to pray...
..."Lord give me strength to be happy."

                         Yours Forever,
                         Karen Wells   (Written: May 1984)

I felt guilty for humbly praying for one thing, yet desiring to have something better. Most notably, I knew I needed to learn to be happy with God's plan. I was developing acceptance that we will never understand God's plan. I was learning that we need to ask for strength to be happy with whatever God sends our way. This was all a part of God preparing me for my injury. There are no unnecessary moments. All are of great value to our spiritual development. Like a sculptor chiseling away piece by piece over a long period of time and forming a beautiful image, God uses every moment to perfect His creation.

The next morning Jennifer came into my room. She carried two items that she wanted to give me. One was the book, *Children's Letters To God*, and the other was a blank journal book. *Children's Letter to God* was priceless. It contained humble messages from children. The journal was to be used for my letters to God. She asked me if I had followed through with my promise to write a letter to God. I said yes. She knew by the look on my face, my experience was positive. I thanked her for her generosity in sharing herself with me and helping me in such a time of need. This was the beginning of many more wonderful spiritual connections with Jennifer, and more importantly with God.

PRAYER HAS EXTRAORDINARY power and is a God given privilege. It is the ultimate of pagers or cell phones, never to be likened by any other form of communication here on earth. God can take every incoming message or call, all at once, twenty-four hours every day of the year, including holidays. He knows our words before we speak them. God reads our hearts.

If I were to compare prayer with our technological system here on earth, during my recovery we would have crashed the entire communications network. There wasn't a piece of technology in this world equipped to handle the volume of prayers that were said on my behalf.

I knew God heard and answered every prayer, despite my earlier doubts. When I was younger, I thought of prayer as one way communication. Early in my recovery, when I asked for life to be as it was before my injury, I seemed to get no response. I thought my prayers were not being answered. I also wondered why God wasn't listening to the multitudes of people who were praying for me. I felt this way because the prayers weren't being answered in the way I wanted; although they were answered. Thankfully, God looked out for my best interests and saw much further into the future. In fact, he had the entire blueprint of my life mapped out. God was watching over me, perfecting His design continuously. Sometimes, He said no when I wanted a yes. Sometimes, He needed to say wait, making sure everything happened just at the right moment. Nevertheless, he always took care of my needs and didn't answer prayers in a way that would have been detrimental.

Prayers weren't always answered in the time frame I had in mind, either. God was silent, often times when I felt I needed Him most. I had to be assured that even when God was silent, he was working. He may have been quiet, but He didn't quit. He used adversity to accomplish His will and I learned to trust.

It's just like when I was a child and went to a sporting event with my parents. They held the admission tickets for the game until right before we walked through the gate. They were afraid I would lose the ticket if they gave it to me too soon. They were also never too late in giving me my ticket. Never did they walk through the gate with all the tickets in hand, leaving me stranded.

God's methods of taking care of us parallel our relationship with our earthly fathers. God gives us what we need, at the right moment, never too early and never too late. I may have sometimes felt as though it was too late, but it truly never was. All of my suffering had a purpose. The pain I endured has and will continue to produce great rewards. My reaction to my pain played a significant role as a training tool. Unlike the old saying, "Don't just stand there, do something," God might say, "Don't do anything, just stand there." The times when I was unwilling to accept His methods of teaching, trying to do my own thing, were my most difficult times.

During my recovery my prayers changed. They didn't change in content alone, but also in the way I addressed them. Prior to this time, I often said common prayers from memory or repeated the same prayers each night upon going to bed. I'd typically fall asleep before the last amen. They were meaningful because of tradition, having said many of them since I was a little girl. But I was just saying the words, rather than praying from my heart. I'd wake up the next morning not remembering much beyond the first few lines of my first prayer.

After my head injury, I started spending more time praying. This quality alone time with God became important to me. I started to set aside specific time for Him, as opposed to waiting until I found leftover time in the day. Praying came more from my heart than from my mind. From this came a tremendous amount of peace, like sitting down with one's best friend and having a heart-to-heart talk. There was no longer a pattern or formality to my prayers. They were rather simple, but they expressed very genuinely how I felt.

I praised God for His grace and asked for comfort in all aspects of life. All too often, the asking came before praise. As I learned and grew stronger in faith, praising became instinctual. My most common prayer was, "If it is Thy will Lord, please make my desires be fulfilled. If it is not for my own good, please help me to have faith and trust in the path You have chosen for me. Guide me on this path so I do not stray. Please give me the strength to accept Your will with a loving heart."

I received constant reassurance from my family and friends that God hadn't forgotten me. Each time my mother said to me, "Karen, God's watching over you and will answer our prayers," it felt as though the promise became stronger. It made it a twofold promise, one from my Heavenly

Father and one from my mother. It still required faith, but it was easier when faith didn't stand alone.

Stories were told of how countless churches had me on their prayer lists. Friends, both locally and across the country, shared my need of prayers with others. I was overwhelmed with the number of people who came up to me and said they had been praying for me during their worship services. Sometimes, I'd know who the connection was within the church, while other times I didn't have any idea.

Word about my health traveled fast, from Traverse City to Atlanta, Georgia, where my brother and sister lived. Much to my siblings surprise, other people knew how I was doing before they told them.

It often felt as though everyone in the world was praying for me, which was very comforting. It also seemed that if this was the case, then God would get the hint sooner or later that He needed to help me out. I have the feeling He finally said, "Enough already. Okay, I will fix this leak."

M OM VISITED ME everyday. In-between my naps we talked, while she did her cross-stitch. Each morning I looked forward to her arrival. Although we didn't do very much, this time with Mom was very special to me. Having her sit in my room gave me peace, as a child is comforted when afraid. It reminded me of when I was little and had nightmares. I'd call out in the night, and she'd come lay by my side until I fell asleep.

During my recovery, I often felt like I was living in a nightmare, only everything was reversed. The nightmare occurred when I was awake. Falling asleep gave temporary relief, an escape from reality.

Jennifer recognized she was helping me get through this difficult time, and asked to have me as one of her patients each day she worked. Therefore, I came to know Jennifer quite well, as she spent most of her free time visiting with me.

The first priority on my postsurgical agenda was to take my first shower. There was nothing like taking a refreshing shower after having to go several days without one. I thought I was strong enough to take a simple shower. But Peggy, my nurse that day, insisted I go down to the shower room at the end of the hall, where I could sit down while showering. Realizing how weak I was once I got in the shower, I appreciated Peggy's suggestion. I came close to passing out, even while sitting. I was much weaker than I thought. At least I didn't have to worry about washing my hair. I didn't have any.

Each day when Mom arrived, she'd walk the halls with me, as I started to build my endurance. One day while we were walking, both of us happened to glance into room 856 at the same time. We were surprised to see an elderly man laying in bed on his back, sleeping very soundly, with his mouth wide open, snoring. He looked just like my grandfather. Mom and I looked at each other and said at the same time, "Doesn't that look like Grandpa?" It was an eerie feeling, since this was how we remembered Grandpa spending much of the last two months of his life in the hospital.

As we walked, we crossed paths with other patients. There was a woman who walked with her husband, who Mom and I greeted each day. Everyone on Meyer 8 had some form of neuro injury or disorder, giving us an unspoken bond. One evening, after Mom returned to the hotel, I saw this woman in her room and introduced myself. Her name was Mary Jo. She invited me to sit with her and talk. We talked for almost an hour about various aspects of our recoveries.

We compared scars, as they were clearly visible. The residents had removed the bandage from my head, clearly revealing a scar stretching from ear to ear. I had only a little patch of hair left on the back of my head, where my head must have been resting on the table when they shaved it in the OR. Mary Jo's smaller scar was mostly covered by her longer hair. She described her surgery to me, a ventriculoperitoneal shunt revision after having problems with the reoccurrence of hydrocephalus. The shunt is one that extends from a ventricle inside the brain, all the way down to the peritoneum, a lining of the abdominal and pelvic cavities. This was the shunt Dr. Cilluffo wanted to put in me prior to my decision to change to Dr. Hoff as my surgeon.

I was curious how she felt about having this in her brain, since I had been terrified of having it put into mine. While she seemed quite at ease, she wasn't happy with its need to be replaced due to its malfunction. Dr. Long was also her physician. We spoke of how thankful we were to have the best neurosurgeon. Others frequently said to us, "How did you ever

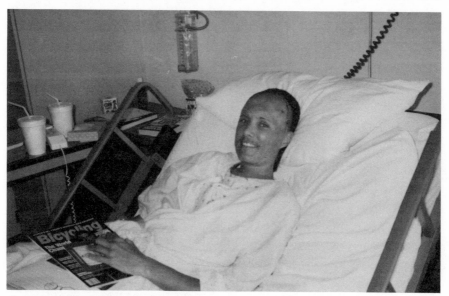

One week after the third craniotomy.

get Dr. Long to be your doctor?" Dr. Long didn't take every patient who asked. We both agreed we felt special and honored to have him as our surgeon.

Our conversation rapidly moved towards inspiration and our spiritual strength. We freely shared our feelings, happy to talk with someone who shared a similar challenge. We agreed that each new day was a very special gift. Our discussion motivated me to write a poem that night. I wanted to give it to Mary Jo before she was discharged the next day.

Today's Gift
Each day when we awake,
    With the coming of daylight;
May our eyes open to the beauty,
    Unwrapping the gift of life.

A gift given to us from God,
    A special gift given to no other;
Its contents yet unknown,
    Like any gift one to another.

We may never understand its value,

Or whether to say thank-you or why;
But we do know where it comes from,
    And that it is one of a kind.

This is our gift for today,
    Very different than tomorrow's;
It may bring peace, it may bring joys,
    Or hardships, challenges, or sorrows.

Dear Lord, help me to open this gift,
    With child like anticipation;
Even playing with the box,
    When accepting the contents with trepidation.

Please give me strength to cherish each day,
    Your generosity is beyond comprehension;
if I open my eyes to see what's there,
    The brightness is blinding, the darkness a lesson.

Yes, life's a gift,
    To me from You;
To share with those around me,
    Just as You did too.   (Written: July 1994)

I gave this poem to Mary Jo the next morning. She was pleased to
know she had inspired me to write, and happy that I shared it with her.
This was the first time my life crossed paths with someone, connecting at a
unique personal level, knowing when we said good-bye that we probably
would never see each other again. Yet, these friends will never be forgotten, for they played a very important role in my life. A friendship is significant, no matter how long or short its duration. I believe once a friend
always a friend, even though physical or emotional separation may occur.
Our lives will never be the same having connected with another.

I met another woman while I was on Meyer 8. Anna Pearson, an
elderly patient, was having tests performed on a tumor in her neck. We
met one day after my mother and I walked into the patient lounge. Anna
was standing near the window, taking in the beautiful skyline view of Baltimore and the Chesapeake Bay. I commented on how wonderful it was to
be able to enjoy such a view. I'll never forget the smile that blossomed on

Anna's face when I talked to her. She said, "Oh yes, this is a great place to call home." Anna was from Baltimore, and proceeded to point in the direction of her home. This was the beginning of another wonderful friend-ship. Each day when I walked the halls, I'd look for Anna. When Mom wasn't with me, I'd sit and listen to Anna's stories, delighted to hear about her life.

M Y LOYALTY TO my career was such that even brain surgery could not diminish it. Both before and after surgery, while I was in Balti-more, I continued following up on business contacts and marketing my program. The hospital sent a lap top computer with me, so I could fax proposals and documents to clients. I did not miss a beat. Some might think it was an obsession, working in the midst of recovering from brain surgery. I, on the other hand, was trying to keep my job and maintain the quality of my department. I enjoyed my work.

M Y FRIEND, MARY Crenshaw, traveled all the way to Baltimore from Richmond, Virginia to be with Mom and to visit me for a few days after my surgery. It was good to see Mary, a special person in my life, and a relief to know Mom wasn't alone. They enjoyed their time with one another. Mom met people at the hotel who shared rides on the shuttle, but they weren't the same as a longtime friend. Everyone on the shuttle shared stories of their loved ones in the hospital, and became a part of a unique family. I enjoyed hearing Mom's stories each day. I felt as though I came to know these people, too.

The bond that is formed from these interactions is very close. I thought it was very special when Mom said she was going to another building of the hospital (Hopkins has 56 buildings) to visit a relative of someone she met at the hotel. The patient's family had to go home for a few days and were concerned about leaving their mother alone. So Mom offered to visit her.

Each day, as early as 6:00 a.m. the residents did rounds, checking on all the patients. There was a group of eight residents who followed my case. I always wondered how I ever passed their neuro evaluation so early in the morning, when I was still half asleep. After a thunderous knock, they'd come barreling into my room, asking without hesitation, "Karen, how are you doing today?"

On days when I was awake and feeling well enough to give them a hard time, I'd reply, "If I were awake I might be able to tell you," or "I don't know, I haven't been awake to find out." They appreciated my humor and upbeat attitude. They must have liked me, because I came to notice they started coming to my room last during their rounds. This gave me an extra hour of sleep.

I came to know all of the residents by name, as each of them ended up having some form of individual contact with me during the course of my treatment. Dr. Perry belonged to this team. I came to know and like him very well. He was one of the most sensitive young doctors I ever met. I'll never forget Dr. Zydman. The first day he walked into my room I thought a pro football player had put a white coat on and was playing doctor. He filled the doorway, as he was at least 6'6" and 350 pounds. He reminded me of a grizzly bear, but was extremely gentle and soft-spoken.

The longer I remained in the hospital, the more I came to recognize the residents' authority and also the possibility of their mistakes. I learned the latter when a group of them, not my usual group, walked into my room. They asked to see my incision, pointing to my abdomen. I was lying there with a big white bandage wrapped around my head, and they were pointing to my abdomen. I had to tell them I didn't have an incision there, it was on my head. It was difficult to do this with a straight face. They seemed a bit puzzled and started asking questions about my surgery. As it turned out, while they learned about the characteristics of my case, I learned to be cautious with their actions and words. They were still students.

Dr. Long made rounds everyday as well, including weekends. He'd come in and sit down, as a friend or father would. He acted as if he had all the time in the world. He was very pleased with my progress and impressed with how good I looked. His positive outlook and confidence was refreshing, and gave me mountains of hope.

I was discharged nine days after surgery, when Dr. Long felt I was strong enough and clear from any risks of infection. He said it was okay for me to fly home and he'd call me as a follow-up appointment. He was proud to see I hadn't leaked since surgery and was confident of his success. I asked whether the pressure changes while flying would affect my head. He said, "No, you should have no problem."

This was good news. We had been in Baltimore for three weeks. Both Mom and I were ready to go home. Although we met many wonderful people in Baltimore, it was extremely difficult to be gone so long. This was a long time for Mom to be separated from Dad. Plus it's physically draining to go back and forth to a hospital everyday, for any length of time, no matter who the patient is or the circumstances.

I was discharged on a Sunday afternoon. We waited until Tuesday to fly home. Dr. Long suggested I move through the transition slowly. Returning to the Tremont Plaza, where Mom and I began our Baltimore adventure, was strange. It felt as though time had stood still while I was in the hospital.

Upon returning to the hotel, I felt pretty good. After resting awhile, my mother asked if I wanted to try walking outside a little. I had walked everyday with her while in the hospital and she thought it might feel good to walk outside. I didn't know how far I'd be able to go, but was excited that she was suggesting a walk.

The only other factor to consider was my bald head and frightful scar. I forgot the hat I had worn after my first two craniotomies, so I had to go without anything on my head. I didn't mind, but I felt bad for the people who saw my scar. I must have looked like Frankenstein.

We started out slowly. I was worried I'd go too far, and have a difficult time returning to the hotel. Luckily, my athletic training came in handy in situations like this, where I really needed to pace myself and read my physical status.

We made it all the way to the Inner Harbor and sat down at the outdoor amphitheater, where there was different entertainment every hour. We enjoyed sitting through several shows, and then Mom asked if I wanted to say hi to the sea lions. I couldn't wait to see them, remembering the joy they brought to us before.

By the time we made it back to the hotel I was exhausted, but proud of my accomplishment. After all, it had only been nine days since Dr. Long was working inside my head.

It felt as though our trip home was somewhat of a metaphor for my recovery. After five long years of battling headaches and flying high and low on the medical roller coaster, it was time to go home. It was time to go home to my new life, without a leak. It was time to start fresh.

Nineteen

Home, But Not So Sweet

Because the Lord is my Shepherd,
I have everything I need.

PSALM 23:1 TLB

Y RETURN HOME WAS filled with mixed emotions. It was wonderful to be greeted by my father at the airport, but I also faced the loss of Akita. The look in Dad's eyes, when he first saw me walk through the door, was very touching. Having been caught up in my own fears, stress, and grief, I hadn't taken enough time to think of how it must have been for him, to sit and wait alone during my surgery. My guess is, it was even more difficult being one thousand miles away.

Of course, I talked with Dad on the phone after my surgery, but that wasn't the same as seeing someone in person. As I walked through the gate, his eyes expressed, "Thank you Lord. Thank you for bringing my baby home to me again." I saw tears well up in his eyes before he gave me a big hug and held me tight.

It didn't hit me that I wasn't going to see Akita again until we opened the garage door of my house and I saw Akita's water bowl by the step. Within the first ten minutes of being home, I realized I hadn't gone through the grieving process as I should have. Because I was in an environment where Akita wouldn't have normally been, I did not truly grieve her death.

Everywhere I turned in my house, something reminded me of Akita. Her toys were still on the floor, her food in the pantry, her fur, which she shed, on the carpet. At significant times of the day, my thoughts were, "I need to feed Akita," or "I better let Akita outside." It took a long time for this to pass. My friend was gone. The house was too quiet.

I assured Mom and Dad I would be okay by myself. If I needed help, the Hodgins were next door. My parents were hesitant to leave me, but also anxious to get home to have time to themselves. The house and yard were in perfect order, so there was no need for me to do anything physical, except keep walking for exercise. I also wanted to get back into my work routine, as Manager of the Vital Choice program at Munson.

After my parents left, the silence in my home was distressing. I missed Akita, and was afraid to cry, for fear I wouldn't be able to stop. I kept thinking back to that lonely day when life didn't seem worth living, thinking of how Akita had whimpered outside the garage door, wanting me to come out, wanting me to live. How could I ever forgive myself for taking her life? Would I ever be able to put this behind me?

I picked up her picture. Tears rolled down my cheeks like a river. Life didn't seem fair. Why did there have to be so much pain? Despite having tremendous headache pain for five years, emotional pain had far exceeded my physical pain. In five years, I had felt more pain than in my previous twenty-eight years of life. Was it because I avoided pain, stuffing feelings away so they wouldn't interrupt my agenda for life? Why was I suddenly feeling all this after a traumatic brain injury? Were more traumatic things happening to me or was I more sensitive now? If I am more sensitive, is it because I had learned to open up or was it from damage to my brain? Why were all these questions running through my head after arriving home, after being at peace with everything in Baltimore? And finally, what happened to that peace?

The last question helped me re-focus. My peace was from God. He was here with me. I wasn't alone. My mind was just taking over. It didn't matter how much pain I endured. I knew I could take as much as He handed to me. Pain was my teacher, and it's unfortunate I chose not to learn in this fashion during the first twenty-eight years of my life. At least I could still learn while I was young, having many more years to put these lessons into practice. Even if my increased sensitivity was because of damage to my brain, it was a blessing, not a tragedy.

T HE NEXT DAY I began making contacts with my employees at Munson. I wanted to let them know I was home and available through my home office, where I had performed much of my work over the past five years. (Accommodations for me to work from home part of the time were made for me shortly after my accident. It had worked out very nicely. I even increased my productivity since I had fewer interruptions.)

Now there was some uncertainty about my job and whether my accommodations would continue. This added a new dimension to my recovery. For five years I was allowed to work from my home. I brought financial success to the department for the first time. I was promoted. All of this was in the midst of my rehabilitation and recovery from the injury and my surgeries. The point is, I was doing my job successfully, and then suddenly I was told I could no longer do it. I was informed I could return to work only when I could work a minimum of twenty hours per week at the hospital. I was then expected to increase to full-time within two weeks. Previously, I was allowed to return to work, even if it was only six to eight hours the first week. I had appreciated the flexibility of hospital policy.

This was a test of my peace of mind. Over five years, I had: survived a brain injury, rehabilitated cognitive deficits, underwent two sinus surgeries, handled a seizure disorder, found out I was misdiagnosed, adjusted to a less active life-style, had a CSF shunt surgically implanted, lost my grandfather, had craniotomy #1, leaked CSF again, had craniotomy #2, leaked CSF again, lost my marriage, battled with divorce, maintained my job, and survived craniotomy #3. Now I was told I would lose my job if I couldn't return under new parameters.

I was furious. After all I had done for the hospital, it was truly a slap in the face. To function successfully in this complex political world, it was necessary for me to possess the capacity not only to express my anger, but also not to express it. Expressing my anger didn't diminish it, it simply released it.

What was most unfortunate was that I reverted back to feeling as though it didn't matter what I had endured and who had carried me through my trials. My career was still more important. It was again a control issue. Control was being taken from me in the only area where I still had maintained control, my job.

I had relinquished the need for control and was at peace in all areas of my life, except my career. The ironic part was, I really never had control of my career, either. In fact, it had major control over me. It was a competitive issue. My competitiveness was no longer just pushing me to excel, it was manipulating my life. I was caught in its web, blindfolded, unable to break free from two qualities I learned as positive attributes: dedication and determination. My focus was my destination instead of my journey. There were more lessons to be learned.

O NE WEEK AFTER returning home from Baltimore, seventeen days post-surgery, I bent over to pick something up off the floor and fluid poured out my nose. "Please Lord, let this be my imagination. Please," I whispered in shock. I didn't think it was possible. "Dr. Long said he fixed all the leaks. He said flying wouldn't effect my head. How could this be?"

I had glucose test strips in my medicine cabinet, so I pulled them out. I bent over, cupping the palm of my hand under my nose. Fluid filled the palm of my hand. I knew I didn't need to test the liquid for glucose. I knew it was spinal fluid.

After the glucose strip showed positive for glucose, I made a phone call to Dr. Long. My voice quivered as I spoke with the head resident, Dr. Zydman. He sensed I was heartbroken and didn't want to alarm me unnecessarily. He calmly said, "We'd love for you to come back out to Hopkins. We can still help you."

In a panicked tone I replied, "But didn't Dr. Long fix all the leaks or is it because my pressure is too high and it keeps springing leaks?"

"I can't say for sure, Karen, until we have you back out here. How soon can you come?"

"How soon can you get me in?"

"We need you to come as soon as possible. If we wait, there's too high a risk of meningitis."

"Okay, I'll try to get a flight out as soon as possible."

"I'll have a room ready for you as soon as you arrive."

I hung up the phone in a daze. It was happening all over again, a nightmare that wouldn't end. Suddenly the stress over my job didn't matter at all. There were far greater things to channel my energy towards.

Just when I thought I was going to make it without tears, I opened my mail. I received twenty-five get well cards from friends. The first one I opened released the flood gates of my tears. Its cover was a picture of a huge rainbow, and it said, "It takes both sunshine and rain to make life's rainbows." I thought to myself, "God you truly are amazing. Your message is very clear. There is always hope. Thank you."

His messages to me were always there, but I had to be open to see them. With my experiences in seeing His five rainbows the last time I started leaking after surgery, I knew this wasn't just a card from a friend. It was a card from God. It was comforting to have tears of joy and peace, in the eye of a hopeless storm.

All the cards were special and lifted my spirits. I received a card from my dear friend, Joy, who told me she was lighting candles for me at church, as she said a prayer for my healing. There were candles burning for me across the country, and a wealth of energy and optimism flowed through these friends from God. I tapped every source.

Less than twenty minutes after talking with Dr. Zydman, Dee Bennett, Dr. Long's assistant, called to tell me I was scheduled to be admitted Monday morning at 9:00 a.m. She said Dr. Long was first going to put a lumbar drain in me, to see if he could lower the pressure enough for the leak to stop. I told her I'd try to get a flight to Baltimore before then and would call if there wasn't anything available. It was already Tuesday afternoon, so I'd need to work fast to make all the arrangements.

I called the airlines and found I could depart Sunday morning, which would be perfect. I then called my parents to tell them I was leaking again and needed to return to Hopkins. I was disheartened by their response.

When I said, "I'm leaking again," there was no empathy in my mother's reply.

She said, "Oh, what does that mean?"

I wanted to scream, "It means more surgery Mom, what do you think it means?" But I didn't. I obviously had a lot of anger for what was happening to me, and projecting it onto my mother would not be fair. Instead, I simply replied, "I'm going to be admitted Monday morning at Hopkins. Dr. Long wants to put a lumbar drain in me."

After a moment of silence, Mom said, "Can't this be done some other time? Your father and I are going to Nebraska to the Marshall wedding. We're not going to miss that."

As she spoke these words, I held my breath. I took a deep breath before stating, "No Mom, it can't be done some other time. This is critical to my health. I need to go as soon as possible. They want me there Monday."

"Karen this doesn't fit in our schedule."

"Well it doesn't fit in mine either, but I have to take care of myself, Mom. My flight leaves Sunday morning."

"How will you get around? Where will you stay Sunday night? How will you get from the airport into Baltimore? You can't do this alone, you just had brain surgery."

"I've already made reservations at the Brookshire Hotel. They have a shuttle from the airport, as well as to and from Hopkins. I guess I'll have to go alone. I'll be okay."

"I need to talk to your father. We'll call you back. Love you. Bye." Click.

I hung up the phone and cried. "Dear God why does it have to be so hard to openly and honestly express our feelings to one another? We're family and yet sometimes I feel worlds apart from them. I know it's because all of us are devastated by this whole mess, and are unwilling to share our feelings. Why does my anger stand in the way of being the first to initiate appropriate communication?"

I didn't know what to do. Whenever I felt lost, I called my best friend and sister, Kay. It happened to be Kay's day off work so she was home when I called. I told her the whole story. She was most empathic, dumbfounded to hear I was leaking again, and startled by Mom's response. Nonetheless, Kay always sheds a positive light on everyone and plays the role of mediator quite well. She offered to be with me in Baltimore for a few days. It was her slow season at the store and she thought she might be able to get a few days off. Knowing she couldn't be with me a long time, she suggested Lamar might be able to arrange a few days away from work as well.

What a relief this was, to think I might not have to be alone. I'd do it if I had to, but to have someone with me would give me great comfort. I didn't have any idea what to expect with the lumbar drain. I knew they'd be draining CSF out of me through my back, but I didn't know how much, how I'd feel, or how long they were going to do this.

My father called me back later that evening. Dad never calls unless Mom won't talk to me, which didn't surprise me after our earlier conversation. It's basically the childhood routine of, "Go talk to your father." I always liked talking to Dad. Even as a kid I never minded Mom making this suggestion. It wasn't that Dad always said yes when Mom said no. It was just easier to talk with Dad, because there were less conflicting emotions in the conversation. We could always talk about the specific issue, rather than bring other factors and details into it.

When I heard Dad say, "Hello Karen, how are you doing?" I knew what to expect. Dad always ends up in the middle of things, wanting to be supportive of everyone. He usually repeats Mom's words, despite having conflicting feelings of his own. I didn't know what Dad felt on this day. He restated Mom's comment, "Karen this doesn't fit in our schedule. We've had this trip planned and we're going to Nebraska."

Without allowing him to go further, I told him my plans were already made. I couldn't change them, due to the critical nature of my health. I then told him Kay was trying to make arrangements to be with me in Baltimore. He seemed surprised by this, but I'm sure, relieved. He told me they'd be over to see me before I left.

Their inability to give me emotional support at this time hurt more than their choice to go to Nebraska. I don't believe they knew what to do in this situation.

I was being hit by so many unexpected complications, it was difficult for any of us to react appropriately. By this time, my medical condition was beyond defying the odds. It had turned into a medical nightmare that would not go away.

Kay called back the next day. She said, "Karen, Lamar and I made arrangements to be with you at Hopkins. We staggered our stays, so we could cover a longer period of time. I also talked with Mom. She said they'd plan to drive to Baltimore after the wedding, if it looked like you were going to be there for a significantly longer period of time after we left. How does that sound?"

I choked back my tears and said, "Great, I can't tell you how comforting it feels. I was dreading having to be alone."

"Lamar will arrive Sunday afternoon and leave Thursday. I'll fly in Wednesday and leave Sunday. That way he and I will be there at the same time for a few days."

Lamar called that night, to get directions of what to do once he got to the airport. Our flights arrived roughly four hours apart, so we planned to meet at the hotel.

My parents came over the next day to visit. The tension was evident. I was stressed, not only about the tension between us, but also about leaking again, and fear of the unknown. I ended up having a seizure that day, while they were at my house. This was the first time they witnessed one of my seizures. I know it was terrifying for them. This was a difficult note to say good-bye on. I'm sure they were scared, knowing I'd be traveling alone, especially after seeing the seizure. But, they assured me they'd be in touch and said good-bye.

M Y FLIGHT SUNDAY morning was at 6:00 a.m. We were delayed an hour, which was going to cut my layover time in Chicago quite close, four minutes. When we landed in Chicago, I really had to hustle to catch the flight to Baltimore. Given the long distance between the commuter terminal and the main terminal, I knew in order to make my flight I was going to have to run. The only physical activity I'd performed since surgery was walking around the hallways in the hospital at a relatively slow pace. It was going to take greater effort than that to make my flight.

I started to run down the concourse, despite feeling the weakness in my legs, a shortness of breath, and light-headedness. When I arrived at the gate, there was not a soul sitting or standing in the area, except for the flight attendant at the door of the gate. She looked at her watch and said with a smile, "Four minutes. You made it in four minutes. That's at least a ten minute walk. From now on, I'm closing the door after four minutes, now that I know it can be done." The flight attendants from my first flight must have called ahead to tell them I was on my way.

As I arrived at the gate, I started to get a bit dizzy and nauseated. I didn't read the flight information at the gate when I arrived, but went straight to my seat and sat down. Suddenly, my body felt extremely weak. I asked the woman sitting next to me, "We're heading to BWI, aren't we?"

She said, "Yes, Washington National," not knowing BWI was a different airport in the Washington D.C./Baltimore area.

I thought to myself, "Oh no, what happened? I made reservations for BWI." I pulled out my ticket. Sure enough, the agency had booked me to arrive at Washington National (but depart from BWI). It was too late to change. We were already 20,000 feet in the air. I'd just have to figure out how to get from Washington National into Baltimore.

When we arrived, I was confident my luggage didn't arrive with me; after all, it couldn't have passed through O'Hare like I had. This was a blessing. It saved me the energy of carting it around, as I made my way to Baltimore.

I asked for directions on how to get to Baltimore. They sounded something like this: "Take the Metro shuttle to Washington National station. Then, take the Metro to Union Station. Go to the bus station and take the Washington Flyer bus to BWI Airport. From there, you can catch the Baltimore shuttle, and it should take you directly to your hotel. We'll deliver your luggage to you this afternoon, wherever you want it."

This sounded like a comedy act. I thought to myself, "You have got to be kidding. How am I ever going to find my way?" I didn't have a clue as to what she had said. There was no way for my short-term memory to recall these directions.

I pulled out my Franklin Planner, and said, "Can you repeat that for me, please?" I could tell she wasn't too thrilled about having to restate everything. This was where my shaved head and ugly ear-to-ear scar came in handy. I didn't have to do much explaining about my condition. She could tell there was something wrong with my brain. (At least she didn't ask if I had been bitten by a shark.) As I took notes, she repeated the directions, and I was on my way.

I got off the first shuttle, after the driver announced Metro Station. When I got off the bus there wasn't a station in sight, only an empty sidewalk in the middle of nowhere. I walked ten steps in one direction, turned around and walked ten in the other, realizing I didn't know where I was supposed to go. I glanced up at the bus driver, who was laughing with me, as I realized how dumb I looked. He pointed down the stairwell to the right.

Once I was in the station I asked a woman how to get a ticket to wherever I was supposed to go. She was very helpful. I passed my ticket through the mechanical ticket taker at the turnstile. At the same time, I heard the same woman say, "Sir, sir, make sure you pull it out after you go through so you can get off the train." I laughed to myself. At this point, I wasn't about to explain to her I wasn't a man. I thanked her and went on my way.

I boarded the Metro and started looking at the map, so I'd know where to get off. Suddenly I heard it again, "Sir, sir....where are you headed?"

I thought, "What the heck?" I lowered my voice a notch and said, "Union Station," turning quickly in the other direction to read my map, praying she wouldn't start flirting with me. I really wasn't in the mood to explain details to her.

When I got off at Union Station, I was directly in front of the White House. I sat down on a park bench for a few minutes to catch my breath, before venturing onto the next leg of my adventure. A thought crossed my mind, "And Mom thought flying into a strange city was stressful. At least we ended up where we thought we were going. If she only knew where I was right now and what I was doing, she'd have a coronary." I thanked the Lord that this happened to me alone and not while Mom was with me. I also asked Him to protect me through the rest of my journey.

I found the bus station, only to discover I needed to take this bus to another station in order to get a bus ticket, board that bus, which would take me to BWI Airport. What's one more leg among many? I finally arrived at BWI Airport, where I was supposed to arrive an hour and a half earlier. If I'd been delayed two more hours, I could have met Lamar when he arrived. Instead, I headed for the hotel. I needed to rest.

I hadn't considered the check-in time at the hotel. Even with my delays I was two hours earlier than check-in, and thus had to find a place to lay down near the Inner Harbor to kill time. Despite being alone, it was comforting to be safely back in Baltimore, solely because it was the home of Johns Hopkins Hospital. Sitting on the wall at the Inner Harbor and watching the entertainment reminded me of when Mom and I were there.

It felt as though she were there with me. Of course, I had to go visit the sea lions and tell them I was back. I finally figured out why these animals meant so much to me. They were the first animals I made contact with after leaving Akita with the veterinarian. They filled a void at a very critical time in my life.

As soon as I could check into the hotel I did. I desperately needed to rest. Within two hours Lamar arrived. It was so good to see him. There's no other feeling like having big brother there to protect and comfort little sister. I've held Lamar in the highest regard for as long as I can remember. While it often seemed as though he wasn't connected with me throughout my recovery, I know I remained in his prayers and his love for me never wavered. While the circumstances for us to be together weren't ideal, it was still good to spend quality time with him. There were very few opportunities like this. It was also a convenient time to teach him more about my injury and its impact on my life. This gave him the opportunity to see firsthand a small piece of my medical roller coaster, and for a brief stretch, to ride it with me.

We spent the evening at the Inner Harbor. I couldn't wait to show Lamar what a neat place it was. We spent most of the evening talking about my previous surgeries and experiences. It was a chance for Lamar to ask me questions he always wondered about, but never took the time to ask over the phone. He showed great interest in my recovery, and was quite distressed by some of the truths about my condition.

Before heading back to the hotel, we walked over to the aquarium. I introduced Lamar to my sea lions. He appeared to enjoy them as much as me.

The next morning, we took a taxi to Hopkins, arriving in admitting at 9:00 a.m. I asked the receptionist if there was a chance I could be placed on Meyer 8 again. Within ten minutes they escorted us to Meyer 8. As the elevator door opened, Krista, Jennifer, and Tracy, three of the R.N.'s on Meyer 8, gave me a warm welcome from the nurses station. Although saddened by the circumstances, they were happy to see me again.

Much to my surprise, I saw Anna Pearson walking down the hallway, on her way to the patient lounge. She hadn't been discharged, since I left two weeks ago. She gave me a big hug, as I briefly told her why I had to return. Jennifer, having heard I was returning, requested to have me as her patient. She escorted me to my room, number 856. This was the room where Mom and I saw the man who looked like Grandpa. I felt as though God was still giving me messages from Grandpa. My mind flashed to my favorite Psalm, the 23rd. This always reminded me of Grandpa, because he sang it with us word for word at my wedding. The first verse was very appropriate at this time. "Because the Lord is my Shepherd, I have everything I need!" (Psalm 23:1 TLB)

I introduced Lamar to all my friends on Meyer 8, the nurses who took care of me last time. It didn't take long for word to spread across the floor that Karen's brother was extremely good looking—and single. I'd like to think everyone was making a special effort to see me frequently, but I have a sneaking suspicion they were interested in seeing Lamar. Neither of us minded, we loved to talk.

Before long, Dr. Sampath came into my room to place the lumbar drain in my back. I wasn't expecting him to do this procedure in my room, but it relieved some of my anxiety, since I concluded it must not be real invasive. (This was before it was explained to me what he was about to do.)

He'd do a lumbar puncture, similar to when they tested the fluid or did the radioisotope studies. Then he'd feed a tube into my spinal canal to drain CSF out of my system, similar to after my second craniotomy while in NICU. Memories of the pain in my head from that drain quickly surfaced. He said they'd leave the drain in as long as they needed to stop the leak, but no more than three days. Three days was their protocol. I'd need to stay in bed, except to use the rest room, and lay at a minimum twenty degree angle. The nurses would change this for me, if I desired, because there would be a need to recalibrate the system each time I moved.

I curled up in a ball on my side, the position for a lumbar puncture. Lamar was able to stay and watch, but a bit reluctant when he saw the size of the needle come out of its package. Typically, it was very easy for doctors to perform a lumbar puncture on me. Since I'm so thin, they can find their landmarks easily. Not this time, however. Dr. Sampath poked and probed around in my back with his needle like he was spearing for fish while ice-fishing. He struggled with his ego a bit more than the needle, unwilling to accept responsibility for his inability to perform this procedure. I tried to lay as still as possible. He touched a few more sensitive nerves, before giving me a warning to hold on and prepare for one final, big jab with the needle. As he pushed the needle further, it touched a major nerve, sending an electrical shock down the back of my right leg. He proudly said, "I'm in." What a relief I felt, not realizing I was already soaking wet with sweat.

Throughout this ordeal, Lamar watched with difficulty, at times closing his eyes. This gave Lamar a new appreciation for the types of things I had to endure.

Dr. Sampath fed the tube into my back and CSF began flowing freely into an attached bag hanging at my bedside. He secured the drain and asked Jennifer to calibrate the system.

Now this system was not the most sophisticated system around. It was all manually calibrated. Lamar and I weren't impressed when we saw a carpenter's level brought into my room to level the collection bag to my earlobe. Although this seemed pretty archaic, it worked.

They started the drain at 15cc of CSF per hour, which is a significant amount of fluid over the course of a day. When this fluid loss is combined with leaking fluid out my nose, it makes for an even greater headache.

Lamar and I enjoyed our time together, talking, reminiscing, and solving life's most difficult problems. We always have deep conversations about life, love, and relationships. He's a very sensitive man, in touch with his feelings and not afraid to express them. We've both been down the road of holding our feelings back, only to have it lead to emptiness in our relations with others.

Our time together was also filled with laughter. The funniest episode happened when I was going into the bathroom. I commented on how thankful I was not to have to use the bedpan. Lamar very innocently said, "Yea, I don't think I'd be able to go on that thing, either."

"Yea, I always have to at least sit up in bed when using it," I replied. "It's impossible for me to use it lying down. I always feel like urine is going all over the bed anyway, let alone trying to us it while laying flat. I have a problem getting a good seal. Because I'm so thin, my butt doesn't fit right on it."

"I think anyone would have a problem sealing it, by the looks of it. My question is...why is it shaped like a banana?" I knew immediately what Lamar was thinking, and I started to laugh uncontrollably. I laughed so hard, pain shot down my leg from the movement of the drain in my spinal canal. Lamar's question was sincere, which made it even funnier. He obviously didn't have much experience with hospitals, just enough to have seen the spit basin, a banana-shaped pan. Once I regained my composure and explained to him that it wasn't a bedpan, he joined me in laughing at our conversation. I never admitted to him that I once thought the same thing about the spit basin. That made it even funnier for me. Great minds think alike. Lamar learned all sorts of fun things while sitting with me in the hospital.

As a patient, I never lacked entertainment. The team of residents came in one day. Their designated lead doctor for the day said, "Well, the good news is we've looked at your chest x-ray and your lungs look clear. We're going to let you go home today."

My reply was, "Who's chart have you been looking at? It's certainly not mine." They looked at me, dumbfounded. I had not had a chest x-ray, nor was I going home that day with my lumbar drain. I continued, "Do I get to take this home with me?" They were very embarrassed, as they filed out of my room and back to the charts they had gathered.

Three days later, my leak still hadn't stopped. Dr. Long decided to keep the drain in longer and increase the amount of CSF draining. They had already bumped it up to 20cc per hour, now he asked for 25-30cc per hour, if I could tolerate it. It was more difficult, as the pain increased through my eyes. I often felt as though my eyes were going to pop. This quadrant of my head had been the predominate location of my headache pain since the day of my injury. The whole frontal region of my head felt as though it was crushed.

Kay arrived midweek. What a joy it was to have both my brother and sister with me. We had two days together, sharing stories of Lamar, and my experiences. Every morning before coming up to the hospital, Lamar went jogging around the Inner Harbor and visited the sea lions. He showed Kay the area, and introduced her to the sea lions, as well. These animals had become a part of our family.

After Lamar left, Kay and I spent quality time together. You would think we'd run out of things to talk about while spending all day just sitting next to one another. We never did.

One day, while Kay and I were talking, Dr. Ben Carson walked into my room. I was shocked to see him, since the only connection he had with my case was that he was the reason I went to Hopkins. Dr. Carson introduced himself and commented on how Fran, my nurse, mentioned to him my interest in meeting him. I briefly told him the story of how he was instrumental in connecting me with Dr. Long. I thanked him for being such an inspiration and for taking the time to visit me.

After he left, Fran came in and told us how Dr. Carson's assistant had tried to tell Dr. Carson that he didn't have time to see me. Dr. Carson refused to listen, feeling the importance of taking time for someone. He is an amazing man.

Dr. Long came to check on me later that afternoon, giving Kay a chance to meet him as well. We laughed when he said, "Karen, I never knew how you looked with hair, because we keep shaving it off."

Before he completed his statement I pointed to Kay and said, "Now, you know." We also talked about the drain and what it was doing or not doing. He was still debating how long to keep me on it, and whether to increase the amount of fluid being drained. As they increased the amount of CSF being drained, however, I became increasingly uncomfortable and sick.

One day, during a conversation with Jennifer, she spoke of how she could handle most any messy situation as a nurse. The one and only thing she struggles with is vomiting. Feeling quite nauseous the very next day, I rang my call bell. When Jennifer checked to see how much CSF drained since the previous hour, she was startled to see 40cc. No wonder I was feeling so bad. There probably wasn't any left in me. She suggested I sit at the side of my bed to see if the nausea would go away. As soon as I sat up, I lunged for the spit basin, heaving my lunch. I still didn't feel relief as Jennifer took the filled basin from me, handing me the empty wash basin for round two. Not only did I feel bad physically, but I also felt bad for Jennifer.

Jennifer stopped the drain for several hours, which gave my body a chance to catch up with its production of CSF. It also gave me a break from extreme pain and nausea. She ended up resetting the drain to take off 30cc per hour, which was still difficult to handle, but not to the point of vomiting. The leak still did not stop.

After five days on the drain, without success, Dr. Long decided to take it off. He needed to explore other options. Meanwhile, it was time for Kay to leave. Even though Mom and Dad were planning to arrive soon, it was extremely difficult to say good-bye. I knew I was heading down the road to another craniotomy, consequently, saying good-bye was emotionally exhausting. This type of a good-bye is so very different than a "Good-bye, see you again soon." As Charles Swindoll says, "The lens of fear magnifies the size of the uncertainty."

MOM AND DAD arrived two days later. Our interactions were tense from the moment they arrived. There were numerous unknowns, for all of us, and none of us knew the appropriate way to deal with them. I believe my parents thought I was hiding information from them, because I didn't have any answers. In the past, I had filtered information I gave them; this time, I truly didn't have the answers. Dr. Long didn't, either.

I resented the fact I felt my parents didn't trust me. I had been carrying this resentment throughout my recovery. I never lied to them, I just withheld information that could have caused them unnecessary anxiety. When they asked specific questions, however, I always told them details. Nonetheless, I sensed their continuous doubt. Each time they questioned and requestioned why something was happening or not happening, I took it as personal criticism. I felt as though they doubted me and my doctors, and there was no way to satisfy them. I believe the only way they could have been satisfied was to have me back, the way I was before my injury. They wanted desperately for a physician to fix me, and Mom and Dad couldn't understand why this hadn't happened. They were going through all the stages of grief, just as I had. Unfortunately, none of us was sympathetic to the other's grief. A huge wall had formed between us.

Our conversations were vicious circles. Words were taken out of context (in both directions) and then later used as daggers to throw at one another. Anger mounted to uncontrollable and unhealthy levels.

Each of us felt threatened and defenseless. We were desperate to survive, and didn't have the appropriate survival tools. Mom and Dad were afraid of losing their daughter, either through disability or death. I was concerned about a number of possible disabilities, though not afraid of death. We weren't armed with the most essential tool to get us through the battle: communication.

It was as though our family had been thrown into a raging river full of white water, rocks, and tree stumps, all leading to a deadly waterfall. We were thrashing to save our own lives, not capable of seeing one another. We were tossed against the rocks, beaten by the tree stumps, and terrified, while only catching our breaths long enough to worry about one another. We knew we were all in it, heading in the same direction, but we weren't capable of doing anything to help the other. We could only help ourselves, and pray.

It's true you most hurt the ones you most love. There was never any love lost in the heat of our anger, but there was definitely pain. The longer it took for my leak to be fixed, the harder it was for my parents and me to deal with our emotions, let alone interact with each other.

A FTER DELIBERATING WHAT to do next, Dr. Long finally decided to go back into my head, to find the remaining leaks. He knew he needed help, however, and brought Dr. Holliday back onto my case. Dr. Holliday came to my room to talk with me about my leak. He was accompanied by Dr. Howard Francis, an Otynlaryngologist doing a fellowship with Dr. Holliday. Dr. Holliday wanted to go over the details of my leak again, to refresh his mind with the history of what had failed so far. He questioned where the fluid was coming from, my left or right nostril. Was it only when I bent over, and how much volume? Dr. Holliday then told me that he and Dr. Long would perform another craniotomy, as soon as it could be scheduled.

My heart started racing. No matter how much I suspected or felt prepared, the confirmation still had a heart-wrenching impact. I thought to myself, "I can do this. I've done it before. I've just never done it only four weeks apart. Am I going to be strong enough to handle this?"

My first two craniotomies were four months apart, and it was more difficult to recover after the second one. I didn't think I was even fully recovered when I had my third surgery seven months later at Mayo Clinic. Now, we were talking about a fourth craniotomy only one month after my third. My body was screaming for a break, yet I wanted to get this behind me.

I told Dr. Holliday the sooner we could do the surgery the better. As he walked out the door, the phone rang. It was Kay. What a relief to hear her voice. I told her the news about more surgery. Like after all the other times I said these words to her, there was silence. I knew the impact of hearing this was devastating. In fact, I think I was getting more comfortable with surgery preparation than my loved ones.

My recovery often felt like a full-time job. The emotional effects were relentless and required endless monitoring and attention. For the physical side, I took a more clinical approach. I knew all the medical details of my case: the terminology, and the anatomy and physiology. Most every doctor involved in my case respected my knowledge, and used it to their advantage. Even though I let go of my need to be involved in the clinical side upon arriving at Hopkins, physicians and nurses automatically offered detailed explanations of what and why they were doing things. I appreciated the respect I was given.

Surgery was scheduled for Friday, August 19, 1994, which gave me four days to prepare. Two days prior to this, the same day I found out I would have a fourth craniotomy, I had asked my parents to return to Michigan. The stress of having them with me seemed to outweigh the comfort. It was a very difficult thing to say to them. I hoped the message would get my point across, that I could no longer handle the tension between us and deal with brain surgery, too. Meanwhile my heart was screaming, "Mom and Dad I need you." No one, however, is taught how to handle this type of tragedy, neither as a survivor or as a parent. I was no better at asking for the type of help I needed than they were at providing it.

I asked Terri, the social worker on Meyer 8, to help me with the difficulties I was having with my parents. She was most helpful. She explained how there was a need to clearly communicate to my parents what my needs were, asking them to help me in these areas. She also agreed with me when I said I thought it would help if I could talk to my father alone.

I then called my parents' hotel and Mom answered. I asked her to trust me, and to stop going behind my back to talk with physicians. I was met with great anger. Her anger had risen to an agonizing level. No matter what I said, she wasn't going to hear it. I asked her to let me talk with Dad. If this mess was going to get worked out, it would require Dad's help.

I asked Dad if he would come to my hospital room the next day, Thursday, so we could talk alone. He didn't give me an answer either way, but indicated it wouldn't be easy to do this. I said I thought it was the only way each of us could reach a comfortable place before my craniotomy on Friday.

That evening I asked my nurse if I could go down to the chapel. She said she'd take me down on her way to dinner. When I entered the chapel, it was empty. It was a small, dimly lit room with an altar, kneeler, and chairs along the back wall. I knelt down, bowed my head, and began to pray. I prayed for God to help us. I prayed for Him to allow my parents and me to be at peace with one another, before my surgery and forever thereafter. I was horrified by the thought of going into a craniotomy without my parents' support. I was scared of the potential for seizures during surgery. Tears rolled down my cheeks as I prayed and I listened. "I need help God. Please help me." Eventually I looked up at the altar. I couldn't believe what I saw. On the mosaic tiled wall was Psalm 23, "The Lord is my Shepherd I shall not want..." This was my message that God had heard my prayer. This is my favorite Psalm, one that pops up in the most strategic places. I didn't know what His answer was going to be, but I knew everything would be okay.

I was still very uptight that evening and was feeling a little discomfort in the area where my hamstring muscle attaches to my butt. My body was not used to such a sedentary life-style. I knew it was going to be difficult to lay on my back for several days after surgery. The best thing I could do for my muscle was to keep walking and stretching. Fran, my nurse for that evening, offered to bring the stationary bike from the Epilepsy Monitoring Unit into my room, so I could exercise my strained muscle. This was a wonderful suggestion. I hadn't been able to do anything more than walk in the halls for over a month.

As soon as they brought the bike into my room, I got on and started pedaling. It felt so good to move, even for only a few minutes. I couldn't last more than five minutes, but it was the answer to my hamstring problem.

I made sure to tell Fran the bike must be moved out of my room before my parents arrived the morning of my surgery. They already expressed to me their opinion on my need to slow down and not exercise as much. This was the last thing I wanted my parents to see. The bike, however, remained in my room until I was discharged, stimulating many comments. Most people would say, "Only Karen," or, "Only an Exercise Physiologist would have a bike in her hospital room."

The following day, my father walked into my room around noon. Tears filled my eyes as I silently thanked the Lord for bringing him to me. After all the years of standing silent, my father was finally taking a step forward to help. My father has always loved me more than I'll ever know.

We talked for four hours. He asked questions. I answered. I asked questions. He answered. We shared our feelings. We shared everything about our lives and how it related to where we were that day. We understood one another, and accepted that it was okay to agree to disagree. Both Dr. Long and Dr. Holliday came in separately while Dad was there. This gave Dad an opportunity to ask questions of them as well.

At the end of our conversation, when we were about to say good-bye, I asked where Mom was. She was downstairs in the lounge. I asked if he thought it was okay for me to go see her. He was hesitant, but then said he thought it would help.

As we walked to where Mom was sitting, my heart started racing. I took a deep breath and said, "Hi Mom." I was met with silence. I said it a little louder, thinking maybe she hadn't heard me.

In a somber tone and without looking up at me, she said, "Hi."

I took another deep breath and said, "Can I have a hug?" She laid her cross-stitch down, stood up in tears, and gave me a big hug. As we hugged I said, "I don't want it to be this way."

She held onto me as tightly as she could, and said, "I love you. I don't want it like this either." We embraced for a long time, neither of us wanting to let go, a symbol of our lives. Neither of us ever wanted to let go of the love we had for one another. When faced with the threat of this love being torn apart, through no control of our own, we fought. Instead of focusing our energy on fighting for my health, we fought one another.

After wiping our tears, we walked to the cafeteria to have some frozen yogurt. Our conversation remained on the surface, but that was okay, because I had what I most needed in front of me, my mother and father.

Twenty

Setting Anchors Deep

We can't direct the wind,
but we can adjust our sails.

ANONYMOUS

I KNEW THE ROUTINE well: nothing to eat after midnight, awake at 5:00 a.m. to shower, and then IV antibiotics start. Afterwards I'd walk the halls, trying to reduce stress and strengthen muscles, knowing I'd be immobile for at least a few days after surgery. The phlebotomist from the lab came to draw my blood, finding an empty bed. Brenda, my nurse through the midnight shift told him, "Just look in the halls for her. She's out roaming."

I was prepared physically and mentally. The night before, I went to the chapel and prepared spiritually. I praised God for bringing peace to me and my parents. My faith was strong. God was going to be with me.

Mom and Dad arrived around 6:00 a.m., knowing I'd probably go to the OR around 6:30 a.m. Mom walked a few more laps with me, before I was ready to settle back into bed and relax with prayer. The hours before surgery paralleled the many hours I had spent with pre-game or pre-race preparation. I warmed up by walking, then it was time to take my mind through my mental preparation, visualizing the operation and crossing the finish line. As with any competition preparation, I displayed only confidence.

Everyone from the OR was familiar with me. Even the transporter called me by name. I was impressed (although it hadn't occurred to me

314

that he should know the name of the person he was taking down for surgery).

My parents followed us down to the surgical floor. This was a very stressful time for them, so they planned to explore the hospital, to distract their minds, while I spent a minimum of six hours in surgery. We said good-bye, confident we would talk to one another ten to twelve hours later.

I was taken to the OR. As I laid there, contemplating what was about to happen, Keith walked up to my gurney and said, "You can't get enough of us down here, can you?" I was so relieved to see him. He had become another one of my many angels. God was placing them everywhere, making sure I felt at ease.

I said to Keith, "Make sure you just take a little off the top this time," as I rubbed the top of my head. He laughed, knowing my whole head was going to be shaved. We chatted until they started hooking me up to the monitors.

Before sticking the monitor pads all over my chest and side, they pulled my gown and sheet down to my waist. I laid on the operating table, bare chested. One of the anesthesiology residents walked into the OR and said, "Is *he* ready?"

As I was chuckling to myself, my favorite neurosurgical resident came to my rescue. Dr. Perry pulled the sheet back over me and said, "Yes, *she's* ready." I think he was a bit embarrassed. I thought it was pretty funny.

During this surgery, Dr. Long and Dr. Holliday went through the same incision. Most people made jokes about how my incision should have been closed with a zipper the first time. After Dr. Long got into my skull and under my brain, Dr. Holliday did most of the work. He exposed the frontal and ethmoid sinuses, looking for the leaks. He also made an incision in my abdomen, where he took pieces of fat and muscle fascia to repair the leaks. Since Dr. Long sealed the right frontal sinus in the previous surgery, Dr. Holliday proceeded to look for leaks in the remaining left frontal sinus, and right and left ethmoid sinuses. Finding leaks in all of these areas, he sealed them with the grafts from my abdomen. He then closed the dura and replaced my skull, using microplates to secure it into place.

Seven hours after entering the OR I was taken to NICU, where I re-mained asleep for quite some time. Typically, after general anesthesia, I don't wake up easily on my own. Before I finally regain consciousness, usually the nurses must talk to me, call my name, and move me. Then, the awful part comes. I feel like a chunk of ice. My whole body shivers and shakes.

I experience discomfort, but it's always localized to a specific part of my body. This was different. This was total distress that engulfed my entire body. Nothing anyone did helped relieve the cold. They snuggled me tight with heated blankets, hung heat lamps over me, and massaged each limb, attempting to increase my circulation.

A nurse took my temperature. It was 89.6 degrees. I asked her, "Why does it feel worse this time, compared to previous surgeries?"

"You were in surgery for more than seven hours and they lowered your body temperature during that time to reduce bleeding. The longer the surgery, the lower your temperature goes. It was especially important this time, due to the extent of work done in your head. You've just come through a very difficult surgery. You'll warm up soon. Hang in there."

I put every visualization skill into practice. I started picturing myself running near the Inner Harbor, where it had been reaching 100 degree temperatures when Mom and I were waiting for my first craniotomy at Hopkins. I pictured myself sweating profusely, feeling the high level of circulation throughout my body. I tried to relax each muscle, feeling relief from intense shivering. Every muscle in my body was as hard as a rock, bracing against the discomfort, shivering instinctively. Eventually, my ef-forts helped. I felt the warm flow of blood slowly rewarm each segment of my body.

Dr. Francis came in, anxious to perform neurological tests on me, to make sure there was no further damage from surgery. Dr. Long came in shortly after and described the surgery to me. He said he and Dr. Holliday went deeper into my skull than they had ever gone with anyone. They wanted to make sure they found every leak. He was very pleased with how I handled the surgery, and was confident this was the last of our problems with CSF leaks.

Dr. Francis had observed my surgery. He was very interested in my case because it was so atypical. My case was going to be written up in medical journals, and had already been presented at seminars and conferences to neurosurgical associations and groups. This was Dr. Francis's opportunity to see everything firsthand. I sensed his concern that I might have more neurological damage, due to the critical nature of my surgery. They were most concerned about my vision, because this time they had worked closer to my optic nerves.

As Dr. Francis began testing me, I noticed a calendar on the wall showing one date at a time. It read August 12th. (It was really August 19th.) When he asked his second question, "Do you know what day it is?" I cracked a smile and replied, "The 21st." He questioned my response and my related smile. I confessed I had cheated, by reading the calendar. He laughed and appreciated my honesty, but questioned my transposing the numbers since the calendar read "12." I told him that since my injury, I often transposed numbers. He continued his testing. I only had slight difficulty with the visual segment of the test.

During my first night in NICU, I felt blood run down the side of my head, into my ear. This was frightening. It felt as though my incision wasn't closed all the way. It wasn't, because they had placed another drain in my skull to relieve the pressure. I rang for the nurse. She immediately started wrapping more gauze around my head to stop the bleeding. It did stop, but I still had a hard time not thinking about the blood.

I dozed off to sleep for a few minutes. I awoke to find a nurse checking my monitors and writing my vital signs in my chart. As soon as she saw I was awake, she commented on me being from Michigan. She was originally from Michigan and was anxious to talk with me. Within a brief time I discovered she grew up in a suburb of Detroit, Oak Park, where my friend Joy was currently living. As soon as she said Oak Park, I felt Joy's presence. What a neat way to be connected with a dear friend who was a thousand miles away. Several other little occurrences like this made me feel very close to home.

The night was long. It was difficult to get comfortable. The pain in my head throbbed like a heartbeat, rhythmic and strong. Opening my eyes intensified the ache, rising in severity every time I moved my eyes. I abandoned my attempt to see the doorway of my room. It exceeded my threshold of pain. I feared sneezing or coughing, knowing the increased pressure in my head would magnify the pain tenfold. I laid motionless from the chest up, fearing the discomfort of any head movement.

It was unusual for me to have trouble sleeping after surgery, but this was one night I couldn't sleep. Typically, when I couldn't sleep it was because I couldn't quiet my mind, but tonight it was more physical. My mind was at peace, while my body was fighting for survival. My blood pressure dropped, and my heart rate slowed. Two nurses were at my side, while others continually rushed in and out of my room. Dr. Perry came to check on me frequently, testing my neuro functions.

Slowly I started to feel very sleepy, as though energy was being siphoned. I concluded from all the attention, my condition was deteriorating. I needed to work hard to keep my body awake, for it was slowly losing its source of physical strength.

I lost consciousness. I could not rebound from the loss of blood during surgery, and my already low blood pressure. Dr. Perry and the nurses injected me with medication to increase the productivity of my cardiovascular system, to get more blood flowing into my brain. It didn't take long for me to respond, the monitors showed a gradual rise in rate and pressure.

After regaining consciousness and learning what happened, I realized why I had been so uncomfortable. I had been struggling for control, fighting the impossible. I had been able to relax my body, which gave me the illusion I was in control. There was, however, a limit to my capabilities. I needed to relearn how to separate that which I did have control of and that which I did not.

I T WAS A relief when I was finally returned to my room on Meyer 8. Although I had come to know the nurses in NICU quite well, Meyer 8 was beginning to feel like home. Shortly after Jennifer took my vitals, she helped me get out of bed, for the first time in three days.

I was very weak, but determined to get moving again. I had never felt tiny in my life, but with my muscles atrophied from being so sedentary, I felt tiny. My thighs were once full of power and strength from climbing hills on my bike. Now, they weren't much bigger than my calves. Once I was up and walking, all I could think of was the Energizer Bunny. Keep going, and going, and going. I wasn't going to let anything keep me down.

My vision difficulties persisted, prompting a referral by Dr. Long to the Wilmer Eye Center at Hopkins. In the afternoon of my first day back on Meyer 8, Gary, the transporter, came to take me to the eye center. Gary was a young man who I came to know quite well. He did many of my transports to and from the Radiology Department. I enjoyed talking with each of the transporters, especially after a comment was made by one of the nurses. She said to me during my very first week at Hopkins, "The only people around here that won't talk to you are the transporters. They're a breed of their own." I thought this was a strange comment, and definitely a challenge if I ever saw one.

Gary was my first transporter. All I had to do was ask him a question about himself and he talked all the way to Radiology. I never met a transporter who wouldn't talk to me. As far as I was concerned, they were just as valuable to my team of health care providers as any other staff member. I'm sure they appreciated the respect I gave them.

After Gary took me to Wilmer Eye Center, I was left in the waiting area to see the ophthalmologist. I had been in bed for three straight days lying only at a slight angle. I wasn't used to sitting up and having the CSF pressure change in my head. The time it took to get to the eye center was long enough. The pain in my head started to magnify. I was moved into the exam room, where the doctor proceeded to keep me in an upright position. It was unknown whether the double vision I was experiencing would persist or diminish with time. The trauma from surgery had a slight impact on this area. I was very thankful it was only slight, but for the moment I was a hurting puppy. I needed to lay down to relieve my pain.

The doctor completed her exam and wheeled me back out to the waiting room. I thought I was headed back to my room, and therefore could withstand a few more minutes of sitting up. This, however, wasn't the case. Once I was put in the waiting area, I sat there for a long time. Five, ten, fifteen minutes went by, and no one came to take me back to my room. By this time, I was extremely nauseated and about ready to vomit from the intense pain in my head.

I finally lost patience. I wheeled myself up to the registration desk and interrupted someone mid-sentence, "If someone doesn't either get me back to my room or let me lay down somewhere, I'm going to toss my lunch all over your floor." Just then a transporter walked up and the receptionist pointed to me and told him to hustle me back to my room.

The next few days were critical. After having experienced three previous surgeries that failed, I was very cautious with my level of confidence. I worked each day at building my endurance by getting up and walking. Most of my energy was spent taking a shower and getting dressed into a clean T-shirt and scrubs.

Each morning I looked forward to the housekeepers coming into my room. While they cleaned, I'd chat with them. They too, played a very important role in my recovery. By the time I was discharged, we were good friends.

When I wasn't walking, sleeping, or eating I sat in the patient lounge ten feet away from my room. It was a place where I could meet other patients and their family members or talk to the hospital staff. Other times, I was assisting the nursing staff on Meyer 8.

It was apparent the entire staff on Meyer 8 was working hard at lightening the worries and fears of patients and families. Before long, nurses started referring me to other patients, to talk with them. Oftentimes it was before their upcoming surgeries. I tried to lessen their worries and transfer some positive energy to them. I really enjoyed responding to these requests. I truly didn't do it because the nurses asked me to, I was doing it because I was made aware of someone's need. I was able to meet some very interesting and wonderful people. I formed lifetime friendships with many. It felt good to help others, and it felt good to be so highly thought of by the nurses. But most of all, it felt good to feel needed.

I'd knock on a door if it was closed, or step to the foot of their bed if it was open and introduce myself. I'd ask how they were doing and make small talk with them for awhile. Eventually, I'd ask them about their condition. By this time, they'd usually pour every conscious feeling out to me, opening the door wide enough for me to speak of faith in God and the hope that is ours forever. By the time I left, I could already feel the impact I had on their lives.

O NE OF THE first people I met was Mel Taylor. Mel was sitting in the
patient lounge when I struck up a conversation. He had surgery to
remove a pituitary tumor. Mel was a black man from Baltimore, who was
in his early fifties. He was a very big man, yet gentle, reminding me of a
life-sized teddy bear. Mel and I became good buddies on Meyer 8. We'd
talk for long periods of time, about everything. Mel was very anxious to
go home, as we all were, but his ambition was a bit premature.

Mel was discharged the same day as my fourth craniotomy. I was disappointed when I found out he had been discharged, because we hadn't
said good-bye. But by the time I returned to Meyer 8 from NICU, five
days later, Mel had been readmitted to Meyer 8. The fluid he had been
leaking from his nose after his surgery was CSF. The surgery was performed
through his mouth and nose, also the location of his leak. His doctors
were confident it would seal on its own, given the nature of the procedure.
When Mel returned, he was diagnosed with bacterial meningitis.

Mel and I had some things in common. Not only did both of us leak
spinal fluid and have horrendous headaches, but we were both also placed
on the lumbar drain. Two weeks after I was off my drain, I asked Mel how
much fluid they were draining from him. He said, "5cc, and the headache
it's giving me is almost intolerable." Even though Mel was a very big man,
and probably twice my body weight, they had taken over five times as
much fluid, 25-30cc, from me.

This was my first clue that something probably wasn't right with my
CSF production. I wondered if it was possible that my body had adapted
to leaking CSF by increasing its production of CSF. This might explain
why after Dr. Hoff and Dr. Long seemingly fixed all the leaks, I began
leaking again. Maybe it was like a leaky basement, as Dr. Cilluffo had first
described. If the volume and subsequent pressure was too great, no matter
how many times they stopped the leak, it was going to find a way to make
a new path out.

I asked Dr. Long if this could be possible. He was indecisive, not
knowing for sure what was occurring. A way to measure this phenomenon
didn't exist, so it remained only a theory. But, this theory began to sound
more believable, when I began to leak again.

It was only a few days after my fourth craniotomy. I was apprehensive to bend over and test whether I was leaking. I needed to try it. The longer I avoided the dreaded test, however, the longer I could avoid the truth. Unlike any of the other times, this time I was suspicious I was still leaking. I don't know why, but I had a gut feeling. After putting some realistic thoughts into it, I recognized the need to find out as soon as possible. The longer I waited to test it, the longer it would take to eventually fix it, if there was still a leak.

I bent over in my hospital room, as I had so many times before. CSF ran out my right nostril, not in the amount it had before, but it flowed. I was right. There was still a leak in my head. When I reported it to my nurse, and then to Dr. Long and Dr. Holliday, they were each noticeably shaken. They knew how badly I wanted to go home and have this behind me. They too, wanted it behind them.

The fluid tested positive for glucose, verifying it was CSF. It was back to the drawing board. Dr. Long and Dr. Holliday began discussing what should happen next. There were several conversations with me and without me, talking about whether to do another craniotomy, attempt to seal the leaks from below the skull, or do something with shunts. While I couldn't picture myself being strong enough to go through another craniotomy so soon, it seemed to me like the only choice.

While I waited for my doctors to make a decision about my leak, I received many conflicting messages. Communication between my attending doctors and the resident group was obviously lacking, making me feel as though I was riding a wild roller coaster.

It was especially nerve-wracking the day Dr. Holliday came to see me in the morning. He said he was planning to do another surgery by the end of the week. He was leaning towards an approach through my mouth and nose, so as to reach the sphenoid sinuses. These were the only sinuses that had not yet been explored for possible leaks.

Dr. Long saw me in the afternoon. He said he wanted to perform more tests before he went back into my head, and that he still needed to talk with Dr. Holliday. He was interested in finding out what Dr. Holliday's thoughts were on going in from below. He said he was also tossing around the idea of sending me home for awhile, so I could regain my strength before they'd do more surgery. He knew I was getting weaker. This was my ninth week in Baltimore, with only a few days in between at home after my first surgery with him. He knew I was very anxious to go home, but my desire to have everything repaired as soon as possible outweighed those anxious feelings. He agreed the sooner the better to repair everything, reducing the risk of meningitis. If I could keep working at building my strength with exercise, he knew I could handle more surgery.

By evening, the residents came through and told me I was going to be discharged the next day. Talk about a whirlwind of messages. I didn't know what transpired between Dr. Holliday and Dr. Long once they left my room, but all indications told me they were both leaning in the direction of keeping me there and doing more surgery to repair the leak.

I didn't know what I was supposed to do with this most recent information from the residents. Should I believe them? I didn't want to. My heart cried out to God, "No...please let this not be true." Part of me thought I needed to believe them, after all, they were wearing white coats. Another part of me remembered the mistakes they had made before. I had to work hard to convince myself to be patient, and to wait until I spoke with Dr. Long the next day. The problem was that the residents would come in again at 6:00 a.m. to tell me I was discharged, before I could speak with Dr. Long.

I made a phone call to Dr. Long's nurses Mary Kay Conover-Walker R.N. and Susan Schnupp R.N., with whom I had developed good rapport. I left a message on their voice mail about what was happening. Fortunately, Mary Kay worked late that night, took the message, called me and said, "Don't go anywhere until you talk to Dr. Long." I felt a bit awkward telling the residents the next morning that I wasn't going to leave until I talked with Dr. Long. They were defensive, but once they found out from Dr. Long that I was right, they sheepishly came back to tell me, "Dr. Long is still discussing with Dr. Holliday what will be the next step." I was very thankful I was still capable of managing my health care. Otherwise, I would have gone home with a chronic CSF leak. Who knows what would have happened next.

There were countless situations of this nature, that I never shared with any family or friends, including my parents. I learned this lesson early in my recovery, when I started receiving conflicting opinions from doctors and other health care professionals. My entire recovery was atypical. Nothing happened in a usual fashion. If the odds of something happening were very low, it was almost a given it would happen in my case. This included interpretation errors of radiology studies, not seeing skull fractures, and hitting the measure of error in laboratory tests. It included physician errors, hitting the tiny percentage that a test can't determine results, and having this happen every time the test is performed. The list could go on and on.

People tend to believe the most positive opinion of medical results, not considering or not knowing all the details of the whole picture. This was where Dr. MacKenzie became invaluable to me. I could always count on him to see the whole picture and to advise me on what to believe and discard.

In communicating information about my test results to others, I needed to filter everything. If I didn't, not only would they ride the emotional roller coaster with me, but I'd spend most of my time trying to help them make sense of the mess. Some people placed doctors right up there with God. To get people to understand that health care professionals make mistakes, would be difficult. When a test result came back negative, or a CT scan was read negative, there's no question in their minds these were accurate. This was hardly the case with my injury. Therefore, the communication of results had to stop at me, or be filtered before sharing details, for the sake of my support system.

The first instance that taught me to filter information was when I was told by my first general practitioner that I was perfectly okay and able to return to work. This seemed pretty believable to everyone, because my injury wasn't visible. Beneath this favorable diagnosis, however, sat the reality of a shattered skull, CSF leaking, and cognitive deficits.

Using my parents as an example, they thought I was perfectly okay, as I relayed the advice of my physician. When I continued to have problems, my parents questioned me. When I started seeking additional care, they thought something was wrong with me psychologically. Eventually, they realized there were further complications, and then they tried to convince me to go to the University of Michigan for medical care. But, from this point on, I always had to wonder what they were thinking and believing. It always felt as though they doubted me over a doctor, thus I began protecting myself from this stress.

We never communicated effectively, relying primarily on nonverbal communication. We danced with what was appropriate and what wasn't, tiptoeing through the delicate phases. We were at odds with one another from the onset of my injury, but never was there love lost.

I had an advantage of being able to freely talk with the health care professionals about my condition, because I worked in the medical field. My extensive knowledge of human anatomy and physiology help me understand what was happening to me and why. I was also more aware of the frequency of error, both human and technical, than the average nonmedical person, and thus responded accordingly. I sought multiple opinions when critical decisions needed to be made. I was fortunate to be capable of managing my care.

Other examples of my need to filter information were when Dr. McCaffrey told me "You don't have a leak," and when I was told, "The fluid tested negative for beta II transferin and therefore CSF." If I would have told anyone these details, they would have believed them. They would have thought I was crazy to be searching for a neurosurgeon to do a craniotomy on me to fix my leaks, when I had been told I didn't have a leak. As it turned out, after I pursued finding Dr. Long, several leaks were found and repaired. Instead of being faced with a lot of questions and doubts from others, I chose to selectively tell details. It would have just exasperated the situation, because I imagined they'd say, "Oh, that's wonderful, you don't have a leak." And yes, it would have been wonderful— if that were the end of the story. Unfortunately, it wasn't. Holding this information back gave me a tremendous load to carry alone, but I'm confident it was the lighter of two loads.

As I REGAINED strength, I was able to move around more and meet more patients on the floor. One day, I met Jim and Judy McGeoch in the patient lounge. Their teenage son, Brian, had suffered from severe epilepsy for many years. He was now in the Epilepsy Monitoring Unit on Meyer 8. They were monitoring his seizure activity for a full week, in a special room equipped with twenty-four hours per day electroencephalograph (EEG) monitoring and video camera. The EEG monitor consisted of several electrodes placed over the entire head, attached by wires to the monitor. This required the individual to remain in bed for the entire week of monitoring. The video camera is used to record how the seizures look.

Jim and Judy were the most delightful people. We became friends very quickly. Each day I'd ask for an update on Brian, and they'd follow my progress. We joined one another's support team.

While sitting in the patient lounge with them one day, I saw a man walking the halls. He was walking alone and in street clothes. The only way I could tell he was a patient was by the arm band hanging around his wrist. Later that evening, when he walked past my door, I introduced myself. His name was Bob Lambert. He was having a biopsy of a growth in his brain the next day. Bob said doctors suspected it was an abscess. He had a heart attack a few months prior to coming to Hopkins, and the doctors led him to believe there could be a link between the two. Bob was extremely nervous about his surgery, and needed someone to listen. He sat in my room until 1:30 a.m. He told me about his life as a retired history teacher from the Naval Academy. We talked about our families, as well as our faith.

He had been a member of the Catholic church all of his life, until the last few years, when he had become involved in building a Baptist church. He spoke of this church with great pride, but seemed to be connected with it in a very business like way, not spiritual.

I was shocked to hear Bob say, "If this thing is malignant, all I have to do is not take my heart medications, run up and down the stairs a few times, and that will do the trick to check me out of here." I tried to get him to talk more about his faith in God and the strength of that relationship. I asked him how he was going to weather this storm, using the analogy of what the Navy does when weathering a storm. He replied, "They throw out the anchors and batten down the hatches." I asked him where he thought his anchors were, as he went through this medical storm. He hesitated, then asked what I meant. I explained how my anchors needed to be deep in Christ our Lord, in order for me to weather a storm. This stimulated more discussion on how faith has helped me stay positive. We concluded our conversation by speaking of how important it was to be surrounded by people who loved us. It was obvious each of us had been overwhelmed by the care of our friends and family. We were appreciative of each other's support, and the neat connection we had developed in only a few hours.

The next morning as I was eating breakfast, I said a prayer for Bob, knowing he was in surgery.

While eating, I also heard the voice of a patient down the hallway. She kept saying, "Who's there?" Coinciding with this voice, was a repetitive knocking sound. I put the puzzle together. A nurse was pounding pills into tiny pieces, and the patient thought someone was knocking on her door. I chuckled to myself, thinking these circumstances were a bit humorous.

The patient, Mrs. Fishman, was eighty-two years old. She had a malignant brain tumor. After this first incident, I heard her more often. It was no longer humorous. She was hallucinating. The nurses tried everything to help calm her, and even tried to get her walking again, but Mrs. Fishman wouldn't get out of bed. She felt she was too old to recover. I never saw anyone visit her. I'm sure she was lonely.

I discovered one evening it was Mrs. Fishman's 83rd birthday. As my nurse walked with me through the halls, I asked if I could go into Mrs. Fishman's room to sing happy birthday to her. As I walked into her room, she laid in a fetus position, afraid. As I sang happy birthday, her eyes opened wide. We talked. We spoke of how we were each medically challenged and about who was taking care of us. She was a little disturbed with the nurses, complaining that they were not attending to her every need. It opened the door for me to talk about who was attending to all our needs, our Heavenly Father. As I started leaving the room she said, "Oh sonny, (I still had a shaved head) please come talk to me tomorrow."

The sun had barely risen above the horizon when I opened my eyes. I heard this rhythmic squeaking from the hallway. I turned by head to see what it was, and unexpected tears filled my eyes. Mrs. Fishman was moving towards me with her walker. She sat down and the first words from her mouth were, "Please tell me more about who is taking care of me." I was in awe. She had not been out of bed since surgery, and here she was determined to hear the Word of God.

It wasn't long before two nurses, with panicked looks on their faces, glanced into my room, as they combed the halls looking for Mrs. Fishman. Upon seeing her sitting beside me, they said, "We should have known all along where to look for her. We always find our missing patients sitting in Karen's room."

The connections I was making with people during my extended stay at Hopkins made me wonder if this was why my stay was so long. I felt God's presence and the work of the Holy Spirit amidst these encounters. Most of these people I will never see again, here on earth, yet I know I touched their lives. They touched mine.

The friendships I made were not restricted to the walls of the hospital. There were several that developed from a Lutheran connection. The same church in Baltimore that my mother and I attended together, started to take me under their wing. Ellen Commarato and two teachers, Carla Melandy and Susan Haar, from Atonement Lutheran grade school, came to visit. They didn't know me. I didn't know them either, but we came to know one another quite well. They brought a great deal of support to my recovery, with their humor, prayers, and understanding. They visited me as if we'd known one another for years. They went out of their way to connect with me, giving so much of themselves to help me through this process. The children from their grade school made numerous cards to decorate my walls. The wall in my room became quite a showcase of love and support, known to everyone as "The Wall."

The pastor of another church near Baltimore, Pastor Paul Koelpin, stayed in touch with me the entire time I was at Hopkins. I'll always remember the story he told me of a young girl who was drawing a picture of the Ascension. When she was asked who the two people in the airplane were, she said confidently, "This one is Jesus, and this one is Pontius the pilot." I was very appreciative of all those who went out of their way to share their faith, hope, and laughter with me. They helped renew my faith and to focus on the unseen as is written in 2 Corinthians 4:16-18 NIV. "Therefore we do not lose heart. Though outwardly we are wasting away, yet inwardly we are being renewed day by day. For our light and momentary troubles are achieving for us an eternal glory that far outweighs them all. So we fix our eyes not on what is seen, but on what is unseen. For what is seen is temporary, but what is unseen is eternal."

Two days after Bob Lambert went into surgery he returned to Meyer 8 from NICU. I was walking past his room when he called to me. He asked me to come in and talk. It was late in the evening and his family had already left for the day. I sensed a little anxiety in his voice. I walked in, sat down, and asked how he was feeling. A saddened look on Bob's face gave me instant feedback. He said, "It's malignant." I was struck by the cold, terminal feeling this word brought to my heart. I didn't know what to say. Bob needed a comforting friend to help him see hope. Two nights ago Bob had carried a conversation many hours into the night, today he was speechless.

I began by asking what was going through his mind and whether his family knew yet. He repeated his physician's recommendation over and over again, "Radiation." Then he started talking about his family and how important they were to him. The one thing he longed to do was to go home and sit on his back deck, where life was very peaceful. He said this was his favorite place. I asked Bob what kinds of things he would do to keep his mind off of his battle with his health. He described his interest in photography, and proceeded to tell me of the time when he saw a great opportunity for a picture. He said, "The lake was beautiful, with the trees perfectly reflecting off the calm water. I almost walked away, but instead, I turned back and took the picture. The best picture I ever took was one I almost walked away from."

I immediately turned what he said into an analogy. I asked Bob if he realized what he had just said. He did not know what I meant. I said, "Bob, just like the best picture you ever took was one you almost walked away from, so might the best part of your life be ahead of you. Don't walk away."

He was silent again. He knew why I said this, acknowledged its impact, and promised to weather the storm.

Courage is not the absence of fear. It is taking action in spite of fear. It is moving against the resistance fear has created, moving towards the unknown and into the future. Stepping into the future is like stepping into the darkness. The gift of hope lights a candle, instead of cursing this darkness.

E ACH AND EVERY step of my journey was invaluable. Each point had lessons to teach and more seeds to plant, creating new growth. It often felt like a weight training workout. I'd resist change, then slowly release my resistance, feeling the burn and discomfort of letting it go, only to have greater strength. It may have been more like a yo-yo at times. There was a lot of pull and release. But as long as life was handing me lemons, I was making lemonade.

The fifth attempt to repair my CSF leak was finally scheduled, after Dr. Holliday and Dr. Long wrestled with the options. They decided to go back into my head to try repairing the leaks from the bottom side up.

I was anxious to get it over. I had a greater focus on the process, rather than my destination, making it easier to handle the emotional stress. By this time, I knew we were never given a warranty on our bodies, but we were given a lifetime guarantee. God never said we wouldn't get broken, injured, or scarred. What He did give us is most valuable, a lifetime guarantee of eternal life. No matter how many years we last on earth, or how much we must endure, we'll be fully restored with eternal life.

During my recovery, death was never a frightening issue for me. I felt God's presence all around me. The Lord was walking in front of me, to light my way; behind me, to give me strength; and beside me, to fill me with guidance and abiding love.

New parents often say, "It's too bad we're not given an owner's manual with this baby." During my recovery I discovered we really do have owner's manuals, the Bible. I started studying the Bible with greater interest than ever before, finding great comfort in everything I read. It placed a whole new perspective on my relationship with God. It helped me to talk with other people about God. I wasn't as hesitant or uncomfortable with the subject, trusting that the Holy Spirit would give me the appropriate words. He did as evidenced with my interactions with other patients.

I found the hospital setting to be a prime location to speak with others about their spirituality. People's vulnerability while being a patient brought down barriers that normally might be erected. It opened doors for easy conversation, at a level most often reserved for close friends. I enjoyed this opportunity, as I longed for spiritual connections with others. I made the most of each day, working to capture every opportunity to talk with people, but most often, it just happened without any effort on my part.

A few days before my next surgery was scheduled, I overheard Fran, one of the nurses, talk about a man who had a bike accident recently. She asked me if she could introduce me to him, since we had something in common. She knew I would jump at the chance to meet him. Sylvester "Andy" Anderson was admitted after he fell from his bike, causing a compression of his vertebrae. The swelling was placing pressure on his spinal cord, causing paralysis. When he was first admitted, he had no feeling or movement from the neck down. Within a week as swelling dissipated, he slowly regained sensation above the waist.

Fran introduced me to Andy the next morning, while I was doing my daily after breakfast walk around the halls. He was a very nice man, with a very positive outlook. We shared cycling stories, particularly the stories of our accidents. Andy and I were thankful we weren't given each other's challenge.

He hadn't been able to get out of bed yet, not even to sit in a wheelchair, and was getting very anxious. I suggested he ask the neurosurgical residents the next time they came to see him if he could be put in a wheelchair. The residents made rounds twice a day, so later that evening Andy would have the chance to ask.

I sensed a bit of frustration in Andy's voice, as he talked about how long it was taking to see even a little bit of progress. I started talking in cycling terms and asked him to remember how it felt to climb a hill on a bike. I reminded him, "For every hill you climb Andy, there's always a descent. You're climbing a mountain right now, but keep your focus on how it feels when you crest that mountain and are able to power down the opposite side." He could easily relate to this.

It was refreshing to share stories of racing and training with someone, while dancing around the topic of competing in our current challenges. I learned of Andy's achievements in cycling, and it was easy to see he wasn't going to have difficulty with the physical determination and perseverance needed for rehabilitation. His positive outlook was also very strong. I knew Andy was not going to be satisfied with his present condition and would work his tail off to regain his physical capabilities. If Dennis Byrd, the football player who had close to the same injury as Andy, could walk again, I knew Andy could too.

Before leaving Andy's room, I reminded him again to ask the residents if he could get out of bed and sit in a wheelchair. I told him as soon as he could get up, I'd be more than happy to push him around, escorting him wherever he wanted to go.

That evening, when I was walking the halls, I glanced into his room and saw that Fran had just put him into a wheelchair. Andy had a huge smile on his face as I gave him a big cheer. She pushed him towards me and said, "He's all yours. You two have fun, but no racing in the hallways." We were like two kids at Christmas, overflowing with excitement. We didn't go far, but just wheeling through the halls of Meyer 8 and into the patient lounge was fun. It didn't matter where Andy went, anything was better than laying in bed.

The next morning, as I walked past Andy's room, he was just coming back from physical therapy. I stopped to say good morning and to see how therapy went. I immediately sensed Andy's gloom and asked what was troubling him. He was frustrated that his progress wasn't moving faster, and also by a recommendation the therapist had made. They wanted him to be admitted to a residential rehabilitation center, where he could undergo more intense therapy and also learn to accommodate his disability. They indicated this could be a six month process.

I was glad I walked by when I did, and was able to listen to Andy as he poured out his feelings. Without appearing like a cheerleader for every difficult situation, I gently suggested we talk again about what this would be like in cycling terms. I asked, "Andy, what do you look at when you climb the mountains on your bike, like we talked about?" He asked what I meant by this, so I rephrased the question. "When you are climbing, where are your eyes focused? Are they looking at the top of the hill or are they looking somewhere closer, in front of you?"

He said, "I always focus on what's right in front of me. It's too difficult if I look at the top. It would feel impossible to climb." Just as he said, "...impossible to climb," he realized the connection to his rehabilitation.

I continued by saying, "You really need to approach your rehabilitation the same way you climb a hill, focus only on today, not tomorrow or six months from now. It's too overwhelming to look that far ahead." A spark returned to his eyes, as he related to this analogy.

Each day we talked a little more. Before Andy was discharged to the rehabilitation center, I told him to remember one more thing. "When cycling, we take turns being in the lead position and drafting off of someone else's wheel. Now is your turn to draft Andy, and allow your friends and teammates to pull you along. There will again be a day when you will be out front helping them, but for right now, suck a wheel." I knew his personality all too well. It was similar to my own, afraid to ask and allow others to help. I said good-bye and wished him well, hoping we would stay in touch, if only for the times when he needed encouragement.

There were some miraculous things happening during my stay at Hopkins. I began to wonder if maybe this was a part of God's plan for me to be connecting with all these people. It felt as though He was working at it both ways. They needed the support I was giving, and I needed the reassurance of God's presence from seeing these connections unfold. It wasn't just a few. There were many, and it was happening daily.

Two friends of Kay's happened to be in Baltimore, while I was still at Hopkins, and came to visit me. Joey and Barbara were delightful people. They gave me a sense of the presence of my sister. Within a few minutes, I felt I had known them for a long time, as we openly talked of our faith in our Lord. Before saying good-bye we held hands and prayed together, after only being together for approximately thirty minutes. This wasn't something I would have ever been comfortable with before coming to Hopkins. God was sending me angels in so many different life forms, I would have been a fool to not open myself to His gifts.

Friends I hadn't talked to in fifteen years, not since graduating from high school with their daughter Dana Foster, called me out of the blue at Hopkins. The Easterwoods kept in contact with my brother, and were aware of my condition. Their call shocked me, but the message was very clear. As they too spoke freely of God's love and presence in our lives, I felt as though God made the call Himself.

These are only a few examples of the many circumstances where God was revealing Himself to me. Because of my history of concentrating on· how I could control things, I'm sure He wanted to make sure I saw the picture very clearly. It was vital, especially now after finally acknowledging I never had control, for Him to show me His omnipresence and His control. Combine this with my daily fear of the unknown. He knew I needed constant reassurance. These events left not a shadow of a doubt.

Twenty-One

She Ain't Heavy, She's My Sister

There is a destiny that makes us brothers;
None goes his way alone:
All that we send into the lives of others
comes back into our own.

EDWIN MARKHAM

I T WAS THE MORNING of the fifth attempt to repair my CSF leak. I had
a good night's sleep, even with the anticipation. Everything was the
same; another day, another operating room. The OR transporter
came to get me earlier than anticipated, before my parents arrived. While
I feared not being able to tell them, "I love you," before surgery, I had a
hunch they'd find their way down to the surgical area and find me. They
also knew this routine.

While laying in the holding area of the OR, my father walked in with a
surgical gown, hat, and mask on. Relieved to see him and wanting to help
him relax, I said, "Hi doc. Are you performing the operation this time?"
Although he laughed, I could tell he was out of his comfort zone. Yet, he
wouldn't have missed the opportunity to see me before surgery for anything. Only one person was allowed into this area, which normally was
totally restricted, so my mother couldn't come in. I'll never know how
they decided who would come see me, but I'm sure Mom's persistent generosity prevailed.

Keith appeared again, making sure I knew he was there with me. I thanked him for letting my father into the holding area to see me. Then I said, "We really have to stop meeting like this."

After watching everyone hook me up to the monitors, the anesthesiologist said, "You'll start to feel sleepy." The lights started to dim, everything in the room became a blur, and the faint buzz in my ears intensified. What seemed like seconds later was ten hours later, when I awakened in the NICU.

The eight hour procedure was successful. Dr. Long and Dr. Holliday clearly saw another area where CSF was leaking, only this time they were able to see it from the underside of my skull. While watching it freely drip into the right sphenoid sinus, they acknowledged the complexity of my case. Who would have ever thought it would take five craniotomies to repair the damage.

Using the Caldwell-Luc antrostomy approach, they were able to go through my mouth and nose to reach underneath the base of my skull and seal this area. Once again, they took fat and muscle fascia from my stomach to plug the holes, after scraping out the mucosa membranes from within each sinus. Filling all but the left maxillary sinus with this tissue, they used a fibrin glue mixture of cryoprecipitate, calcium, and thrombin. During the operation there was a need to stretch the third cranial nerves, the trigeminal nerves, to reach the location of the leak. I also had significant blood loss.

It was difficult to wake me in NICU. They intentionally slowed down my return to consciousness, because of the extreme nature of the surgery. When I finally woke up, it felt like my face had been beaten several times with a baseball bat. There wasn't one area from my ears forward that didn't radiate pain. My cheeks were like chipmunks and my lips difficult to move. I was reluctant to open my eyes a second time, after my initial exposure to light. Beams of dim light pierced through my head like daggers when I opened them. The pain penetrated my eyes, even when shut.

As with all my surgeries, the first thing to enter my mind upon regaining consciousness was a prayer of thanks for my safe keeping. It didn't matter that this was the worst postsurgical experience of all. I still was thankful. I concluded they must have made it into the center of my head where the sphenoid sinuses are located. I prayed the depth of the surgery would reflect its success. I couldn't picture myself going through any more surgeries of this nature.

As I opened my eyes, my NICU nurse came in. She introduced herself as the nurse manager of the NICU, Ski. To minimize my pain, she told me to remain as still as possible as she checked my monitors. I tried to ask her how the surgery went, but had a problem moving my lips. Ski reached over and swabbed my lips and tongue with a giant wet Q-Tip. As she did this, I realized I couldn't feel it rubbing against my lips.

She next had me perform the neuro function test. When testing my trigeminal nerves (facial nerves), it was apparent I lost a significant amount of feeling. I had no sensation from below my lower eyelids down to my lower lip. It was most noticeable to me when I tried to talk and couldn't move my upper lip. It felt as though I had just had major dental work done and the Novocain hadn't worn off yet. With my eyes closed she touched several areas around my face, including my nose. She said, "Tell me when you feel something." After a minute I opened my eyes thinking she had left the room. I hadn't felt anything yet. Finally, Ski touched my lower lip. I could feel this.

My jaw was also very sore, from being pried open for so long. It felt as though they tried to see how many hands could fit into my mouth. This discomfort made it difficult to open my mouth to talk or put items into my mouth. My mouth was very dry, so Ski managed to fit ice chips into the crack between my lips.

After surgery, it was very common for me to become nauseated from the anesthesia. I was very thankful I had no sense of taste. The crack between my lips wasn't very wide. Whenever I'd get sick, it felt like I was going to rip every patch they laid and blow through every leak they repaired. It was a very frightening feeling, especially when there's no other option but to get sick. I felt the same way if I had to sneeze or cough. Any added pressure in my head scared the daylights out of me.

Dr. Daniel Hanley, the Neurologist in charge of the NICU, kept a very close eye on me for the first forty-eight hours. I had a tremendous amount of blood loss during surgery and my body was struggling. Similar to after the previous surgeries, my blood pressure and heart rate remained very low. This time my blood count had also dropped. My hemoglobin was

9gm/100ml (normal = 12-16gm/100ml) and my hematocrit was 20 percent (normal = 37-48 percent). Because my body was very healthy, they hoped it would start making red blood cells on its own and avoid the need for a transfusion.

After a few days, when I was stable, they moved me back to my room on Meyer 8. I couldn't believe how weak I was the first time they got me out of bed. I thought I was weak after all the others, but this was no comparison. I got short of breath just walking to the bathroom, which was only three feet away. The nurses kept a close eye on me, not allowing me to get out of bed by myself. Instead of increasing with time, my hemoglobin decreased. The doctors first thought I might still be bleeding in my head.

Head CT scans were run with contrast dye. Results showed the extensive work from surgery but no abnormal bleeding. This was a relief.

Dr. Long recommended I work with the dietitian to increase my iron intake. Karen, the dietitian, started working with me. But it was difficult for Karen to get high amounts of iron into my diet, since for many years I preferred not to eat red meat—one of the best sources of iron. If there was any hope of building my hemoglobin up naturally, I had to make an exception to my preferences. I continued to eat lots of vegetables, concentrating on leafy greens. I had some difficulty with peas one day, not remembering how limited my movement was in opening my mouth. The crack between my lips was obviously smaller than the heaping spoonful of peas I was trying to shovel into my mouth. My upper lip shaved all but the bottom layer of peas off, as I slid the spoon into my mouth. Peas rolled everywhere, down the front of me, into my bed sheets and on the floor. I started laughing, feeling only my lower lip break into a smile. Who knew what my upper lip was doing.

Besides eating chicken and turkey for lunch and dinner, everyday at 3:00 p.m. I'd get a special delivery in a brown paper bag from the kitchen. It contained a large roast beef sandwich, the highest source of iron. Most days I ate some of it, but other days, I must admit, it got flushed. On top of this, I was receiving large doses of an iron supplement. All this was throwing my whole system out of whack. High iron doses are very constipating. So on top of all this, I had to load up on the bran and prune juice, to keep things moving. As it was, I still felt uncomfortable having a bowel movement, afraid of the increase in intracranial pressure.

Despite our efforts, we still weren't seeing an increase in my blood count. I remained very weak. I had to keep selecting one task to do when up from bed, such as brushing my teeth or washing my face. Anything more would have surely put me on the floor. In fact, it did one day.

After a few days of demonstrating my ability to move on my own and use my better judgment, the nurses said I could get up without assistance to move within my room. If I were going to walk in the hallway, however, I still needed assistance. The next day, when I got up to brush my teeth, I must have taken longer than usual. Getting weaker and weaker, I passed out in the bathroom before I could get back to my bed. When I woke up on the floor, I pulled the emergency cord that dangles near the toilet.

Everyone was quite shaken by this, prompting the nurses to put more pressure on Dr. Long and Dr. Holliday to order a blood transfusion. We had done all we could to avoid it, but to no avail. It was time to give my body some help.

With all the horror stories I had heard, I was apprehensive about a transfusion. My first thought was that maybe my parents could donate blood to me. Before I could ask about this, however, Dr. Long described how much testing needs to take place before receiving *any* blood. They didn't have enough time to test my parents' blood. I needed the transfusion as soon as possible. He reassured me of the reliability of their testing procedures and that the blood I'd receive would be fine. Once the decision was made, it took at least twelve hours to match my blood type. Then, no matter what time of day or night, once the blood arrived, I had to have the transfusion.

At midnight my blood arrived. I received two units. A nurse remained with me the entire time, to monitor any adverse reactions. Everything went smoothly. I felt the effects of my fresh source of oxygen transporters within a very short time.

The roast beef sandwiches continued to be delivered, so I found a neighboring patient who was happy to have a midday snack. My blood count rose to a near normal level thirty-six hours later. Until then I was required to remain in bed.

I called the nurse for a bedpan one afternoon. Cheryl, the nursing assistant, brought one for me. She stood there as if she though she'd wait until I was done, then take it from me. I told her I wasn't that talented, so she left. Two minutes later, Jennifer walked in and said, "So what's up?"

I said, "I'm sitting on the bedpan at the moment." At the same time the other nurse's aid walked in to take my vitals. I let her do her thing, while at the same time the television lady walked in and asked for payment for the week. As my temperature was being taken, I wrote a check for the television.

The television lady said, "Boy, you are multi-talented aren't you; writing a check, having blood pressure taken, and temperature done all at the same time."

All but Jennifer were shocked when I said, "Not as talented as you think. I'm also sitting on the bedpan."

O NCE I WAS able to start walking the halls, to build my strength, I did. It was lonely having to lay in bed all day, and to get up only with assistance. I wasn't able to meet other patients, as I enjoyed doing. The first person I met was Barbara Hughesian. Barbara is a dwarf. She was at Hopkins for tests on her neck. She was very nice and we struck up a friendship very quickly. She was discharged that same day, but she and her mother were staying at the same hotel as my parents. My parents were able to meet them before Barbara's surgery, which was scheduled for a few days after her tests. (While there were many people I met at Hopkins who I never saw again, there were a few who became lifelong friends. Barbara and Rose Hughesian are two of them.)

Some extra special, lifelong friends are the Kampen family. I met them while recovering from my fifth craniotomy. Kathleen Kampen was admitted for surgery on a tumor located in her brain stem. Krista, her nurse, asked me to stop by Kathleen's room, which was right next to mine, to talk with Kathleen. I waited until later in the day, when it appeared traffic in and out of her room had quieted down. I introduced myself, and seeing that she still had a roomful of family, I told her I was next door, if she needed someone to talk to.

I wanted very deeply to help her and to comfort her if I could in any way. All I could think was, "What would Jesus do?" In reality, I was a stranger; in essence I was a friend. I had experienced what she was about to undergo, and wished there was some way I could transmit the peace within me to Kathleen and her family. I knew, there were no words of comfort for a time like this in someone's life. I had been there. I knew, however, that the presence of those who love you and the richness of God's promise to be with us always, was most comforting.

The next day, as I sat in the patient lounge, with a shaved head, a headband of staples from ear to ear, black and blue swollen face, I began to encounter some pretty astonishing things. I noticed Kathleen's parents sitting in the lounge, as they waited for Kathleen to be taken to surgery. Carol, Kathleen's mother, had a most dreadful look of despair, a look only a mother could understand. I could tell she was fighting a battle within her mind, as she dueled back and forth, tears welling up in her eyes, then fighting them back.

Meanwhile, I was joking with the nurses and housekeepers, as I did most every day. Invariably, the jokes centered around the length of time I'd been at Hopkins and their desire to put a plaque on my door saying, "Dedicated to Karen Wells." I said no problem, as long as it didn't read, "In Memory of Karen Wells." Then I'd tease them about their need to put me on the payroll since I was the Meyer 8 floor socializer. It probably appeared to many people that I was having fun and enjoying myself. I was!

Ken, Kathleen's father, sat with Carol in the lounge. They couldn't help but observe my interactions with others. Their first question to me was, "How long have you been here?" Upon hearing six weeks, each of them took a deep breath. I needed to hurry and explain to them this was not typical of recovery from a craniotomy. I could see Carol was terrified by my answer, as she looked away with tears in her eyes. The pain parents endure when faced with life threatening episodes in their children's lives is beyond what anyone should have to bear. I wished there was something more I could do to comfort them, but I was confident God's presence was seen through me.

After Carol rushed to Kathleen's room to see a nurse who entered, Ken's second question was, "How can you be at peace with what is happening to you? What is your secret?" I was prepared for this question. It

was not the first time it had been asked. Once again, it opened the door
for me to witness to someone the comfort of God's love. I explained to
him I was in the hands of the Lord. I had let go of trying to be in control,
and was very confident God wouldn't give me any more than He and I
could handle. I had separated what I had control over and what I didn't
have control over, praying "The Serenity Prayer."

God, grant us the serenity to accept the things we cannot change,
courage to change the things we can, and the wisdom to know the
difference.

I could only control things like getting out of bed in the morning,
walking to build my strength, and staying positive. What I didn't have
control over I handed to God.

Ken's eyes lit up, like he had just won the lottery. He was excited by
my response, searching for anything that was positive. His daughter was
about to go in for brain surgery. To see someone sitting in front of him
who had not only survived brain surgery, but was happy and illuminating
God's love, showered him with hope. Our conversation continued on a
spiritual level. I mostly listened, as Ken asked all the questions preoccupy-
ing his mind. Why do good people suffer, was his biggest uncertainty. I
could only say I believed there was a time and place for everything. It's all
a part of God's plan. He never intended for us to suffer, but He's most
certainly going to use it somehow in a positive way.

We ended our conversation as Kathleen was taken to surgery. I said to
Ken, "Every time I'm taken into surgery I pray, 'Father in Your hands I
lay.' Keep the faith, Ken, and pray. I'll be praying too."

A few hours later, while I laid in my room talking with my parents, Ken
stopped by my room. Kathleen was still in surgery, but her family was
going down to the Inner Harbor area for a picnic. I introduced Ken to my
parents. He said to them, "I just want to tell you how wonderful your
daughter is. She helped us prepare for our daughter's surgery more than
I'd ever be able to tell you." Not knowing the scope of my interactions
with other patients on the floor, my parents thought, "Who is this guy?"
They appreciated his compliment, nonetheless, for they were already extremely proud of me.

Later that afternoon, while I was sitting in the patient lounge, I met Fran Payne. She was admitted for weakness and numbness in her hand. She seemed embarrassed because she was a patient for such a mild medical problem, especially when she saw the severe levels of medical distress other patients were facing. This was my opportunity to share with someone what I've always believed to be true. There are no minor problems. If someone is struggling, no matter what the severity, I believe it is significant.

Fran gave me one of the kindest gifts I could have received at this time. She asked my nurse if it would be okay to take me for a ride in my wheelchair, away from Meyer 8. I had not been outside of the hospital for seven weeks. Knowing this, Fran planned to take me down to the courtyard, where we could sit, talk, and enjoy the fresh air. What a treat this was! She also took me to the original Johns Hopkins Hospital building, which was now the administration building. This building's architecture was very impressive, but of greatest interest to me was the nine-foot tall statue of Christ in the center of the dome. It was comforting to know that even one of the largest medical institutions in the world was centered around Christ.

I met another patient, Beth Milton, who has become a lifelong friend. Dr. Carson performed her craniotomy to relieve facial pain. I heard she was having a very difficult time with postsurgical pain and tried to reassure her family she'd get through it. I didn't actually meet Beth, until several days later, when she was walking in the hall. Her family must have spoken about me; it appeared she knew me before I had a chance to introduce myself. Beth and I shared the challenge of handling severe, chronic pain. We also shared the difficulties and determination in finding a physician who could help us. We gave encouragement to one another, lightening the load if only for a moment.

I was overwhelmed with the number of relatives and friends who were making a huge effort to stay in contact with me. Everyone rallied around me, carrying me through the painful, lonely, hopeless, frustrating, and exhausting times. I tried my best to keep everyone up-to-date with where I was and how I was doing, but it was difficult, given the number of people with whom I wanted to communicate. I called the Kalis family one evening, not having talked with them in a long time. Just as the phone rang in their home, Shawn Kalis completed their final prayer request as the entire Kalis family prayed together, "God, please let us hear how Karen is doing. Please let her be okay."

When they answered the phone and heard my voice, they were speechless. They knew God answered prayers, but never had they seen results this quickly. For me, it was a message saying not only does God sometimes answer prayers long after we would have liked them answered, but He sometimes answers them much sooner than we expect. Everything was on God's time, not ours.

The next day, one of the nurses came to the door of my room and said, "Karen, do you know someone by the name of Norm, Norman Wells?"

I couldn't figure out why she'd ask this question, but I said, "Yes, my grandfather. Why do you ask?"

"We just received a call at the nurses' station. He's on the phone, trying to get through to you."

I was confused, and for a few brief moments wondered how this could be true. I said, "My grandfather's dead."

The astonished look on her face mirrored mine, until she thought further, and said, "Do you maybe have an uncle...?" Then it struck me. It must be my uncle Norm Howard Wells, who we have always called Howard. But for those few moments, in my mind, my grandfather was calling me. It was a wonderful feeling, an affirmation that my connection with him lives.

T HE FIRST DAY I was able to get out of bed, I tested whether I was leaking. When nothing came from my nose, I was ecstatic. Each day I tested it multiple times, and it still was not leaking. The longer I went without leaking, the more my headache started to return. I thought, "How can this be? Once the leak is stopped, the headache is supposed to go away."

I reported how I felt to my nurse each day, and also to Dr. Long and Dr. Holliday. Their first question upon entering my room was always, "Are you leaking?" They were equally excited to see success. They had covered not only the leaks, but also all the areas in my skull that might have the potential to leak. They didn't seem as concerned about my headache, concluding it was probably postsurgical pain, especially since they had been in my head five times.

I was disappointed. Even though I knew one of the reasons for repairing the leaks was to reduce the risk of meningitis, my primary goal was relief from the headache. Meningitis wasn't real to me, my headache was.

A few days later my head felt like it was going to explode. Dr. Perry became increasingly concerned with my discomfort. Since he knew I was happy with the results, and not one to normally complain, Dr. Perry suspected something was wrong. His close observation and intuitiveness moved him to order a lumbar puncture. This measured my CSF pressure, which had been running low (6.0-10.0cm), due to leaking. Normal levels are 10.0-20.0cm. He also wanted to test my CSF for meningitis, which could very possibly have been the cause of my headache.

Dr. Perry performed the lumbar puncture in my room, and much to our surprise, my CSF pressure was 26.0cm. This answered two questions. First, I wasn't leaking, otherwise my pressure would have been low again. Secondly, too high pressure also causes headaches, and this pressure was well above the normal limits. He still sent a CSF sample to the lab for testing, but indicated Dr. Long needed to address my new problem with pressure.

Dr. Long came by later that evening, and said he wanted to relieve this pressure as soon as possible. Because I leaked CSF for so many years, the ventricles inside my brain had shrunk and were very rigid. The ventricles are cavities inside the brain where CSF circulates. With the dramatic increase in pressure, there was a potential for further brain damage. With the uncertainty of how high this pressure was going, Dr. Long needed to move fairly quickly.

I was scheduled for surgery to open my lumbar-peritoneal shunt the next day. Dr. Hoff had implanted and then clamped this shunt. Dr. Long needed to open the shunt to relieve pressure.

One theory was that there was damage to the CSF receptors that told my body to absorb the appropriate amount of fluid. Fluid was constantly being produced and absorbed. If I didn't absorb enough, pressure increased. Another theory was that because I had been leaking for so long, my body had started to produce more fluid than the average person. The

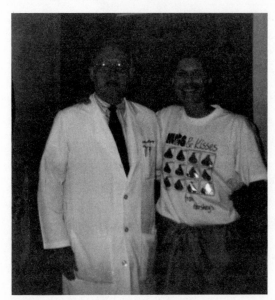

Don Long M.D. and author.

body does amazing things to find equilibrium. Once my leak was stopped, a buildup of CSF was likely.

Opening my lumbar shunt was a simple procedure, and gave me relief within six hours after surgery. Before sending me home, Dr. Long wanted to monitor my progress with the shunt open for at least another week. This was the first time in fifty days I felt the likelihood of going home. While I didn't want to get my hopes up, I was already thinking of what life would be like without a headache. It had been five years since my injury and thus five years living with a constant headache. I truly couldn't remember what it was like.

The next few days were spent healing and resting. I continued working to get back my endurance after the blood transfusion.

My new friends from the Lutheran church in Baltimore continued to visit; and Anna Pearson, the first patient I became friends with, came to see me each day after her chemotherapy treatments. She had been discharged, but our connection was strong enough that she kept track of me. It was a thrill to sit and listen to her stories again. Fran Payne, the woman who took me outside to the courtyard, also came back to see me after she was discharged. I was in awe. I believe each one of these people, whether they knew it or not, was sent from God. They were a part of the team of angels God had recruited to help me.

My parents persevered for this entire time, living at the hotel out of suitcases, and visiting me everyday. Their energy was dwindling, but never once did they complain. Once my shunt was opened and they knew I was not leaking, it was time for them to head home. I knew they were exhausted from all of the emotional stress. Riding the medical roller coaster didn't allow for much relaxing.

Kathleen Kampen did well with her surgery, although the tumor was a benign, inoperable, pineal tumor. Each day thereafter, we talked about our progress and burning desires to go home.

Kathleen was discharged within a week of her surgery. On the day she was going home, her father, Ken, came into my room. He said, "Karen, I want you to know that we are only forty-five minutes from this hospital. If you need anything, we will help you. If you need a place to stay before you can fly home to Michigan, you can stay with us. We will take you to the airport when you're ready. We want to help you in any way we can."

I was bewildered. I had known these people for less than a week, and he was opening their home to me. I felt myself being drawn to them. They were such loving and caring people. It seemed as though it was God's way of really driving home His message... "You are never alone." My parents had already left for home, but were hardly leaving me alone. They saw how I was surrounded by so many angels.

There was about a week between the time Kathleen and I were discharged. Carol and Kathleen called me frequently to check on my status. They seemed just as excited for me to be able to go home as I was. Eight weeks and three surgeries after being admitted for the lumbar drain, Dr. Long finally gave me the nod to go home. I had patiently waited for this day, and now I was nervous that it was happening. Before Ken offered to help me, I worried about how I'd get to the airport and how I'd arrange my flight. Would I stay in a hotel for a night or two, like I did last time, or should I try to fly home right away?

As soon as Ken said they'd help me, my worries diminished. I didn't want to impose on them and I was anxious to get home, so I made flight reservations for the day after I was to be discharged. Jennifer offered to drive me to the Kampen's home, where I'd stay overnight.

Walking out of the hospital was exhilarating. I was extremely weak, but nothing could stop me from leaving. Even though I never felt restricted in the hospital, I felt a new sense of freedom. My mind adjusted to my body's needs during my lengthy stay, never once feeling the need to do more than I could handle physically. I never felt the need to leave, until the day I was discharged. That's not to say I never had the desire; I most certainly did. My desires were brought to peace, knowing the importance of healing.

I spent the night with the Kampens. The next morning, I couldn't believe how weak I was just from getting ready. I was very light-headed and my whole body felt like a dish rag. I was determined to make it home, however. I appreciated Carol's generosity in helping me to the airport.

Upon arriving at the airport, Carol realized I probably couldn't carry bags or walk a great distance. She dropped me off at the terminal and went to park the car. While I waited for her, it was a struggle to stand. I couldn't see a place, other than the curb, to sit where Carol could see me. I wasn't thinking very clearly either, not remembering I could go inside the terminal and Carol would find me there. I feared losing Carol. She was my strength. I knew I had none of my own.

My independent personality stepped forward, as I tried to do what I needed by myself. While standing in line to check-in at the ticket counter, Carol immediately saw I was struggling. She helped me to a nearby bench saying, "Sit here. Don't move. I'll take care of everything." I didn't have a problem allowing her to do this, perceiving my own frailty. Carol requested a wheelchair for me, and also arranged for someone with a wheelchair to meet me in Chicago to take me to my connecting flight.

As we headed towards the gate, I wondered if I'd make it through security, with all the plates and screws in my head and the shunt in my back. I did. Unlike the first shunt, which was detected when walking through the magnetometers, everything in me was made of a nonmetal material.

We arrived at the gate just in time for pre-boarding for those needing assistance. The flight attendant at the gate said to Carol, "I'll take her aboard and get her settled." Just at that moment, it struck both Carol and I we had to say good-bye. Neither of us was ready. In fact, I couldn't believe how I was suddenly overcome with heart-wrenching feelings. I looked at Carol. Her expression suggested she was feeling the same. Carol asked if she could take me on board the plane to help me get settled. They said okay.

We were delaying the inevitable, but at least it gave us some time to adjust to our feelings, rather than be torn apart. Saying good-bye to Carol was like saying good-bye to a member of my own family. These feelings took me by complete surprise, having only known Carol a short time. It was as if I had known her all my life. I felt a huge lump in my throat and tears filled my eyes. I knew I was not a stranger, as once again I saw that look in Carol's eyes, just like on the day of her daughter's surgery. We hugged, wiped our tears, and promised to keep in touch.

The entire flight home I pondered all that had happened to me. My journey still didn't seem complete. I had promises to keep. However this time, my promises were of a completely different nature. No longer was I the hard driven, competitive woman who had promises only to herself. This journey had taken me to a different place in life, where promises were to other people, and first and foremost to God. I had a completely different sense of value for my life.

My life was now seen for its true, priceless value, the most precious gift one could ever receive. No longer was my focus on my physical life, how I could become faster or stronger. I began concentrating my energy on what role I could play in helping others to reach new levels of faith, hope, and love.

I was thankful for this journey. Had I not been riding in that race five years before, only God knows where my life would have gone. It most assuredly wouldn't have gone where God wanted it to go. I highly doubt it would have gone where I ultimately wanted it to go. With God's guidance, I turned a tragedy into an opportunity. I had a choice. I could run from it or I could learn from it. I chose the latter.

There was no need to return to my past, except to take it with me into the future, as a source of growth. I left home very much at peace with handing all the pieces over to God. As I returned home, I made sure all

the pieces, even the ones that were put back together again, remained in
His hands. I learned that's where they belong.

I T WAS SUCH a good feeling to be home, but also strange after being
gone so long. It's often difficult as a homeowner to not do things
around the house that require attention. My priority was getting my strength
back, not making up for lost time. My work situation was still a cause of
stress to me. My doctors were going to permit me to work from home on
a limited basis as I did before, but this was no longer acceptable to my
employer.

The first weekend I was home, I was so excited about going to church.
I couldn't wait to praise and worship God for taking care of me and for
fixing my leak. I also couldn't wait to see my friends who had supported
me beyond a dream. I got up early, showered, ate breakfast, and drove to
church. I couldn't figure it out, the parking lot was empty. Then it hit me.
It was Saturday, not Sunday.

I contacted the Kampens to let them know I had arrived home safely.
We talked on the telephone weekly to see how all of us were doing post-
surgically and emotionally. I also started sending them various things I
had written during the years of my recovery. I prayed it would help them
get through their difficult times, just as much as writing helped me.

I also sent them a cassette tape of music. I have enjoyed for many years
selecting special songs with a common theme and recording them on one
tape. I very carefully chose songs with words that meant something to me,
and in this case the songs were ones relating to how I felt about the Kampens.
The cassette also had some songs with inspirational words to help them
hold onto hope. One of the songs was written by John Denver, "The Gift
You Are." It was a special song for me to share with them. The words fit
perfectly how I felt towards them. Another one was "He Ain't Heavy,
He's My Brother." It felt as though they had said this to me when they
had so generously taken me into their home. I wanted to say it back to
them, as I longed to help them in whatever way I could.

I stayed in touch with several other people I met at Hopkins, patients,
their families, and nurses. I received letters and phone calls from many,
checking on my status and thanking me for the support and love I shared.

I was thrilled to receive a letter from Bob Lambert, thanking me for the time I spent with him. In his letter he spoke very positively about his recovery, despite already having difficulty with cognitive skills. His tumor was causing brain damage and cognitive impairment. I wrote back promptly, continuing to encourage him to throw his anchors deep in the Lord.

The numbness in my upper lip and cheeks persisted, making it challenging to eat and talk. I had to drink from a straw for over six months, until I could get used to not feeling a beverage against my lip. I shaved countless teaspoons of food into my lap, before I learned my height restriction. Many hours were spent in front of the mirror, saying words which required upper lip movement, learning to say them differently. Generally any word that required my mouth to close was difficult to say. With the passage of time, all things improved, although numbness remains.

My connection with the Kampens was beyond human understanding, and most certainly a part of God's plan. It was unlike any other friendship. We were truly soul mates. They were gifts, angels from above the dark clouds that hung over each of our lives. We each sought ways to lift one another up. We wanted to lessen the heartache, divide the pain, and double the joy. We shared a common path, one heart, one love for life, one guided by our Lord. Just as Barbara Johnson has said, "There is no better exercise for the heart, than reaching down and lifting someone up."

I found myself pouring my heart out to them, strongly devoted to helping them through their struggle with Kathleen's tumor. It was not so much the struggle with the tumor, as it was the wrestling with feelings that came along with it. I prayed for my experiences, perceptions, humor, and smiles to somehow help them. After all, they were sent to me as angels, maybe I was being sent to them as an angel. Only God knows.

AFTER BEING HOME for only a few weeks, my headache became progressively worse. At first, I attempted to tolerate it. My CSF leak had successfully been fixed, so it seemed strange that my headache came back. I waited six weeks before calling Dr. Long, hoping it was only postsurgical pain. It was apparent my CSF pressure was not stable. I could tell if pressure was too low or high by the way I felt in various positions. If I laid down, my headache dissipated somewhat. Anytime my head was elevated, while standing, sitting, or laying on a pillow, my headache was intolerable. Based on experience, I knew this meant I had low pressure. Fluid flowed back into my head if I was laying flat or bent over with my head below my back, giving me relief.

I called Mary Kay, Dr. Long's nurse and told her about my condition. This was upsetting to her, as I had become her friend, in addition to being her patient. She made sure Dee Bennett, Dr. Long's assistant set up a telephone appointment for me. She knew it didn't sound good. Dr. Long asked me to have an MRI done on my head at Munson, so he could see the size of my ventricles. Dr. MacKenzie ordered the MRI, and I had it done the following week. I was still used to being able to have it done the same day it was ordered. Unlike Hopkins who has close to thirty MRI's, Munson has one and there's always a long waiting list.

The films were Federal Expressed to Dr. Long. He called me as soon as he received them to request that I return to Hopkins immediately.

On this day the sunset was the most brilliant shade of red. It was fun to watch God paint the sky. I remembered the saying, "Red sky at night, sailor's delight." I knew my return to Hopkins would be okay. Again, I knew I'd be in good hands, God's hands. He placed me on this road to further growth and gave me some of the tools I needed. It appeared I needed to pick-up more of life's lessons as my journey continued.

Twenty-Two

Angels To Watch Over Me

Some people come into our lives and quickly go.
Some stay for a while and leave footprints
on our heart and we are never, ever the same.

SOURCE UNKNOWN

THE KAMPENS INVITED ME back into their home, offering to help with my return trip to Hopkins. I expected to be in Baltimore one week to ten days, at the most. It was the first part of December and I had made plans to spend Christmas with my parents and sister in Florida. Although I was frightened by my need to return to Hopkins, I was excited about the opportunity to spend time with the Kampens. I planned to make the most of every minute with them, since our last time together was under such duress.

I flew into BWI Airport, where Carol and her youngest son, Stephen, picked me up. It seemed to me there was another reason for me to return to Baltimore other than for regulating my CSF pressure. I didn't know what it was; it was just intuition.

I was stunned when I saw Kathleen. I didn't know her before her biopsy surgery, but I could tell by looking in her eyes she wasn't her normal self. Her eyes were always opened wider than normal, her pupils dilated, and movement slow. Her gate was abnormal and she had poor balance. She seemed depressed, although easily humored. I really wasn't sure what was normal and what wasn't, until I asked Carol and Ken. They were extremely worried about her, but not certain what to do. It was evident their primary needs included figuring out how to help Kathleen, and to have someone listen to, care for, and support them. I knew I could manage the latter, and was confident we could find out the former.

Unfortunately, I didn't have much time to spend with the Kampens. Things happened very quickly the day after my arrival. I was admitted to NICU at Hopkins. Dr. Long was very concerned with my pressure change. The more fluctuation I had, the greater the possibility of additional brain damage.

Stephen and Kathleen drove me to the hospital and waited with me until I was taken to NICU. I first had to undergo several tests, including an MRI with contrast; blood tests; x-rays; and an eye exam. The eye exam took the longest, due to a slight problem in communication with the resident ophthalmologist. She had difficulty speaking English and needed to take my medical history. I knew it was going to take me hours to give her my history when she started asking me how to spell words like spinal fluid.

While waiting for my admissions blood test, Gary, my favorite transporter, walked by. I recognized him right away, but wasn't sure if he recognized me. Not only did he recognize me, he called me by name. I was impressed. It was very comforting to know that people knew me. It was as if I was home and being admitted to the same hospital where I was employed. Jennifer met me in admitting and took me to NICU, our conversation helped me relax.

Dr. Long requested that Dr. Hanley, the neurologist in charge of the NICU, perform a study on my CSF pressure. While it was in some ways similar to the lumbar drain, it was much more restrictive. A resident doctor from the neurology team came to get my history and prepare me for the study. He said Dr. Williams, who works with Dr. Hanley, was going to do a lumbar puncture and place a probe-like instrument into my spine. This probe would be attached to the monitor beside my bed. This monitor was calibrated, the same as the simple manual calibration method of the lumbar drain, but had a machine that electronically recorded data. It was a little more sophisticated, but an archaic beast nonetheless. I was surprised at how much of the data still had to be manually recorded. I would have thought this would be computerized, but the demand for moni-

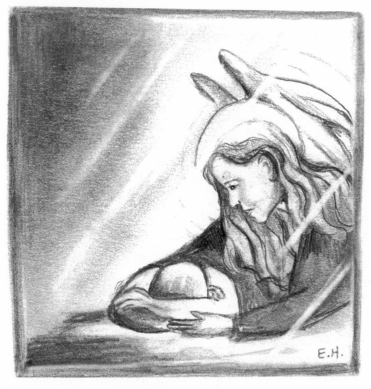

Angels watching over me.
Illustrated by Emily Helman.

toring CSF pressure hadn't been that great until I came along. I would have rather not been so special.

The procedure to hook me up went smoothly. After twenty plus times, I became quite used to doctors sticking needles and instruments into my spinal canal. I was also very fortunate never to have any complications. I was hooked up to several corresponding monitors, such as an electrocardiogram, pulse oxymeter, blood pressure, and respiratory monitor. Not only was I restricted to bed, but I was also told to limit my movement. Having a probe in my spine had its risks. It wasn't the most comfortable experience. Each time I'd move I could feel tingling in different parts of my body. It was more uneasy mentally than physically, wondering what the potential for spinal cord injury was.

It was a new experience for both myself and the nursing staff in NICU. Very rarely do they have the pleasure of caring for patients who can talk to them. I managed to keep them entertained, and they all felt it was a pleasure to have a smiling face greet them each day. One thing I heard over and over again from health care professionals and others who crossed my path was how they respected me for never complaining. My reply was always, "I don't have to look very far to find someone who is worse off than I am. I can't complain. I've been very blessed."

Once the nurses from Meyer 8 heard I was back at Hopkins, they started coming down to visit. Ken and Carol came to visit in the evenings, just as if I were their daughter. We had a chance to talk a little about Kathleen, and the related feelings they were wrestling with. I didn't know how it felt to be a parent watching a daughter deteriorate, but I did know how to listen, and to support a friend in need. They had so much love to share, it beamed like the sun from them. It hurt me to see their anguish. I couldn't help but think of Ken's question, "Why do good people have to suffer?" He was referring to Kathleen, but I was seeing the two of them fall within this category as well. I would have done anything to take their hurt away, but there wasn't anything I could do except be there for them. I believe this is why God sent me back to Hopkins. Everything I endured over the next six months was worth it.

THE WATER WAS running in the sink in my room in NICU. I'd been sitting on the bedpan for quite some time, with no success. Unfortunately, this monster of a machine wasn't going to follow me to the rest room when I needed to go. A bedpan or bedside commode were my only options. Usually the sound of water running helped me, but not this time. My bladder was about to burst, so we were trying all the tricks to get things moving, before having to resort to the dreaded catheter. I thought the sound of the water changed a little. It sounded more like a waterfall, but I thought I was probably imagining a waterfall, praying a similar phenomenon might happen to me. My nurse had disappeared, leaving me alone to contemplate. As time passed without relief, I was getting more and more frustrated.

Suddenly, a platoon of nurses came running into my room. I knew I needed help, but I didn't think it was so critical to justify five nurses. It sounded as though they were running through puddles. They were. The sink had plugged, overflowed, and was flooding the entire NICU. As I laid there on my back, all I could see was the ceiling.

The housekeeping crews were called in. Of course, they asked me what had happened, as if I had a major accident. I only wished it were true.

After things calmed down, Dr. Hanley came in to discuss the results of my CSF pressure monitoring. I already knew from watching the monitor that my pressure was 0.0-2.0cm, an extremely low level. He confirmed my analysis, and said there was a need to alter my shunt to increase my pressure. He said Dr. Long would come by in the morning to let me know what his plans were for surgery.

After having been connected to the monitor for five days, it was finally removed from my spine.

After being removed from the monitor, I was moved up one floor, back to my penthouse on Meyer 8. I was greeted by all my friends and caught up to speed with the latest news on the floor.

It was early Friday morning. Dr. Long came to see me and said he wanted to clamp my shunt again. He said, "No wonder you're in pain with this headache, you're close to bone dry up there. We need to go in and clamp the shunt again to see if the pressure will come back up to a comfortable level. We'll plan to do it first thing Monday morning, if that's okay."

This would mean I'd have surgery seven days before Christmas. My hopes of going to Florida for Christmas were looking slimmer. Even if I was physically able to travel, to be able to book a flight into Orlando this close to the holidays would be impossible. I didn't, however, have a choice. I needed this surgery.

Before leaving the hospital, I made several phone calls to people who I befriended during my lengthy stay at Hopkins. I talked to Andy Anderson, the cyclist. He was addressing my Christmas card when I called. I was so excited to hear his voice. This meant he was out of the rehab center. He told me he was walking. He had regained most of the feeling in his legs, was still doing physical therapy, and had made substantial progress. He had even been on a stationary bike. It was so good to talk with him and to reminisce about our days together on Meyer 8. He thanked me for all the encouragement I'd given him, admitting how depressed he was at the time. We both reiterated to one another the critical role our faith played in our recoveries.

I talked with Mel Taylor, Beth, Anna, Fran, Judy and Jim, as well as a few of the others I had met. They were happy to hear from me, and I felt a renewed sense of peace after talking. We were in essence "family."

The phone call I avoided making was to Bob Lambert. Of all the people I had met, he was the one who was most terminal. I wanted to call, but was scared of the unknown. After being in the Baltimore area for several weeks, I finally called. Gladys, his wife, answered. She immediately asked how I was doing and where I was. She said she received my Christmas letter and read it frequently for inspiration. She had been intending to write to me since receiving it. She needed to tell me Bob passed away December 11th. My heart sank. It was the same feeling I had when Bob told me his tumor was malignant. I had met so many sick friends at Hopkins, Bob was the first one who died.

I only spoke with Bob a handful of times, yet I felt as though I had lost a dear friend. Gladys went on to tell me how much it meant to Bob and their whole family, for me to connect with Bob as I had. She said the letter I received from Bob was the last letter Bob had written. She described how much I meant to Bob. She said he fought to the very end and died peacefully at home. Immediately my mind thought...Bob didn't walk away, he weathered the storm, and he died in the place he most loved. I was confident his anchors were deep in the Lord.

I WAS DISCHARGED for the weekend, until my surgery Monday morning. I returned to the Kampen's. It was a pleasure to be with them, especially during this special time of year. They didn't do anything out of the ordinary to make me feel like a part of the family, other than be themselves. I immediately felt as though I was family.

Most of my focus turned toward helping Carol and Ken discuss their feelings about Kathleen's condition. Everyone was getting very frustrated with Kathleen. It appeared she was giving up on overcoming her benign

tumor. There wasn't anything more heartbreaking than watching someone deteriorate before my eyes. It was dragging all of us through each
stage of the grieving process, whether we knew it or not. I knew this
process all too well.

Thinking back to our phone conversations, I realized the Kampens
were in denial, they didn't just have a positive attitude. It was easy for me
to confuse the two. When I was discharged from Hopkins for the weekend, I joined them in the stage of anger. Anger was being projected onto
Kathleen for not taking an active role in her recovery. At times, I wanted
to grab hold of her and say, "You have so much to be thankful for. God
never gives up on you, so don't you ever give up on God." But I didn't do
this. I just sat back, observed Kathleen and her family, and facilitated conversations.

Jennifer also became friends with the Kampens. I asked her if this was
normally what happens with people who have pineal tumors. While she
maintained that the seriousness of this tumor was not to be taken lightly,
she questioned Kathleen's emotional response. We all knew Kathleen's
faith was strong, and thus her stubborn, lazy, attitude didn't fit. She seemed
to be very depressed.

The Kampens are devout Catholics, so it was very easy to talk about
faith and how it fit in the picture of recovery. (I am Lutheran, but this at
no time affected our conversations.) God's lesson was that He doesn't
discriminate, and thus I shouldn't either. I never had before, but it wasn't
tested as much as it was during my time with the Kampens.

I always enjoy going to church and worshipping with my family and
friends. It magnified the feeling of oneness with the Lord and thus with
each other. Being in church provided an optimal environment, but that's
not to say this experience couldn't happen elsewhere. "For where two or
three come together in my name, there am I with them." (Matt. 18:20
NIV) I believe you cannot become more spiritually and emotionally inti-
mate with a loved one than when you pray, sing, worship, or kneel next to
them. It is the most divine connection I can attain.

My endearment with the Kampens went to this next level when I worshipped with them at Sacred Heart Catholic Church. It became a very
angelic relationship. While kneeling beside them, praying for God's peace

to be among all of us, I felt God fully embrace me. Never before had I felt His presence in this way, even though I knew He was steadfastly holding me each minute of every day. I never opened my eyes to this spiritually and emotionally, keeping my knowledge of His presence at an intellectual level. My faith was in my head, more than my heart.

Being alone in a strange city, many miles from home, with a critical medical condition, made it very clear to me how I needed God's presence. I knew all my comfort and hope came from God, though I felt it come through books I read, cards I received, phone calls and messages from family and friends, sermons I listened to, and my small Bible study group. All of these were symbols of God's presence, but I never translated it into a visual picture of God holding me. I saw it as God's way of communicating with me, as if He were standing in heaven, transmitting His love, comfort, protection, and guidance through these people and things. I intellectually knew He was in my heart and soul, but never stopped to feel the everlasting warmth that radiated through my body because of His presence.

My experience with the Kampens pulled many pieces of my spirituality together. It then became a personal relationship with God, rather than just worshipping my Creator, Comforter, and Savior. I felt the warmth of Him holding me and carrying me over the largest mountain range of my life. I came to understand that all I had heard, received, and read came directly from His voice and His hands.

God was orchestrating this huge concert and every instrument was finely tuned. I often thought the music was not to my liking, but my ears were not yet trained. What my eyes could not see, my ears began to hear.

BEFORE RETURNING TO Hopkins for surgery, I often sat quietly at the Kampen's and tried to picture what my life would have been like if I hadn't met them. There was no question in my mind, it would have been impossible. They were truly His angels. To walk alone during my recovery would have been like walking without God—impossible.

I was about to enter the six most difficult months of my recovery. I wouldn't have believed it at the time, but what I already went through was only training and preparation for what was to come. It was a tough year for Jesus at age thirty-three, when He suffered and died for our salvation. It was about to be a tough year for me as well at age thirty-three.

I was admitted to Johns Hopkins Hospital the same day as my surgery to clamp my lumbar shunt. Carol drove me to the hospital and stayed with me until I was taken to my room on Meyer 8. The surgery was a simple procedure. Keith found me on the OR schedule and made sure he requested my room. I came through it with no complications and felt pretty strong shortly after surgery.

In fact, after the nurses settled me in bed and left to tend to their other patients, I noticed a survey from the recovery room sitting on my night stand. I filled it out. At the bottom it said to give it to the nurses at the nurses station after it was completed. I got out of bed and walked down to the nurses station. Melissa, the nurse who was just coming on the afternoon shift looked at me like she was seeing a ghost. She screamed, "Karen, what are you doing?"

"I'm bringing this survey to you or anyone who wants it."

"I just came out of report and they said you just returned from surgery."

"Yes, I did."

"What are you doing walking around?"

"Like I said, I'm just bringing this survey to you."

"Oh my word, only Karen Wells would do something like this. We better get you back to bed. Let me hang onto you."

I didn't think anything of it. I felt fine and thought I'd feel even better by getting up and moving. No one told me to stay in bed. They just assumed patients would stay in bed immediately after surgery. I was the exception, defying all odds and always eager to get moving again. This was so contrary to patients who bask in the attention from the nurses.

Within a few days, I could tell there was again too much pressure building up in my head. It was so painful to lay flat in bed I was nauseated. The original problem of hydrocephalus was still prevalent. There was too much CSF in my brain pushing on the ventricles to the point of damaging my brain. A lumbar puncture confirmed Dr. Long's suspicions. I was scheduled for more surgery, December 22, 1994, four days after he clamped the shunt. Dr. Long decided to put a valve on the lumbar shunt, regulating

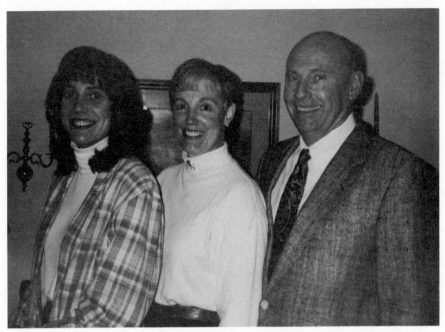

Kathleen, Carol, and Ken Kampen...my angels.

the amount of fluid released. Because a clamped shunt created high pressure and an open shunt was too low, he opted for something in-between.

This confirmed that I was not going to Florida for Christmas, and that I'd probably spend Christmas in the hospital. I felt okay with this, praying for only one Christmas gift. I wanted the surgery to be successful and to free me of my headache.

The night before surgery, the Kampens planned to attend a Christmas concert at their church. Knowing my love for music, they told me to ask Dr. Long if he'd let me go outside of the hospital for a few hours to attend the concert. I felt like a kid in school asking for a pass to go to the rest room. I asked Dr. Long. He had no problem allowing me to go. He knew I was in good hands. It took a lot of time to drive multiple trips to and from Hopkins, but Ken and Carol made sure I got to the concert and was able to enjoy it with them.

After I realized I wasn't going to have time in between surgeries before Christmas to shop for a gift for Kathleen, I asked Carol to shop for me. I wanted to buy her a lightning bolt pendant to wear on a chain. A few days before this, Carol had noticed the lightning bolt I wore on a necklace, along with my cross. She asked what it symbolized. It appeared she liked the motto, but made no further comment than to say, "That's nice."

I thought it would be a very nice gift for Kathleen, hoping it would inspire her to remain positive during her recovery. Carol seemed confident she could find one, not telling me she had already bought one for herself.

The next morning I was taken into surgery for the valve to be placed on my lumbar shunt. It was Thursday, Carol's day to work, so I was on my own. I never expected any of the Kampens to follow me through the rigorous roller coaster of tests, appointments, and surgeries, but amazingly enough they attempted to be by my side every minute.

Having surgery with no one to say good-bye to and no one waiting for me when I came out was a lonely experience. It was just me and God, and I was holding onto Him tightly. I was thankful it was a simple operation, which lessened my fear. This was the first time I was without family or friends, and while I knew when I flew back to Maryland that I'd be alone, I didn't know how it would feel.

I knew this was something I had to do for myself. It would have been selfish of me to have expected my family to go with me again. It's difficult enough to be a support person for a few days, not to mention a few years. It would have been easy for even me to give up and say I was tired of having to fight this medical monster. Instead, I persevered, kept my focus on the rainbow, and said lots of prayers. I didn't want to hurt anymore. As long as there was hope, I needed to keep going.

On this day of surgery, I wondered why God had temporarily removed my support system. What did he have planned? I had just learned to feel the warmth of His love through others, and now they were not able to be with me. Did this mean God wasn't with me either? Not at all, I concluded. He was teaching me to feel His presence inside me. It was just He and me, and I still felt the same warmth, comfort, and love.

Throughout my recovery, I learned to be at peace with myself, to be content sitting in silence. I used to always be moving, doing something, and in control. I needed to be productive. On this day, I was not able to move, sitting alone in silence, hardly in control, but hoping I was doing something productive. I was pleased with how comfortable I felt.

I was taken into surgery, where my shunt was opened and a high pressure valve was replaced with a low pressure valve. Surgery was without complication, and after spending an hour in recovery, I was returned to my room. As soon as I was alert, I called my parents to tell them everything went well.

Because of the damage to my ventricles, it was difficult to know what was going to help me. A normal person with hydrocephalus is relieved of their problem with a shunt, without much difficulty. I never pretended to be normal. Because of so many unknowns, my case was different. Dr. Hanley completed the analysis of the CSF pressure study. Although, even with these results, there were no definitive answers. Dr. Long and he admitted there had not been a great deal of research on cases like mine. We were breaking ground. It was a matter of trial and error.

One evening, I heard voices singing down the hallway. It was a group of Christmas carolers. What a beautiful sound! It touched me in a special way. While I accepted not being able to be with my family for Christmas, it was extremely difficult for me emotionally. Given the closeness of our family, with many miles between us, holidays are very special to all of us. It is a time to worship together and feel oneness with God, reaffirming our oneness with each other. I was sorely going to miss this, and dreaded how I'd feel Christmas Eve and Day.

I walked down to the nurses station to hear the carolers more clearly. As I sat there, I flashed back to eight years prior to this, when I was with a group of carolers singing through the halls of a hospital. Tears flooded my eyes unexpectedly, as I listened. What goes around, comes around. We each take turns giving and receiving in this world. It was okay for me to receive.

I always was a bit uncomfortable accepting things from others. My independence stood out, and I felt I should do things for myself. Throughout my recovery, I learned to accept people's generosity. I always kept in mind what my friend Nancy Rowe once said to me, when I asked how I could ever repay her. She said, "Do something like this for someone else someday. Pass it on."

The night I was listening to the carolers I thought, "How in the world would I ever repay the Kampens?" When I saw how much they were doing to help me, I didn't know if I was capable of passing it on. I prayed that God would use me to help them in return.

As I sat at the nurses desk, a young doctor said to me, "You're the triathlete from Michigan, aren't you?" I was shocked. To my knowledge, I had never seen him. How did he know who I was? It turned out he had taken care of me several times while I was in NICU. Each time an incident like this happened, it made me feel close to home.

The morning of Christmas Eve, Dr. Long said I could return to the Kampen's. He didn't want me leaving for Michigan, but he didn't want me in the hospital for Christmas either. I was delighted by his decision. Carol and Ken came to pick me up, taking me home to spend the holidays with their family.

I T WAS A very special Christmas, in spite of not being with my family. The Kampens helped me feel as though I had been a member of their family all my life. I was very comfortable with them, not feeling the least uneasy about spending Christmas with them.

The hardest part was seeing Kathleen's condition, which was slowly deteriorating. I feared it was permanent. I was sad for Kathleen and her family, and scared to death that it could easily happen to me.

It was a rather somber Christmas, though everyone worked hard to turn the circumstances in a positive direction. Before going to Mass, we enjoyed a wonderful dinner together, with Kathleen's twin sister, Joanne, and her husband Eric Durrel.

I didn't try to hold back my tears as I sat in church, unwrapping endless gifts. I first unwrapped the gift of my Savior, the one who was holding me and providing eternal hope. I pictured myself holding baby Jesus in my arms. No gift can ever compare, but each gift was tied to another. Next was the gift of my family, and my tears continued to flow. My heart yearned to be with them, as I remembered the feeling and symbolism of passing the candle flame one to the other, while singing "Silent Night." The gift of eternal hope and God's love is shared with one another. Finally, there was a beautifully wrapped gift with a tag that read: To my beloved daughter with whom I am very pleased. From: Your Heavenly Father. I was sitting among them, my adopted family, the Kampens. This was the truest meaning of Christmas: gifts of self. I recognized giving of self being when one feels the gift without actual presence. The gift of Jesus and my family was already branded on my heart forever.

I've always felt the extravagant gift giving that takes place at Christmas was too excessive. It meant more to me to give a gift of self, to give of my time and love. This Christmas opened my eyes to how these gifts are with us always. Even when in spirit, they are present, as was the case for me while in Maryland. They can be unwrapped at any time, just as I did while kneeling before my Heavenly Father. The value of these gift's will never diminish.

After Mass, we returned to the Kampen's to exchange gifts with one another. I was looking forward to giving the lightning bolt to Kathleen. I wrote a letter to accompany it. Her double vision didn't allow her to read, so I sat next to her and read it aloud to her and everyone else.

Dear Kathleen,

   May this lightning bolt forever remind you of our friendship, and to live every moment of life to its fullest potential. Live for today and take no regrets to tomorrow, for just as quick as lightning can strike, life can change for better or for worse.

   Always remember, your tumor is only a tiny piece of you, by no means the whole. God's the only one who has the recipe to our life. His choice of ingredients, which will form our life, and His plan/recipe is always for the best. We can never separate ingredients, they are all mixed together. "And we know that in all things God works for the good of those who love Him, who have been called according to His purpose." (Romans 8:28 NIV) It's up to us to do the baking however. While we often times would rather eat the dough than bake it, we need to keep moving forward by doing our part. Sometimes we may feel burned, while other times we feel just right. But we must remember, it's okay to feel this way, because we can have confidence that there's no mistake in the consistency of our lives, each ingredient serves a purpose. The hard part is...God continues to add ingredients throughout our entire life, so we never know how things will turn out. But we can move through life with optimism because of His promise, "Lo I am with you alway, even unto the end of the world." (Matt. 28:20 KJV)

And the beauty of life begins when we mix our lives with others and have enriching friendships, just like we have done.

Kathleen, I have a great deal of admiration for your great courage and determination in your recovery. I admire your strength and faith as well. You have the ingredients to bake a beautiful life for yourself, for your family, and for God. You give so much of yourself to others, which will continue to add new ingredients to your life. Everything goes full circle. I know I have helped you in some ways, but you must realize that you have helped me in more ways than I could ever describe. Thank-you for being such a very special part of my life. I feel like you're my sister. You will always hold a very deep place in my heart.

Love, Karen

Everyone was in tears. I had to stop reading a few times to swallow the lump in my throat. Kathleen didn't seem moved. Part of me questioned why, while the other part of me knew her brain's emotional center was not operating correctly. I prayed for it to touch her in some way, if not on this day, on a day to come.

Christmas morning we traveled to Carol's brother's home, where we celebrated Christmas with her entire family. They, too, welcomed me into the family, and many more friendships began. Within a few days, Carol and Ken's oldest daughter, Christine Kolenda, came with her husband and two children for two weeks. Even with a full house, never was there a time when I felt I was a burden.

One evening, I felt a sharp piercing stab of pain shoot through my eye and head. Prior to this, my headache had been its usual, constant throb. The new valve hadn't relieved my discomfort. I laid down on my bed, to see if I could get some relief. The sharpness of the pain subsided initially, but returned within five minutes, with greater intensity. I was in tears. The pain was tremendously intense. I could do nothing to relieve it. Carol came to check on me, finding me in complete distress. She asked Christine, who was a nurse, to come and check on me. They both tried to get me to relax, seeing how my whole body was tensing, trying to resist the pain. Finally, I fell asleep, waking the next morning to my usual headache. The piercing pain had subsided.

Christopher, Christine's husband, drove me to Hopkins for an appointment with Dr. Long a few days later. Dr. Long recommended going back in for more surgery, to replace the valve again. He wanted to admit me immediately and perform the surgery the following day. I wasn't prepared for this, but then again I was never truly prepared for anything that happened. Much to everyone's surprise, especially their four year old, Lauren, Christopher returned to the Kampen's without me. The love we shared had filtered down to the children. Even to them I was family.

During surgery the next day Dr. Long discovered the valve that he had placed on my shunt two weeks earlier had disconnected itself from the shunt. The intense pain I felt several nights ago was most likely when it detached. The shunt must have drained huge amounts of CSF into my peritoneum, with no regulation of fluid flow. Like a break in a dam, the initial rush of fluid undoubtedly caused the piercing pain.

Dr. Long reattached the valve and stitched me back up. I was beginning to think this incision in my abdomen might also have benefited from a zipper. This was the seventh time it was opened.

A couple doctors who had been on the fringes of my case, saw me laying in the recovery room. They stopped to say hi and to ask for an update on my case. I couldn't believe I was a regular at one of the biggest hospitals in the world. I'd rather have been a regular in another setting.

One week later, I reported to Dr. Long. There was no improvement in my headache. I could, however, feel that it was positional. When I laid down, fluid went back into my head and relieved the headache somewhat. Once I sat up, or even put my head on a pillow, the pain increased. Dr. Long asked Dr. Hanley to do a lumbar puncture to remove fluid as a quick test of whether we were really talking about high pressure or low pressure. After discussing these factors with Dr. Hanley, Dr. Long decided to go ahead and change the valve to a medium pressure valve.

Surgery was scheduled for a few days later. For the eighth time, Dr. Long went back into my abdomen to adjust my shunt. My stamina was dwindling, even though I kept trying to build it back up while recovering at the Kampen's in-between each surgery. Again, the surgery went well, and a few days later I was released to go back to the Kampen's to recover.

I was getting quite discouraged by the fact there wasn't any change in my headache, yet I had been through four surgeries in four weeks. I still held onto hope and kept praying. Family and friends stayed in close touch with me, calling and sending cards and gifts. It became a joke at the Kampen's that whenever the phone rang it was probably for me, as I was getting more calls than they were. My mail often outnumbered theirs. They were dazzled by the overwhelming support I received from people who loved me. I knew I had a wonderful family, and was overjoyed by their support. They really helped carry me through these challenging weeks.

I kept my sights on God, through daily prayer and devotion. A very important part of each day for me was attending morning Mass with Carol and Kathleen. This was a wonderful way to begin each day. Never before had I prayed so hard, pleading with God to relieve me of my pain and to reverse Kathleen's condition. I valued my conversations with God, but this time it seemed as though He was silent. He was waiting for something, I didn't know what, but I kept my faith.

It was my sixth week in Maryland, oscillating in and out of the hospital, back and forth with the Kampens. Having set a goal of writing a book about my journey of recovery, I started writing. I kept a journal since the day Margo suggested I do so. This not only was very therapeutic, but it eventually became the foundation for this book.

I also tagged along with Carol when she took Kathleen to doctor's appointments, CT scans, and MRIs. I tried to give her as much support as possible. I felt very comfortable talking with Carol about anything, and it was effortless building this exceptional friendship. I valued every minute of our time together, the fun times, the difficult times, and the silent times. I had tremendous respect for Carol. She was a mother of five children and grandmother of six. She poured love into each and every one of them. On top of that, she poured love into me, too. People who didn't know us thought we were related, especially when they saw Carol with me so much at the hospital.

Carol was the type of person who always put others before herself, giving unlimited amounts of time and energy. There are very few people I have met, besides my own parents, who are as tenderhearted as Carol, which made it that much harder to see her filled with pain. Despite trying to conceal her pain and heartache, I could still detect her distress. I worked hard at trying to get her to open up and to get her feelings out. She needed someone to listen, to encourage, and to shed a positive light on life.

Carol's life reflects her very strong faith and close relationship with God. I believed she appreciated our spiritual talks as much as I did. I discovered talking about spiritual issues and feelings renewed and strengthened my faith.

Ken, on the other hand, was not involved in as many discussions, because he was working. He had, however, a heart of gold. I could tell by our discussions how much he cared. While he revealed less of his emotions than Carol, he still loved and cared just the same. He was a very sensitive man, who felt the distress of the medical fiasco. I appreciated his patience and willingness to share so much of his home and family with me.

I shared the Kampen's worries about Kathleen, as she continued to deteriorate. There was also a concern of whether or not Kathleen would be able to return to her position as a kindergarten teacher at a Catholic school. I was outraged when I heard Kathleen describe her trial day. She described how she was judged by other teachers, including a temporary teacher, who happened to be very interested in staying in the position permanently. The method that Brother William used to evaluate her status was inappropriate. On top of this, Kathleen was placed in a very awkward position after school. The panel of teachers who had evaluated her gathered to discuss whether Kathleen should be allowed to return to her job. I was furious. I felt the urge to stand up for Kathleen, as if to stand up for my sister.

That evening at dinner, as we talked about the situation, Kathleen cried for the first time since her surgery. All of us wanted so badly to protect her from feeling the pain, but I knew this would hurt her more than help her. She needed to go through the pain to get to the other side. That evening I wrote in my journal, "I've been there. I know what it's like, and I still can't help her." It was a very helpless feeling.

These feelings were not unique to this situation alone. I found myself always trying to think of ways to help Kathleen, whether it be for her condition, work, motivation, and personal life. I encouraged her to walk for exercise, which would help increase her endurance and reduce her fatigue. I took every opportunity I could to talk with her, trying to inspire and encourage. I was scared she was truly giving up. Kathleen listened, but most of it was not heard.

Kathleen was helping me, without doing anything. Just being with her was a constant reminder that no matter what type of struggle I was encountering, there's always someone worse off than me. At least I had been able to rehabilitate from my brain damage. Kathleen's condition first appeared to be permanent, with an inoperable tumor pressing on vital areas of her brain. I praised and thanked God for His grace and many blessings, asking also for my friend and sister to be healed.

The hardest thing I had to do with Kathleen and Carol was go to Kathleen's school, where she taught the previous year, and take down all of her things in her classroom. It was a somber day, and the reality of her condition met us face to face. The only one who believed she'd have a chance of returning to teaching again was Kathleen.

It was such a helpless feeling, seeing Kathleen struggle with balance, speech, vision, fatigue, and other adverse effects of the tumor. Caring deeply, all of us went through the grieving process, initially denying it was happening. Then, we moved into the anger stage, before trying to bargain with God to make her better. Fortunately, we never moved into the acceptance stage, because there was more hope for Kathleen to recover than any of us ever dreamed possible.

I HAD ONE more surgery on my lumbar shunt six days after Dr. Long installed the medium pressure valve. After I felt its failure, Dr. Long replaced it with a low pressure valve, the last option available. He was avoiding the inevitable, having to put in a ventriculo-peritoneal (VP) shunt. He admitted he feared doing this because of the condition of my ventricles. Their size would make it almost impossible to feed a shunt into one of them without causing further brain damage. He also knew, however, it would help me. The lumbar drain was not draining properly because of gravitational forces.

The trauma from undergoing five surgeries in five weeks was taking a toll on my body. Before the fourth lumbar shunt revision, I had my first seizure in over five months. I was in bed, then the next thing I knew I was on the floor near the bed and Carol was trying to get me to respond. I was flooded with emotions. Of all things to happen, I didn't want to add this burden to the Kampen's plate. It was already full. I couldn't remember if I had prepared them to know what to do if I had a seizure.

I was tired, but not completely exhausted as I am after really bad seizures. I tried to stay as alert as possible, so as not to scare Carol, but my emotions took over. I began to cry. It was a culmination of all I endured and my fear that I wasn't even close to having it be over. Feeling the effects of the seizure was a dramatic reminder of the reality of my condition.

Before my next appointment, Dr. Long asked Dr. Hanley to join us. Unlike most doctors who leave the exam room when wanting to consult with another doctor, Dr. Long and Dr. Hanley sat on both sides of me, and included me in their discussion. I felt so thankful to have such down-to-earth doctors, who were also the best in the world. They were trying to decide whether we had reached the point where the benefits of a VP shunt outweighed the risks. Given the tiny size of my ventricles, it was going to be difficult for Dr. Long to locate them, without having to probe multiple times through my brain. The risk of brain damage was high, and there was no certainty the shunt would relieve my headache.

Both doctors saw what the pain was doing to me. The quality of my life was very low and would only deteriorate more as the pain persisted. With my consent, they decided to go ahead with the surgery. While I appreciated their careful consideration of all factors, I was ready for the next step. I was ready to be relieved of pain.

Dr. Long asked his nurses and assistant to make the arrangements for my admission and surgery. It was Monday. They said I'd be admitted Thursday, for surgery on Friday. This would give me a few days to prepare mentally and also allow time for my brother to get a flight to Baltimore to be with me. After discussing the practicality of traveling, my family decided it'd be best for Lamar to come. This was a big relief for me, as well as Carol.

Carol was starting to feel the pressure of being the care giver for two "family members." Even though I wasn't really a member of her family, there was no difference in the way she cared for me. Not only was she caring for two, she was caring for two who were faced with very critical conditions. Even though she'd still be waiting while I was in surgery, Lamar's presence would relieve her feeling of complete responsibility.

Before leaving the clinic, I asked Mary Kay about Kathleen's condition. She was very concerned and tried to call Dr. Solomon, Kathleen's neurosurgeon, before I left the exam room. She left a message for him to call her, wanting to tell him about Kathleen's condition, so he might initiate an evaluation of her status. I prayed something could be done to help Kathleen and thanked Mary Kay for her intervention.

Prior to this, I was terrified to have a shunt in my brain. This fear went all the way back to when Dr. Cilluffo recommended it. There were people who were strategically placed along my journey who had VP shunts. This allowed me to talk with them about it. Kathleen had a VP shunt. A few years prior to the discovery of her tumor, she was diagnosed with hydrocephalus. The VP shunt corrected her problem, without complication.

I was about to adopt another new mechanical device into my body, remembering it would only be a piece of me, by no means the whole.

Twenty-Three

More Mountains To Climb

Adversity introduces a woman to herself.

Anonymous

I T HAD BEEN FIVE months since Dr. Long had sealed my CSF leak. The success of this surgery prevailed, despite my uncertainty about the ongoing problem with CSF pressure. The best way for me to prepare for brain surgery number six was to pray. Each morning I went to Mass and prayed to God for His peace.

Over the previous two weeks I had experienced a few breakthrough seizures and was worried about having a seizure on the operating table. My prayer was answered. While on my knees before my heavenly Father, I realized that never before had my faith been stronger. My faith had moved from my head to my heart. Too often our mind forgets the love, hope, and promise of our Savior; while our heart never forgets. Before my head injury, my mind knew who Jesus was. Now, my heart had a relationship with Him.

My surgery was scheduled for early Friday morning. Lamar came to my room at 6:00 a.m. This gave us time to talk before I was taken to the OR. Carol also came to be with me and to wait during surgery with Lamar. When she arrived, she relayed a message to me. I received roses from a friend a few days before surgery. There was one white one among several red. As she was leaving home she noticed only one rose had opened so far, the white one. Without saying anymore, I got the message, hope.

As I was wheeled to the OR, I prayed for God to guide Dr. Long's hands while he fed the shunt into my ventricle; and for a positive outcome in its effectiveness of ridding me of my headache. I hummed the lyrics to a song that goes, "...and He walks with me, and He talks with me, and He tells me I'm not alone." I pictured myself looking into the face of Jesus, and He had a most comforting, huge smile. In response to my thought, as my gurney came to a stop near the OR, a big smile came over my face. Just at that time Keith walked up. "Don't you ever stop smiling?" he asked.

"Not unless I have reason to," I responded. Given the scope of God's love, I believed there were no valid reasons, only ones we created. As it says in Luke 12:22,23,25, "Therefore, I tell you, do not worry about your life, what you will eat; or about your body, what you will wear. Life is more than food and the body more than clothes...Who of you by worrying can add a single hour to his life?"

While waiting in the holding area, I asked Keith only one question. "How do they get the shunt threaded all the way down to my abdomen from my brain?"

Keith's answer was simple, "You don't want to know."

I said, "I can only imagine how barbaric it appears."

"Your imagination is probably pretty accurate."

During surgery a piece of my skull was removed and the shunt was fed through my brain, into my brain's ventricle. Because my ventricles were so small, Dr. Long decided to use the three dimensional, frameless stereotactis, which he normally used to locate tumors. This was the first time he used it for a shunt placement, but his theory proved effective. Instead of having to randomly find the ventricle, this instrument gave him the ability to find the best course for the ventricular puncture on his first attempt.

The shunt was then fed beneath the scalp, down the back of my head and neck, around to the front of my neck, and down through my body. An incision was made just below my neckline, to secure the shunt from any movement. From there, it was fed down the middle of my chest, to the right of my sternum, and tied down through another incision as it met the peritoneum, my abdominal cavity. This was where CSF would drain, and eventually be absorbed back into my system.

A VP shunt performs much like a lumbar shunt, draining CSF out of the spinal canal, into the abdominal cavity. The difference is the VP shunt originates in the brain, whereas the lumbar shunt originates in the lower back. During this operation, Dr. Long also clamped my LP shunt again, so it didn't interfere with the effectiveness of the new VP shunt.

When I woke up in recovery, I felt as though I had been hit by a truck. My head didn't hurt half as much as my neck, chest, and abdomen. All I could think of was my last conversation with Keith. I imagined them using a big hollow pipe with a sharp tip on the end and ramming it through my body beneath my skin. I was quite sure this was the case, and I felt every inch of tissue damage.

I thought I knew what to expect when I regained consciousness after surgery. Carol and Kathleen told me about her surgery and Kathleen's biggest complaint was having to lay flat for twenty-four hours after surgery. "Other than that," she said, "the discomfort was minimal."

It was times like this, when feeling incredible pain, that I felt like Piglet, when he says to Winnie the Pooh, "Pooh?..." followed by silence. Pooh responds, "What is it?," only to have Piglet say, "Oh nothing, I just want to be sure of you." I found myself saying, "God?...," wanting to be sure He was still with me. Most often, when at a loss for words, I need not say anything. God reads my heart. I often needed reassurance of God's presence, but I never had to go very far to get it.

After they returned me to my room, I was told to remain still, though it was not mandatory for me to remain flat, as Kathleen had described. I didn't mind the request to remain still, since movement of any kind was quite uncomfortable. It hurt my chest to laugh, cough, and sneeze. Each time I felt the urge I grabbed my pillow and held it to my chest, trying to cushion the pain.

Lamar's presence gave me tremendous support. He was able to stay until I was discharged to the Kampen's. He knew I was going to be okay under their protective care.

Shortly after my discharge, I began experiencing more seizures. There seemed to be a pattern. They happened more frequently at night while I was in bed. I was becoming terrified of going to bed at night. Carol called Hopkins several times, to get advice on how to help me. Each time a

different resident made recommendations, without any form of communication to other residents or to Dr. Long and Dr. Hanley. Prescriptions
were called into the pharmacy, without consulting my medical records.
One increased my Phenobarbital dosage. Another added a second anti-
convulsant, Klonopin, to my prescription. A third resident added Ativan,
to abort seizures.

After I was given the first increase in Phenobarbital, I was no longer
able to clearly evaluate my need to streamline my care and the prescribing
of medications.

The seizures became more frequent, often in multiples, and on two
occasions going into status epilepticus (a continuous string of seizures).
The more seizures I had, the more the residents increased the amount of
Phenobarbital and Klonopin I was taking. I went from taking 90mg of
Phenobarbital twice per day to 120mg four times each day.

This still didn't control the frequency of the seizures, and the side
effects were incapacitating. I was so sedated I couldn't talk or walk straight.
Never had I been so terrified. I was afraid to close my eyes, for fear of
having a seizure. I noticed frequent jerks and muscle twitches, which scared
the daylights out of me, fearing it was the onset of a seizure. (It was the
side effects of the drugs.) I had always said my greatest fear was of the
unknown. Seizures had a way of intertwining what was known and what
was unknown to exceed all fears. I knew I would have a seizure, but I had
no idea when.

M EANWHILE, MARY KAY had talked with Dr. Solomon, prompting
him to order an MRI for Kathleen. The MRI detected hydrocephalus. Her VP shunt had ceased to function and needed to be replaced.
This was the reason she was having so many problems. Within ten days of
my VP shunt surgery, Kathleen had VP shunt replacement surgery. Her
surgery went very smoothly.

I went with Carol to visit Kathleen at Hopkins one day, but found
myself very fatigued. I needed my usual midday nap. So I laid down on
the couch in the patient lounge on Meyer 8, only a short distance from
Kathleen's room. The room was full of family members of a patient and
they were talking very loud. I attempted to block some of the noise by

covering my head with a pillow. Sometime thereafter, the room must have emptied and someone else walked into the room. They saw me laying on the floor next to the couch, with my head on the pillow. It seemed odd. The visitor asked Krista, a nurse, if I usually slept on the floor. Since my head was still shaved, a new visitor couldn't have known if I was a patient or a visitor. Krista knew me, but didn't know if I might have chosen to take a nap on the floor. She went to ask Carol. Carol immediately surmised I had had a seizure, and ran to help me.

One minute I was taking a nap, the next minute I was in a hospital bed, admitted a few doors down from Kathleen's room. I was admitted for observation, with the hope of getting me into the Epilepsy Monitoring Unit (EMU) to determine the origins of my seizures.

The EMU would not be available until two days later, so I spent time with Kathleen, trying to get her out of bed and mobile. She did very well the first day after her surgery, but from that point on she went downhill again. One evening, while I was in Kathleen's room, the residents came in and were talking about discharging her the next day. They hadn't even seen Kathleen out of bed. She was off balance when trying to walk. She had remained in the hospital for the protocol number of postsurgical days, and so they thought it was time to send her home. I knew there was no way Kathleen should be sent home. She couldn't even stand up on her own. I was furious with their negligence.

The next morning at 6:00 a.m., I made sure I got up before the residents made their rounds. I went into Kathleen's room, woke her up and said, "Kathleen, want to go for a walk with me?" At this point Kathleen was clueless about what was happening around her. For all she knew it was 6:00 p.m.

I hung onto Kathleen and started walking down the hall. Rhoda, one of our nurses, saw us and rushed over to help me. I said, "Rhoda, they're planning to send her home today. Do you think she's ready?"

Rhoda quickly called to the residents who were standing around the nurses' station. She said, "Dr. Davis, I think you better come evaluate one of your patients." Once he saw Kathleen out of bed, trying to walk, he decided not to send her home. It was then determined she needed to go back into surgery. They found that the catheter of her shunt had a kink in it and was malfunctioning.   Once she had a fully-operating VP shunt, Kathleen was on her way to complete recovery.

MEANWHILE, MY CONDITION was marginal.   I was given two medications to help reduce my headache, Visteral and Tylox.   Tylox was a class two narcotic and the Visteral was a muscle relaxer, used in this situation to increase the effectiveness of Tylox.   They were effective in controlling my pain, but it was also very risky.   I was given this combination every four hours, along with my anti-convulsant medication, Phenobarbital.   I tolerated the Phenobarbital for several years, until the variables were changed.   I tried desperately to keep myself on top of things, and stay aware of my condition, but failed miserably.   It wasn't as though I was trying to hide my poor condition from others.   I truly believed I was fine, except for having more seizures and an occasional blunder.

It was a Saturday, the day they were going to move me into the EMU. Carol's mother, Anne Groff, and sister Pat Sullivan, whom I had come to know quite well and felt connected to as family, came to visit Kathleen and me.   I had just stepped out of the shower when they arrived.   I was standing in front of the mirror, next to the bathroom door, putting lotion on. Timing was everything.   At the same time I lost my balance, falling against the bathroom door which then swung open, they opened the door to my room.   There I was, toppling in front of them, stark naked.   I'll never forget the looks on all of their faces.   I'm confident they reflected the look I had on my face—utter surprise and panic.   Carol caught me, quickly reacting in her most lighthearted and gentle way.   I only remember two words being said while this happened, "Oh my!"   While the others backed up and shut the door, so I wouldn't also flash the people in the hallway, Carol made sure my balance was restored.

Later that afternoon, Carol, Ken, Pat, and Mom Groff decided to take Kathleen and I down to the Saturday afternoon Mass on the lower level of the hospital.   I don't have a clear memory of doing this.   I remember only two things: having the desire to go and seeing a room packed with people.

The first time I became aware of my instability was when a comment was made a week later about going to Mass at the hospital and I couldn't recall going.   I started to worry about what was happening to me.

Later that evening, I was placed in the EMU. They first hooked me to the EEG monitor, which was a rather lengthy task. Thirty-two electrodes placed around my entire scalp would detect fluctuations in voltage in different areas of my brain. These electrodes remained intact for the duration of my stay, three days. I was restricted to bed and had a video camera pointing at me at all times.

I went nuts. I felt extremely claustrophobic. No longer was I at peace with submitting myself to the medical care system. I was flaming mad as I pleaded with God, "Why do I have to do this?"

I was literally tied down. I couldn't talk to others, unless they came to me. I had to use the bed pan, which made me very uncomfortable physically, because of my incessant struggle to relieve myself. It was very unpleasant not to be able to take a shower. All things considered, I was not happy with these feelings, even though I knew it was a valuable opportunity to study my seizure disorder. I tried very hard to convince myself to calm down, but was unsuccessful. I stuffed all my rage inside and felt like a ticking time bomb.

There are very few Epilepsy Monitoring Units in the country, thus there was always a long waiting list of patients to be studied. The circumventing factors blindfolded me. I should have been thankful for the opportunity to be studied. All I could think of was my discomfort. I was getting tired of having to put up with all the medical procedures, tests, pains and inconveniences.

My reaction to being in the EMU took me by complete surprise. Previously, I talked with patients who were in the EMU, but I was oblivious to what they were experiencing. Even though I knew what took place, I never considered what it might feel like to be in the EMU.

While I was in the unit, a neuropsychologist started testing me. He gave me the same test as Glen Johnson Ph.D. had given me soon after my injury. I knew the testing procedure all too well. The amount of energy it required hadn't changed. It was a very laborious, fatiguing test. Because of this, he needed to administer it over two days. I was pleased to have the opportunity to repeat the test. These results could then be compared to my previous test results. While hoping to see improvements, I surmised we'd see a decline in my cognitive abilities. I felt as though I had adjusted well to my initial deficits, but it seemed as though some of these modifications were no longer intact. This should have been another clue for me to recognize something was wrong.

During my three days in the unit I didn't have a seizure. This was quite often the case for other patients, too. Therefore, they were unable to obtain any information about my seizure disorder. There was another patient scheduled for the EMU, so they needed to move me to a regular room. I had one more day left of cognitive testing before they'd discharge me.

Dr. Krauss, the neurologist in charge of the EMU, suggested they put me on the EMU schedule for a later date. He was still very interested in monitoring me, with the hopes of determining how to better control my seizures. Unfortunately, I'd have to wait another four weeks to do this.

I have very little memory of the next two and a half months, except for significant events and predominant feelings. My parents drove from Florida to visit me when they heard my condition had deteriorated since the VP shunt surgery. My sister, Kay, flew into Baltimore at the same time.

I remember having the feeling of being "safe" at the Kampen's home and wanting Kay to stay there with me. Much of what I know about what happened during this time was recreated by stories told to me. Kay told me how I pleaded with her to take care of me, telling her of my terrifying fear of the future. Like a two year old afraid of the dark, I was scared to shut my eyes for fear of a seizure. I knew there was something terribly wrong with me, but was incapable of any logical thought.

The astonishing element of this period is that I talked sensibly and was able to care for my personal needs. I was capable of giving directions to a movie theater to my father, remembering correctly how to get there in this strange town. Yet, I didn't remember doing this or being there.

On the outside it appeared as though I was not completely disabled, yet on the inside my brain had shut down many of its primary functions. No one was aware of this, including me.

During this time, an episode happened concerning my career that devastated me. First I was told I needed to go on the disability insurance policy, which meant my income was going to drop 40 percent. I knew this was coming. Then, on the day after I was told that my job was secure, I was told my job was being eliminated. The next day I was again told it was secure. I didn't know what to believe, but I had a suspicion it was going to be eliminated.

I was frantic. How could they do this to me? I had been one of their most loyal employees, giving my energy to them even in the midst of my recovery. This was a royal slap in my face.

I knew the loss of my job, due to my disability, was inevitable. Yet I was devastated. I was about to lose a job that at one point meant more to me than anything else. My reaction revealed that my career was still higher on my priority list than it should have been. I still didn't have the ability to let go of all things. If anything was going to send me off the deep end, it was going to be the threat of losing my job. It was my identity. Losing it seemed to equate to the world coming to an end.

The longer I remained in Maryland, however, the more I was learning that my identity was very separate from my career. All the doctors, nurses, staff, patients, and families I met knew me only as Karen Wells, patient. Most knew nothing more than this. Only a few knew of my competitive success or my occupation. It made no difference to them. Those who knew of my background treated me no differently than those who didn't. This made a big impression on me. I've always made sure to treat everyone the same, no matter what their career, race, gender, or age.

It was interesting to watch the reactions of other people, when they saw me talking with three or four of the housekeeping staff while they ate their lunch in the patient lounge. Some people wouldn't have associated with the staff. I enjoyed talking and laughing with them. Some of my most memorable conversations were with Sheila and Reggie, two very dedicated housekeepers. They were valuable care givers.

I'll never forget the first day I met Sheila. It had only been about a week after a craniotomy. Sheila came in to clean my room, took one look at me, and started laughing. Even though I knew she was laughing at me, I appreciated the joy she brought with her. It was the day I found out I was still leaking. My spirits needed a lift, though it was going to take a crane. When Sheila saw my funny haircut, her reaction was genuine. Only a small patch on the back of my head was left. I couldn't help but laugh with her and tease her for laughing at me. Our friendship blossomed from there.

I treated every person the same, unlike the chicken man, a patient at the same time. This man was caught in an identity trap. His identity wasn't a license to treat people poorly. I was turned off by the mood surrounding this man, undoubtedly because of his success. I didn't believe I had reached this extreme, but the thought of its potential concerned me.

I was banking all of these experiences. They paid great dividends. Observation with an open mind was a great investment.

M Y PARENTS AND Kay left just before I was readmitted to the EMU. It was difficult to see them go, especially when I wasn't looking forward to my return to the unit. I knew exactly what to expect this time, and would have to endure it for an entire week.

I experienced the same abundance of feelings as the first time, despite my preparation. Several of the nurses helped reduce my emotional uneasiness by stopping into my room to visit. Even though many weren't assigned to my room, they enjoyed talking with me. Once they heard I was struggling, they made a point to stop more frequently.

Jennifer came to my rescue one day, bringing with her peace beyond human understanding. She helped me immensely while I was at Hopkins. She went the extra mile, caring for my emotional and spiritual well-being.

The day after I was admitted, after hearing of my distress, Jennifer arrived to cheer me up, encouraging me to hang in there for the sake of the test. It was so good to talk with her. I felt as though I wasn't going to make it through even the first day. She made a list for me of pros and cons of being in the EMU. We talked about how they impacted me and what my options were. She emphasized prayer and said, "Keep writing those letters to God." I told her I wondered what prayer looked like on the EEG monitor. I hoped it wasn't all question marks, but plus signs symbolizing confidence.

God took care of me that day, making sure my support team surrounded me. After Jennifer left, the Kampens arrived. Not more than five minutes after they left, Patti Hennrick, my friend and coworker at Munson, surprised me. She had been at a convention in Baltimore and made a point to take time to visit me. It felt so good to have a friend from home visit. It helped me feel more connected to all who supported me from Munson. It had been three-and-a-half months since I was home, such a long time to be gone.

After Patti left, Carla and Susan came. I recognized how awful the day began and the difference in my perception once friends surrounded me with love. I began feeling guilty, asking God why I felt terrible, even after being surrounded with wonderful friends at such a needy time.

Later, I received a special note from Patti. She wrote, "To actually experience your positive attitude through this whole ordeal, witness your love, concern for others, and in turn everyone's love and concern for you, was such a positive experience for me. You are truly in a caring place, surrounded by good people, and as someone who cares about you, it was very comforting to see." To know others recognized my positive attitude, and were moved by seeing how I survived, warmed my heart. It meant even more knowing how negative I was feeling, yet my positive attitude still prevailed.

The next day was Jennifer's day off work, but she came to see me anyway. She arrived with a couple bags in her hands. She said, "I brought some entertainment with me, but before I reveal the contents, I want to ask your attending nurse if I can temporarily detach you from the monitor." When she returned, she said, "No problem, let's go." I asked where we were going. She said, "To the chapel to pray, and I'll tell you when we're down there what my idea is."

This was such a wonderful gesture. I couldn't think of any other place I'd rather be. On our way to the chapel, I talked to her about my frustrations of the EMU. It was so good to be able to get these feelings out. Then Jennifer told me her plan. We were both going to kneel and pray beside one another in the chapel. While I prayed for my healing and peace, she was at the same time going to pray for my prayers to be answered. I loved this idea.

We entered the empty chapel, knelt down, and prayed our hearts out. Tears filled my eyes, as love and peace filled my heart. I had pleaded with God daily to heal me, strengthen me, and grant me His peace. I had never, however, had someone, knowingly beside me, solely for the purpose to ask God to answer my prayers.

This was a clear demonstration of what was happening all over the country, with other friends and family members. I never went anywhere without someone saying to me, "I'm praying for you."

We returned to the EMU and Jennifer plugged me back into the monitor. Then, one by one, she pulled items from the bags. First, she pulled out a book with only blank pages, for journal writing. She knew I enjoyed writing, and also knew the importance of getting feelings out and not harboring them. Then, she pulled out two posters of wolves, and began taping them to the walls of my room. Next was a video tape of "The Lion King." I hadn't seen it yet. She was very inspired by the underlying messages of the movie and thought it appropriate for me to see.

Next came audio tapes of the Celestine Prophesy. And, since my walkman's headphones were broke, she brought me a new pair of headphones. I couldn't believe all that she had done. She went to a lot of work to do this. I could tell it was all very well thought out and came from deep within her heart. The gesture alone lifted my spirits, and then I enjoyed each of her gifts.

S EVERAL RESIDENT DOCTORS came into the EMU to check on me. I was not familiar with the neurology residents, only the neurosurgical residents. There was a nurse or technician sitting in front of the monitors of all four EMU rooms at all times. They watched the EEG monitors for suspicious abnormalities in the brains of four patients. It was consoling to know they were ready to respond if I had a seizure.

There were additional monitors at the nurse's station, where they could watch with a corner of their eye. I teased them about hooking me up to the monitor by saying, "You weren't getting enough of me. You had to hook me up so you could watch me twenty-four hours a day."

Dr. Krauss came in each day to check on my status. He was one of the only doctors I didn't like. His arrogance turned me off. Even Dr. Cilluffo's arrogance didn't turn me off as much as Dr. Krauss'. At least Dr. Cilluffo was nice. Dr. Krauss was not nice. This contributed to my feelings of isolation while in the EMU. He treated me like his little prisoner, a guinea pig.

I didn't remember much of the day to day affairs that happened during the first few days of my stay in the EMU. I still, however, remembered significant events and my feelings during this time. I remembered being on the verge of tears most every time someone came to talk with me. No matter what I did or what they said, I was overcome with emotion. It was as if I felt I was being punished, sent to my room, and told I couldn't come out for a week. My ability to abstract reason was impaired from my brain injury and thus I knew the purpose for my being there, but it made no sense when reasoning in all the variables. I lost the whole concept of being in the EMU.

When a psychiatrist started coming to my room to talk with me, I realized he thought I was crazy. I was outraged by the questions he asked, "Did your father ever have sex with you? Did your mother ever beat you? Did they do any of this to your siblings? Did your father beat you or your mother?"

I must have just stared at him with my mouth hanging open. I couldn't believe what I was hearing. I had just been to hell and back in six years with a head injury, and he couldn't have cared less about that issue. Throughout my entire recovery I focused only on the positive. I created opportunity from hardship, maintained a positive attitude and grew in faith. I never complained, just persevered. I never asked, "Why me?" I said, "Why not me?" Now someone was trying to analyze me by looking through an entirely different set of lenses, negative ones. He was at the opposite end of the spectrum. No, there was no abuse in my family. In fact, we were showered with love, just as surely as our Lord waters the vegetation of the earth. It was because of this foundation my parents built, I was able to withstand adversity. It was disturbing to have someone attempting to pick it apart.

He didn't ask about my faith. To him this meant nothing. Each time I answered his question by talking of my faith, he repeated the question, as if my answer was invalid. When he finally left my room, he stated his need to talk with Dr. Hawthornwaite about my case, as if I was really out to lunch and he didn't know how to proceed. Then I told him how to proceed, "There's no need for you to come back. God has everything under control." He was stunned by my comment. I was serious. I needed to protect myself emotionally, and he was intruding on my positive pathway.

I had a few seizures while in the EMU, which is what we were hoping for. Data was gathered to help Dr. Krauss make the necessary adjustments in my medications to improve my condition. It wasn't what we had expected, however. When I asked what their findings were, Dr. Krauss said, "We need to reduce your Phenobarbital." I wanted to know the physiological make-up of my seizures and he adamantly said, "You first need to work with the psychiatrist."

"What does he have to do with this?" I replied.

"You need to work out some of the psychological matters involved in your case." He was dodging the issue. He was trying to make it look like a psychological problem, while at the same time I was coming close to overdosing on the amount of Phenobarbital he and the residents of Hopkins had prescribed for me. After seeing my EEG when seizing several times, he knew very well what the problem was. Then in trying to correct his mistake, he was scared I was going to keep seizing from the gradual withdrawal of Phenobarbital.

I also got the impression that because I wasn't a candidate for his research, I wasn't going to be given the time of day. Dr. Krauss became very defensive as soon as he recognized how knowledgeable I was about my condition. He was uncomfortable with my persistence, and the more he resisted answering my questions, the more persistent I became. He didn't want to admit they had found mistakes in my medication prescription. I didn't know it at the time either, but I was smart enough to know there was a reason that he wasn't telling me.

Before any of this occurred, I already had a very low heart rate and blood pressure. When laying down and sleeping, my levels dropped dramatically. A toxic level of a barbiturate, Phenobarbital, that suppresses the central nervous and cardiorespiratory system was added to these factors, compounding my problem.

They started reducing the amount of Phenobarbital I was taking. I remember feeling nervous about this, thinking that the Phenobarbital was for the control of my seizures. Therefore, if I took less, I'd have more seizures. It was a logical conclusion. I didn't consider the danger of being at a toxic level. They kept this information quiet. I was worried about staying in the therapeutic range, and I knew 23-25 was the serum level Dr. MacKenzie desired for me. I kept asking the residents if they were going to test my blood and measure my Phenobarbital level, but I never got a precise answer. When blood tests were run, I'd ask what the Phenobarbital results showed; they never knew. I thought this was strange. As it turned out, they knew all along what it was. They were smart enough to know that if they told me my level was in the 90s I'd go ballistic.

After my parents left Baltimore, right before I was readmitted to the EMU, they had second thoughts about leaving. They were half way home, had driven over 600 miles, and decided to turn around and come back to be with me. They were frightened by my condition when they left, and the only way they could regain some peace of mind was to be with me. Although it was a helpless feeling to see me, they felt better being with me. They wanted to make sure they were available in case there was something they could do to help. I was so glad to see them. I only had a few more days left in the EMU, but their presence made both days much easier. By the time they arrived, my Phenobarbital level had started to come down, allowing me to be more aware of what was happening around me.

I was discharged the day after I was moved from the EMU to a regular room on Meyer 8. My parents took me back to the Kampen's, where I'd remain until my follow-up appointments were completed. Within a week I was again in a state where I lost an entire four weeks. I have no memory, no awareness, not a clue, about what transpired during this time; yet, I talked and made sense most of the time. I have no memory of my last three weeks at the Kampen's.

The next memory I have is after I returned home to Traverse City, Michigan. I can recall only tiny bits of my actions. I had a cloudy memory of going to bed at my neighbor's house, being taken into our new church for the dedication, and my parents being at my house. These three things are the only memory I have of my first week home. I couldn't even say what I felt, it's as if I was comatose.

People have told me stories of events that transpired. After being discharged from Hopkins and returning to the Kampen's home, I was told to take 120mg of Phenobarbital twice each day and 3mg of Klonopin. I thought I had this under control, but something went terribly wrong. This level of Phenobarbital, when mixed with the Klonopin, was still too much for me. Although it appeared to others I was operating semi-efficiently, my brain was under severe cognitive distress. My accuracy of taking the appropriate amount of medication was affected, thus I was no doubt taking more than the prescribed amount. It took a week for me to hit rock bottom.

Carol took me back and forth to Hopkins several times to see various doctors. Dr. Poppagallo was a specialist in chronic pain. He wanted to try DHE, an intravenous medication, which often helps break the cycle of pain receptors. The only problem was he couldn't admit me until May. I was stoned on Phenobarbital the day I saw him and he said come back in three weeks. I suppose since it appeared I felt no pain he didn't see the urgency of treating me. The only doctor I did not see during this time was Dr. Long. Why these doctors didn't readmit me and get my medication back on track I'll never know. I should have never been discharged until my Phenobarbital level was normal. It may have appeared I could take care of myself, but I couldn't. I'm sure my confident personality stepped forward and convinced them I could manage on my own. At this point, there were too many doctors involved in my case. Dr. Long was out of the country, and I was at the mercy of doctors who were not my primary caregivers. The doctor I needed most was Dr. MacKenzie, and he was a thousand miles away.

The Kampens made a critical decision, which was very difficult for them to make, but became my link to reversing my condition. They put me on a flight to Traverse City, via Chicago, where Dr. MacKenzie could take care of me.

I later heard stories of things I did during this time. Some of them I'm able to figure out why, while others remain a mystery. One obsessive behavior was buying books. I collect books, and fortunately the ones I chose are ones I'll read someday. However, the amount of books I bought should last me a lifetime. Whether I sensed my diminished level of cognition, or my need for inspiration and guidance, I'll never know.

I didn't have any idea where my desire to go roller-skating came from, except that some of my behaviors during this time were elementary. I hadn't gone roller-skating since grade school. Carol said I was quite insistent with my desire to go.

I also had an obsession with a pastry called a bagel knot. I remember frequently eating them while at the Kampen's. The story goes that I wanted to take one on the plane to eat for breakfast, along with cranberry juice. The day I flew home, I was wearing a new outfit I had purchased the week before. My new white pants had pin stripes. Carol said she helped me board the plane in the wheelchair, and got me settled in my seat. She told the flight attendant I needed assistance with everything. I was not capable of walking on my own. They had already arranged for a wheelchair to meet me in Chicago to take me to my next flight. During the flight, I must have tried to drink my cranberry juice and missed my mouth. It spilled down the front of me, permanently dyeing my white pin stripe pants pink. Instead of eating the bagel knot, I was determined to take it home and show it to our local bagel shop manager, so he might consider making them.

I made it to Traverse City, where my dear friend Dosie was awaiting my arrival. On our way home she stopped at the bagel shop, which coincidentally was exactly where I wanted to go first. I took the bagel knot in and showed the manager. He was not interested. Dosie told me I said to him, "You're really missing your chance to hit it big with this." (I have no memory of doing this.) Several weeks later, when in the bagel shop and back on my feet again, I casually mentioned to the manager that I had eaten a bagel knot and he might consider making them. He looked at me very strangely and said, "Yes, you brought one in and showed me." I didn't remember, and was embarrassed. I didn't ask him what else I said to him.

I don't remember Dosie staying with me for several days, until I went to my neighbors for the weekend. It was extremely frightening for my friends at home to have me return in this condition. They had minimal information of what transpired at Hopkins and truly believed my condition was permanent. They began grieving the loss of the Karen they once knew, and started trying to accept me in this severely disabled condition. Each of them rallied to help me, thankful for my return home, yet angry at the physicians at Hopkins who had caused this problem. When I had left for Hopkins five months ago, I suffered from a severe headache, but at least my condition had been stable.

Dosie took me to see the movie "While You Were Sleeping." I slept through the entire movie. I don't remember going to the theater. I saw it again several months later and it didn't strike the tiniest cord of memory at all. Dosie's husband, Steve, and their children came over to see us that night. I had never met Steve before. I still have not met Steve.

All of us carried on as though this was a permanent condition. There was no way to know that it wasn't. I was clueless, having absolutely no ability to reason things out or to evaluate my situation. I did seek ways to maintain control, and still manage my care. For example, I must have made an appointment with my optometrist in Traverse City because I was having difficulty seeing. I had double vision. It was primarily drug induced. Once I was back to normal the double vision went away. Currently, I only have a slight problem in changing from one focus to another.

My inhibitions were down. During this time, I made phone calls to my brother, telling him feelings and opinions I never would have revealed to him otherwise. They were about him and my dissatisfaction with some of his behaviors. Having no idea the condition I was in, he was greatly offended.

The only other person this happened with, to my knowledge, was Dosie. I pray that Lamar and Dosie were the only ones I said things to that I normally wouldn't say. Thankfully, they both were very understanding. I never would do anything to hurt either of them.

Several weeks later I found out that I showed anger towards Dosie for attempting to control my medications. For some reason, I was very protective of my medications. I suspect I was reverting back to my old need for control, knowing I was losing control.

There may also have still been a fear of seizures and fear of my anticonvulsant medication being taken away. When Dosie was getting ready to leave and I needed to go next door to Ron and Gloria's, I became resistive. I was confident I could take care of myself. Fortunately, Gloria came over and helped Dosie. She helped reduce my desire to stay home, getting me to consent to go to their house.

My weekend with Ron and Gloria was quite an event. We've since spent many evenings on the back deck, reminiscing. With their medical knowledge, they suspected my condition was medication related. They knew, however, they couldn't change my dosages without a physician. While they knew my condition was critical, they also knew they could protect me until I could be seen by Dr. MacKenzie. So at my expense, which was nothing, they had fun with me.

Gloria knew I didn't eat meat, but made a meatloaf for dinner. When serving the meatloaf, she asked if I wanted some. I said, "Yes, what is it?"

She said, "Meatloaf."

While eating my meatloaf, I again asked, "What is this?"

"Meatloaf."

"It doesn't taste like my mother's meatloaf." The funny thing was, I had no sense of taste. I was probably expecting to taste something, but didn't. So of course it didn't taste like mother's. Five minutes later I asked again what it was.

For the third time Gloria said, "Meatloaf, do you want more?" I told her I did and I made sure she knew I wanted the biggest piece.

There was a different side of me revealed. Like the roller-skating request, my actions one night at the Hodgins took me back to my elementary days. One evening I decided I wanted to go to my house and watch a video. I asked Gloria if it was okay to do this. She said, "No. Why don't you stick around here with us tonight?" She didn't want me out of her sight.

I walked away and went to Ron and said to him, "Ron, is it okay if I go over to my house and watch a video tonight?" I was just like a teenager. Mom told me no, so I asked Dad.

On Saturday, Gloria decided to take me shopping downtown and to lunch. Of course, I wanted to go to no other place than...the bookstore. I was having a very difficult time standing and walking on my own, so Gloria assisted me. In Horizon Bookstore I kept putting my hand down on the book display in the front of the store. Many of the books on the edges of the tables were half on and half off the table. Each time I put my hand down, the whole stack of books fell to the ground. Gloria picked them up as I placed my hand somewhere else, knocking down yet another stack.

I was like a bull in a china shop. I can only imagine how this comedy act appeared. She finally got me to the rear of the store, where I couldn't do as much damage—although I proceeded to do more damage to my credit card. Once again, I bought more books than I ever could afford— or needed.

Our next stop was the drug store. While in Maryland I bought lots of make-up, more than I'd ever use in a lifetime. I've never been one to use a lot of make-up, and why I was using lots during this time I'll never know. I was determined to buy lipstick and nail polish, not just one, but five, almost one of every color. I also wanted red pump shoes. I'm very glad we didn't find any.

When we stopped to pick up my prescriptions at Sixth St. Drugs, Gloria thought it might help me if I had a walker. This helped me get around more easily, without needing as much assistance.

The next day was Feast of Victory's dedication of our newly-constructed church. I was determined to attend. I wanted to see my church family, the people who had showered me with cards, prayers, love, support, and encouragement. I couldn't imagine having to go through life without them.

John and Judy Block offered to take me to both Sunday worship and the dedication. I'm sure I was excited to see all my friends from church, after being away for so long. So much had happened while I was gone, including my friends Mark and Karen Klug having their baby. We were in the same small group ministry. This group was my Traverse City family, and experiencing their pregnancy along with them built my anticipation. Then I left and missed the first four months of baby Paul's life. I'm sure meeting him was a priority for me.

Many people were shocked to see me in such poor condition. They were heartbroken. They had no idea I was in this condition until I came through the doors of the church with my walker. I don't remember doing this, but I was told that during the announcements after church, I stood up and said a few words. I said, "I'm not sure if I'll be able to get through this without crying, but I'd like to thank everyone for their overwhelming support during my stay at Hopkins. I am very thankful for all that you've done for me. I couldn't have done it without you. Thank you."

Several weeks later, when we were finally able to look back at this time and laugh, people were teasing me about what I did in church. Pastor Jim said, "You really impressed the Bishop when you hopped on the alter and started dancing without any clothes on. Then Ruth Schnurr said to me, "You did a nice job of thanking everyone for their support during church."

I thought she was also teasing me and said, "Yea right."

She said, "No, truly, you did stand up and thank everyone." I finally believed her and appreciated having that conversation, because I was about to thank everyone again the next Sunday.

It is hard for me to understand how I could do these things, and have absolutely no memory of them. It was like a big black hole in my life. It's only from people telling stories that I've been able to put some of the pieces of the puzzle back together. I felt like an investigator at first, trying to retrace my steps. I sensed, however, I didn't want to relive each stage. The majority of it I'll never know. For example, how I got through a layover in Chicago's O'Hare Airport, without remembering being there. I suspected a lot happened at the Kampen's home that they'll never tell me about. I carry a lot of guilt for having put them through such an ordeal, but have tried to let it go, knowing I had no control then, just as I had no control after it happened.

Monday morning, when I woke up at the Hodgin's, I tried to stand up from bed and immediately crashed. I fell in such a way that they thought I might have done something to my neck, so they called for an ambulance to take me into Munson's emergency room. Head CT scans came back negative and blood tests showed a Phenobarbital serum level of 90. They sent me home. Nancy Bordine, R.N. a friend and also Home Care nurse for Munson, spent the day taking care of me. My parents were due to arrive later that day from Florida.

The first day my parents were with me I had an appointment to see Dr. Cornellier, my neurologist. She was shocked at my condition and knew I needed immediate attention. She thought I might resist being admitted to Munson, so she called Dr. MacKenzie and told him I needed to be admitted. She was also dismayed by the fact that Johns Hopkins had released me in this condition.

The next morning, when I went to take my medications I couldn't find them. This was one of the best things that could have happened. I went until that evening without taking any medication and thus my Phenobarbital levels started to come down to a more reasonable level. Dr. MacKenzie called and said he wanted to admit me to Munson. I said okay, not asking why. When a woman from the admitting office called, she asked me why I was being admitted. I couldn't answer her. I didn't know. So I called Dr. MacKenzie. He said, "I need to help you control your medications. Your

Phenobarbital level was too high. It's totally your choice whether to be admitted. I'll be honest with you Karen. I'm going to admit you to Center I, the psyche unit." I chose not to be admitted. As soon as I heard Center I, I wondered why in the world he wanted to admit me to the psyche unit. Something from Hopkins was repeating itself. I remembered thinking, "That's all I need is to be admitted to the psyche unit at the hospital where I work." I felt I could regulate my medications on my own. There was no need for someone to do this for me.

Later that evening, Nancy came by to check on me. My parents were at their wits end, wondering how they were ever going to get me to the hospital. We were still wondering where my medications were. Nancy proposed a search, figuring I had been known to put things in wrong places before. We searched the garbage, the laundry, the drawers, and cupboards. Finally, my dad found my medication in my shoes in the closet. Nancy then talked with Dr. MacKenzie to find out what dose he prescribed. He wanted me to take 120mg b.i.d., which was four tablets of Phenobarbital, twice each day.

Before Nancy left, she asked if there was anything more she could do to help. I asked her to make sure my medication box was filled correctly for the next day. She said, "Go ahead and fill it the way you think it should be filled and then I'll check it."

After filling it and giving it to Nancy, she asked me to sit down at the kitchen table with her to look at it. She wrote down what Dr. MacKenzie wanted me to take. She opened the pill box, which is divided into four areas: morning, noon, evening, and bedtime. I put four tablets in the morning box, this was right. I put four tablets in the noon box, this was wrong. I put four tablets in the evening box, this was wrong. I put another four in the bedtime box, this was right. Therefore, I would have taken twice the amount I should have taken.

No wonder I was having such a problem. This was a vicious circle, the more sedated I was the more mistakes I made, and the more sedated I'd become. I placed my head in my hands and cried. Silently I prayed, "God I need help. Please make me better." I said, "Take me to Munson. I cannot be responsible for giving myself these medications." I had been certain I was correct and I very clearly demonstrated I was wrong.

I called Dr. MacKenzie and told him I was ready to go to Munson, only if he didn't admit me to the psyche unit. My parents also spoke with him and told him under no circumstances would they let me be admitted to the psyche unit. He agreed.

It took several more hours before I was packed and ready to go to Munson. We arrived at midnight. We were met by Dr. MacKenzie. I told him of my experience filling the pill box. He assured me we'd get things straightened out.

My progress went very well and I was discharged in three days. My Phenobarbital level had dropped to the 30's and I was feeling significantly better. I was much more aware of what was happening around me and began my investigation of the previous four weeks.

From what I learned, I felt extremely thankful to have made it through such an ordeal without major injury or a real overdose. Dr. Cornellier said to me, "I've never seen anyone survive that level of Phenobarbital. You should consider yourself extremely lucky." I considered myself more than lucky. I considered myself blessed and having been protected by the hands of God. He also made sure my angels were watching over me. God still wasn't ready to let me go.

I wanted to know everything there was about this time, where I was, and what I had said and did. I knew my best source of information was going to be Carol Kampen, but I hesitated to call her. I was terrified that I might have lost them as friends. When I looked at the calendar and saw that it was the second week of May, I was ashamed that I had imposed on them for so long. I loved them dearly, and was extremely angry at myself for not having had control over the situation. I would have never forgiven myself if I had lost their friendship.

I was also afraid to find out what I had done, since I couldn't remember. This was such an uncomfortable feeling. I felt as though I had exposed myself, opening up every door and window I had. I have no idea what I showed them. Thankfully, I have lived a clean life and couldn't have shared too much out of the ordinary. I only feared I might have had a dark side, that had never been revealed before. There was a hint of this with the desire for lipstick, nail polish, and red pump shoes.

I called Carol. She was very thankful, and happy that I was doing better. I shouldn't have doubted there would be a problem between us. Her love never ends. She filled in some of the pieces for me, but left most of them in the trash. There were too many difficult memories for both of us to relive. It was time to move forward. Carol had Kathleen back, and now she had me back. That's all she cared about. This woman had just ridden two major, terrorizing roller coasters for six months. Not only had she hung on for dear life, she also hung onto Kathleen and I when we weren't capable of holding on ourselves. Her strength was invincible. Her faith was flawless. Her hope never ceased.

The trail of evidence I left during my drug-induced period was endless. Over the course of several months, I would find medication hidden in different parts of my home. I found keys in my shoes. I talked with several people who told me I had called them during this time. Many people I spoke to were scared to call me back. My friend, Mary Prange, was one of these individuals. I had called her and tried to talk, but I was severely impaired and unable to speak clearly. Like many of my friends, she thought this was a permanent condition. She avoided calling me, terrified of my condition. She didn't know how to handle it emotionally.

My phone bill and credit card statements were obvious clues. While overwhelming, it was interesting to see the pattern of my calls. The amount of money I spent was outrageous. It seemed as though I thought my condition was terminal.

After getting my mind cleared, I returned to Horizon Bookstore with a huge bag of books. I explained my story to the cashier, who said I needed to talk with the manager. I told the manager I didn't remember being in the store. Although I couldn't afford to pay for all of the books, I didn't have the receipt. She said, "Yes, I remember. I was the one who helped you. We'll be able to find a copy of your receipt and give you a refund." I was shocked when she said she had helped me. Even though I hadn't remembered being there, it was real.

When I returned home from my Munson admission, I unpacked my bag. As I unpacked, I found twelve pairs of underwear, packed in clumps of four. I must have packed three times through the course of the day when I was resisting being admitted. Each time I'd pack, I wouldn't remember what I had already placed in my bag. I also found two hair dryers, two deodorant sticks, and my sunglasses. (Of course I needed the sunglasses. I was admitted at midnight.) I guess I wanted to make sure I had clean underwear, dry hair, and didn't smell.

It was interesting to go through my Franklin Planner and read the things I wrote, the parts that were legible. My handwriting deteriorated and most things were illegible. The most interesting thing I found was a common prayer. "Now I lay thee down to sleep, I pray thee Lord my soul to keep. If I should die before I wake, I pray thee Lord my soul to take." I connected this with my strong fear of going to sleep at night. Most of the seizures happened at night, while I was in bed. Even though I wasn't aware of the reason why, I connected sleep with seizures. After reading this prayer I had written in my planner, I knew two things for sure. One, I continued to pray during this time, I hadn't lost my faith. Two, I felt vulnerable to death in my sleep.

After all this was behind me, I was given all of my medical records. As reported in my EMU reports, I wasn't getting enough oxygen to my brain, which caused an imbalance of neurotransmitters. These neurotransmitters, such as acetylcholine, norepinephrine, and dopamine are what the brain needs to function normally. In other words, my whole system was out of whack. My anti-convulsants were no longer of help to me, but were a danger to me. Once I reached the lower therapeutic range of Phenobarbital, the condition reversed itself. I gave Dr. Krauss the benefit of the doubt, and hoped it was only because of my condition he thought I was incapable of understanding the physiological explanation.

I discovered the reason why they avoided answering my questions. My blood tests showed a serum level of 90-100, a dangerously high, toxic level. My seizures were classified as generalized tonic-clonic seizures, which were eventually controlled by a therapeutic serum level of 23-25.

I also found out I had told the psychiatrist the details of my suicide attempt. Naturally, they monitored me closely, fearing I still had this tendency. They were met with great resistance, as I truly had made it beyond this level. It was all a part of my letting go and giving everything to God. They didn't understand this piece, however, not being spiritually focused.

This led them to think I was intentionally misusing my medication, which was not the case. If they had been more perceptive, and less focused on their fear, they would have been able to see I lacked the ability to correctly administer my own medication. Had the cognitive test reports been processed in a timely manner, they would have immediately seen I couldn't follow directions and was incapable of remembering. All of this explained the reactions of my physicians in Traverse City upon my return from Hopkins.

Many of the pieces fell into place when I read my records. The more I read, the more I was thankful for coming out of it as well and as quickly as I did.

Just one week following the dedication of our church, after having to use a walker and be carried out to the car, I drove to church and walked in, unassisted. Friends attending church that day knew they saw a miracle.

After going through my worst period of recovery, my parents needed time to heal. They needed both time away from me and my medical monster, and time with me to talk about what had happened. They needed to ask questions about specific situations, telling me their perspective and asking for mine. We were able to laugh at many of the events that happened, because we were beyond the tragedy. We had lived on the edge, and if one more thing had gone wrong with my medical care, we might never have been able to laugh. But, since it was behind us, and we had no control of the past, we made the most of our story telling. Just as Lyn Karol once said, "Learn to laugh at your troubles and you'll never run out of things to laugh at."

If felt good to hear them laugh. I feared they would have a difficult time recovering. It was twice as stressful for everyone who was observing my condition, than it was for me. I had no memory of it, only the frustration of not remembering. Whereas they saw everything firsthand, tormented by their fear of my disability.

My mother later shared with me some of their feelings while I was in this state. She said, "Your father and I prayed every night before we went to sleep that God would take care of you and bring you back to us. As we saw your continued deterioration we started to give up on God. We didn't think He was listening to our prayers. We even stopped praying for awhile, because we were so frustrated and doubtful. And then you made the turn-around. God taught us a lesson. Don't ever give up praying. He will always answer our prayers. We learned we needed to be more patient."

My parents are very devoted to God. They were the last people on earth I'd suspect to give up praying. This is how hopeless it seemed. They were already having conversations about whether I was going to end up in a nursing home. They would have never been able to care for me in that condition. They, too, called me their miracle child. They could not be-lieve what a turnaround I had made. All who witnessed this period in my recovery *saw* a miracle. I *experienced* it.

I BEGAN WORKING hard at giving this time in my life to God, accepting that I would never know all the pieces. There was no need to forgive myself, I hadn't had control. I did, however, need to forgive the neurolo-gists at Hopkins for leading me into a dangerous situation and then failing to get me out of it. If Dr. Long had been around and seen me in this condition, he would have made sure it was corrected.

A lesson to be learned: there can be too many hands in the mixing bowl trying to make a cake. Without effective communication and team-work, the cake is sure to flop, especially when everyone has a different recipe.

It was time for me to move forward, to put it all behind me. I'm thankful for everyone who took me under their wing and protected me until I was back in Dr. MacKenzie's care. I'm thankful I survived.

M Y JOB REMAINED an unresolved issue. While I was gone, I was trans-ferred to my disability insurance policy held for me as a manager at Munson. This meant my income dropped to sixty percent, but they still covered me with health care insurance.

During my first follow-up appointment with Dr. MacKenzie, after be-ing discharged from Munson, he indicated he would not allow me to re-turn to work. I was totally disabled. Deep down, I knew long ago that I'd never return to my job. It still didn't take away the pain of losing some-thing I once dedicated my life to. I had given myself to Munson Medical Center, even at the expense of my own health. After all I had been through,

I wasn't about to let this tear me down. I was thankful I had been able to work as long as I did. For several years, Munson was very understanding and willing to provide whatever it took to keep me as one of their managers. I always told people who asked if I was able to maintain my job, "Yes, and the checks that I receive every other week are signed, Jesus Christ."

For whatever reason, it was time to move on. It also felt as though God was telling me it was time to take care of Karen Wells for a change, balancing energy given to others. I needed to find a midpoint, a way to help others, while also taking care of myself. I remained positive, and continued to believe we must live life as though the best is yet to come.

Twenty-Four

It's Never Over

Come to me,
all you who are weary and burdened,
and I will give you rest.
Take my yoke upon you and learn from me,
for I am gentle and humble in heart,
and you will find rest for your souls.

MATTHEW 11:28-29 NIV

NOT BEING ABLE TO return to my job was another turning point in my recovery, taking me to a higher level of maturity. It took over a year of winding upward, back and forth through the dark side and the bright side, but it was a valuable climb. I was fortunate to experience this slow transition, otherwise being tagged "disabled" would have devastated me.

I loved my work. I enjoyed being a care giver, a helper, and most of all someone who inspired and motivated. My entire career was built around an inner drive to succeed. I wanted to build my department, to offer more programs, to impact people's lives, and to be recognized. It was a stronger, higher, faster mentality, that paralleled my athletic upbringing. It became my identity. But there was more to my identity than met the eye, or my consciousness.

When I was young, I learned how the characteristics of athletics would carry me through life, helping me to attain greater success. A work ethic characterized by high intensity and giving 100 percent effort would transfer over to my career. I learned this was how to reach my goals. The theory of playing with pain, "No pain no gain," was going to help me overcome greater challenges in my career and life. The concept of competition, winning and losing, was going to build character and sportsmanship.

I believe many of my athletic experiences helped me through life and through my recovery. I also believe some of them came close to hurting my life, in the same way they complicated my recovery. I've always been a goal-oriented person, but never knew how to pace myself. I always thought I had to go full throttle towards every goal, maintaining an ultra-high intensity. I operated this way in my job, and in sports.

My intensity brought success in the competitive arena. This athletic success, coupled with my intensity, was intimidating. Those who knew of my accomplishments often felt as though they didn't match up. I was like the character Pig-Pen in the Peanuts comic. A dusting of competitive intensity surrounded me wherever I went. Others could see it and feel it. Even though I had no intent for them to feel this way, no matter what I did or said to dust it away, it was always there.

When working with others to improve their fitness, I had to work hard to help them feel comfortable around me. While they admired my level of fitness, they often suspected I was going to ask and expect them to achieve the same level. They felt as though I couldn't relate to their situation, having never had a problem becoming motivated.

I lived and breathed my job. There was never a decrease in my intensity, never time to kick back and just have fun. A walk on the beach or in the woods would have been wasted time, unless of course, I was using it as part of my physical training. This began to change when I started going for hikes with my friend, Paula Helminiak. Paula took a risk the day she asked me to go out to Sleeping Bear Dunes National Park to hike along Lake Michigan. There was a time when she was intimidated by me, feeling my intensity, feeling as though she could never match up. Not only did I want to build a friendship, but I recognized the depth of Paula's knowledge and the potential to learn from her. I welcomed the opportunity to build a new friendship from our working relationship, and accepted her invitation.

It's my belief that Paula was heaven sent. We began our friendship at the time in my life when there was a great deal of uncertainty. I knew something more had to happen in my life, to get me to another level, but I didn't know what it was. If left on my own, I would probably have gone out and tried to do the Ironman Triathlon in Hawaii. Instead, I hiked with Paula, over many miles of trail, talking and taking in the peacefulness of nature.

It was within a couple months of my second craniotomy and I was still trying desperately to control my own destiny, with repeated defeats. I was attempting to manage my health care, by obtaining knowledge about my condition, while maintaining my job, and continuing to increase my success. I was trying to do it all, while recovering from a head injury and recovering from two brain surgeries.

Paula knew of my imminent demise, but was smart enough to know she would be met with great resistance if she confronted me. Instead, we walked and talked. I paid very close attention to her insights and understanding of our world and how we fit in it. I had a great deal of respect for her wisdom. In a very gentle and non-threatening way Paula guided our conversations towards that which is of great interest to her and was lacking in me, balance. I was motivated and excited to listen, but not yet ready to change.

Each time we hiked, I came away with new insight and points to ponder. Even though I wasn't ready to act on anything, I was moving in a positive direction nonetheless. I was moving up the spiral.

The more we talked and the more things happened in my recovery, the more I became aware of how to get rid of the Pig-Pen dust. I knew it was there for a long time, and always tried to get rid of it with a dust cloth rather than taking a bath. In other words, I tried to make people comfortable around me by saying things like, "You don't have to be like me," instead of uncovering who I was, by revealing my inner self.

I started looking around and recognizing others with the same intensity. I watched the stress they carried on their backs and what type of lifestyle they lived. I saw my reflection in the mirror and didn't like what I saw. The very things that I thought were good attributes, learned from athletics, had become a detriment to my life, and ultimately my recovery.

The stress created from my drive to control, my intensity to succeed, and my willingness to do anything to reach it, including playing with pain, was astronomical. It was like carrying an extra two hundred pounds on my body. What an incredible dichotomy! I was the expert, helping people lose body weight, while carrying around my own excess in the form of stress. That which is invisible to the naked eye isn't necessarily nonexistent. It put as much strain on my body as though I weighed over three hundred pounds. This much pressure was surely consuming more energy than I should have been expending especially while my body was attempting to heal.

The body has incredible potential to heal itself, given the proper environment. Studies have shown the hypothalamus, a part of the brain, acts as a bridge between the mind, emotions, thoughts, endocrine system, and peripheral nervous system. Walter Hesse, a physiologist, studied the hypothalamus and found that stimulating different sections of it could produce two different states: deep relaxation or an alert, heightened flight or fight response. The relaxed response is a protective, healing mechanism, promoting physiologic restoration. Our attitudes, beliefs, and emotions affect our body's physiologic responses. Therefore, stress is not the issue, our response to it is. Our reaction to stress can either create a natural restorative environment within our body or a suppressed immune system. A positive response brings about wholeness and balance, while a negative response taxes the body. Those who only react to situations and circumstances fail to empower themselves for further growth; as opposed to people who are proactive and carry their weather with them. It doesn't matter to a proactive person if it rains or shines, they will create an optimal environment for themselves, regardless of the climate.

Paula spoke highly of the principle of letting go. I needed to let go of the stress that was dragging me down to free my body so it could heal. That which I thought I had control over, actually had control over me. Letting go of my mind's need for control would in turn restore control to my body—a mind-body connection.

Within a year of hiking with Paula, the Spring of 1994, I was ready to make changes. I started to see how destructive my behavior was to my life. There was no need to spend energy doing multiple tasks at one time. I needed to slow my whole life-style down. This included driving my car slower, grocery shopping slower, exercising with less intensity, and working a more reasonable schedule for my recovery according to doctors' orders. At first it was easier to do the simple things, like not jumping lines in checkout lanes at the store, not switching lanes while driving, or letting someone go first. These were rather simple tasks, but I was trained to hurry and go faster, so I could accomplish more in a day. Slowing down didn't interfere with my life, it enhanced it.

I suddenly noticed how other people started to become aggravated with me when I was slower and more casual. I sensed they felt I interfered with their life-style, or maybe they wished they, too, could slow down. I'm confident it didn't interfere, but their inability to see what stress was doing to them prevented them from recognizing the benefits of letting go. It was difficult not to fall back into the same pace. I learned to quickly recognize when I reverted back. The weight on my shoulders was just as heavy as it was before.

I took the concept of letting go one step further. If *I* didn't have control, I knew who did, God. It's easier to let go when giving it over to God. Some find it's easier to hand it over to God piece by piece, while others turn everything over all at once. I found it easier to let go of pieces, but it might have turned out this way from circumstances. After having thought I was in control of everything for so long, there were many parts of my life I never realized I managed in this way. With each piece I let go, I discovered yet another that I still was trying to hold onto. I was amazed at the depth of this behavior.

As more and more changes took place at work, my stress levels grew higher and higher. There was a greater need to let go. It still often felt like a tug-of-war game, as I felt pulled back into the fire where I didn't want to be, only to resist and attempt to pull in my direction. I needed to remind myself that it wasn't worth it, that I was more valuable than this. Then I finally let go, sending the rope flying back into the fire without me.

Learning to let go before leaving for Johns Hopkins Hospital was critical to my recovery. I left with a new awareness and without excess baggage. The peace I was able to feel at this time provided an optimal healing environment for my body.

Over the course of the following year, letting go was invaluable. The spiral path was paved for the final test. Would I be able to let go of what once was the center of my world? Would I be able to let go of my job, that which brought success and stroked my ego? Would I feel a lost identity when given the title "Disabled?" I had let go of my need to control my work environment and the subsequent stress, but I was still playing the game. I had let go of my competitive drive, but I still had a hold on my security blanket. It was time to let go of my security blanket, to say good-bye to my job. It was more than okay. It was the best thing that could have happened to me. I walked away knowing I had done a fantastic job. I played my heart out, won some, lost some, had fun, shed tears, but most importantly, I learned and grew from every experience.

I didn't need to be a part of an unhealthy environment any longer. I didn't need to be connected to something that fed my competitive instinct. I didn't need the titles of Manager, Exercise Physiologist or athlete. In fact, with letting go, I have reaped greater success with that which is more meaningful. I've impacted other people's lives in a far greater way, and have been recognized just the same, even with the title of disabled. I had moved to a higher level of consciousness and a greater respect for my place in this world.

THREE MONTHS AFTER coming out of my comatose period, my headache was again intolerable. Dr. Long asked to have my shunt tapped, to determine the level of CSF pressure. I called Dr. Cilluffo's office and talked with Jane, his nurse. I asked her if Dr. Cilluffo would do this simple procedure for Dr. Long. She asked Dr. Cilluffo, who told her to send me elsewhere. He refused to touch me. I recognized his hesitation to do something connected with the work of another physician, especially Dr. Long's. But, it was a relatively simple procedure. None of the Traverse City neurosurgeons would touch me. I was most concerned thinking of what might happen if this were an emergency. Would these neurosurgeons still turn me away? It remains a very disturbing feeling.

I called Sandy, at Dr. Hoff's office. She asked Dr. Hoff if he would do the shunt tap. He was very willing to help and looked forward to the opportunity to see me again. It might have made a difference that he was at the same level as Dr. Long, and they were familiar with each other. It was good to see Dr. Hoff again, allowing him to share in the joy of my repaired leak. He gave countless hours of effort to help me and was deserving of more credit than was recognized. When he tapped my shunt the pressure read 3.0cm. This was extremely low.

Dr. Long called the next day. He knew I was capable of relaying the results. I told him the pressure was again low, at 3.0cm. I also told him the bulb in my head, which allowed me to test the functioning of my VP shunt was not refilling. This meant the shunt wasn't functioning properly. Dr. Long didn't hesitate to tell me to return to Hopkins. He scheduled VP shunt revision surgery for the end of the week. He decided to attach a device to my VP shunt which he called an "up-down valve." This valve would allow me to be more comfortable in both the upright and prone positions, keeping my pressure constant. This made perfect sense, but I wondered if this was going to correct the malfunction of my shunt.

I hesitated to call the Kampens, fearing they wouldn't want to be a part of my continued medical saga. I would have understood completely if this was the case, but it wasn't. They invited me back with open arms, knowing I had bounced back and had my feet back under me. I was overwhelmed, once again, by their unconditional love.

Kathleen expressed a bit of concern to Carol, remembering how I was during my last few weeks with them. She had no memory of our time together before this, during her bad period, when her shunt had stopped working. Carol reassured Kathleen I was not the same person as she remembered.

I was very nervous about how it would feel being back in their home. Would it be the same? Would I feel like one of the family again or had something happened to change this that I did not remember? I prayed that it would be the same. The Kampens meant the world to me and I would never forgive myself, or the doctors who caused my deterioration, if something robbed me of this friendship.

When I arrived in Maryland, Carol and Kathleen met me at the airport with open arms. Everything was okay and I felt like family again. I met a new Kathleen, and she met a new Karen. It was rather strange, since each of us had only a memory of the other's bad period. We didn't really know one another's true personality. It was such a relief to see her doing so well. I was so proud of her. Remembering how resistant Kathleen had been to exercise, I couldn't believe it when I saw her get up at 7:00 a.m. every morning to walk. She was bubbly, energetic, enthusiastic, and lots of fun to be around. Her humor and wit were endless.

The previous winter, when I helped Kathleen and Carol tear down Kathleen's classroom, with little hope she would return, I said to myself, "I'd give anything to be able to help Kathleen put this together again someday." I prayed for God to help her return to teaching. I knew it was the love of her life, just as my job had been mine.

The day after I arrived at the Kampens, I had to complete my pre-op testing. After returning from my tests, my prayers were answered when I went to St. Phillips Catholic School to help Kathleen reconstruct her classroom. She was returning to teaching. It meant so much to me to be with her, helping her start over again. As we walked into her classroom, I choked back my tears. With all the tears shed during the past year, and the blinking beam of sun shining on this day, I'm certain there was a rainbow somewhere, for someone to grasp. The world was filled with hope. We both had come so far, truly blessed by our Lord.

On my first day back in Maryland, I said to Carol, "Please be honest with me and tell me when things are getting difficult for you. I do not want to impose on you in any way or over stay my welcome." I didn't want anything to happen like last time, nor did I expect it to, but I needed to get my feelings out on the table. Carol knew how appreciative I was of all they did for me, and she also knew this trip was going to be a short one. She agreed to be open with me, but cast her boundless, positive spirit on our time together.

My time with the Kampens was important to everyone's healing process. They needed to see for themselves that I was back to my normal self. They needed a chance to ask questions and to talk about some of the bad times we shared; just as my parents. My entire summer was spent helping others heal. I made a point to visit all my friends within a reasonable driving distance. This served a twofold purpose. It helped them heal and it helped restore me as well.

I SPOKE WITH my Aunt Jean and Uncle Howard Wells the night before my surgery. They were concerned that I would be alone going into and coming out of my surgery and offered to drive from North Carolina to be with me. They ended up driving most of the way that same night, so they could pick me up and drive me to the hospital the morning of my surgery. This meant the world to me. They filled the void my parents were unable to fill because of my father's back problems.

Dad had been waiting to see his neurosurgeon at the University of Michigan all summer. Before I left for Maryland, I was able to get his appointment changed to August from October, so it wouldn't interfere with their plans to head south for the winter. My connections with the neurosurgeons at U. of M. came in handy. Then it ended up conflicting with my need to return to Hopkins. I preferred to see my father get help, rather than to travel with me, since he was in so much pain. As it turned out, I wasn't alone after all.

Dr. Long said my surgery went well. He opened the incision in my abdomen, at the sight of the distal end of my VP shunt. This is where he placed the up-down valve. Within a few hours, I was sitting up and attempting to eat lunch.

The next day I was wheeled down to Radiology for a CT scan with contrast. As we moved through the bowels of the hospital, we approached a ladder in the hallway with a man standing at the top looking at the pipes through the ceiling. At the moment we passed him I heard, "Hey, your hair has grown back. How are you doing?"

I looked up at the man and recognized him. He had been on the ladder working in the hallway of Meyer 8 the second time I came to Hopkins and spent two months in room 856. I greeted him each morning and enjoyed his conversation on several occasions. I couldn't believe he remembered me, especially since I didn't have hair then.

I said, "I remember you. The guy on the ladder (a novel statement given he was currently standing on a ladder). I can't believe you remember me." Just as quickly as we crossed paths, we were no longer within earshot.

I wondered if everyone at Hopkins knew me. Doctors and nurses often said hi to me while I walked the main floor of the hospital. Whoever was with me would ask if I knew all these people. Many times I didn't. It must have been my smile that said hello to them first.

I was discharged the next day, Saturday. A follow-up appointment to see Dr. Long was made for Monday morning. My aunt and uncle decided to stay with their friends who lived in Bethesda, Maryland, only a short distance from the Kampen's home. They offered to take me to my appointment. I was very thankful they stayed. Over the weekend it was quite evident the bulb was still collapsing and my shunt was not working. My headache was at an extremely intense level.

I couldn't believe this was happening again, déjà vu of the previous winter. When I saw Dr. Long Monday morning, he was just as disappointed as I was. He said, "I'll have to go back into your head and find the problem. We may have to replace the entire shunt. If we're lucky, there may just be a kink in the catheter. We won't know until we get in there."

I walked out of the exam room and waited for Dee to tell me what I needed to do next. While standing in the corridor, the medical student who was with Dr. Long in the exam room started chatting with me. His first comment was, "Wow you're tough!" I took this as a huge compliment.

Dee gave me my schedule for surgery and pre-op evaluation. I thought, "Here we go again. Will it ever be over?" I knew the answer. Until death do us part. This fits just as well for pain, suffering, and challenges. I asked a similar question during my very first rehabilitation session. "When will it be over?" I thought for sure there had to be a finish line. It would have been so much easier if I could have seen an end in sight. It took several years before I realized there were no finish lines on earth. I'd never get to a point where I could finally say, "I no longer have a brain injury." The only end would be death, and I chose life just as surely as it chose me. So, instead, I set my sights on heaven, only an earthly finish line, yet the ultimate starting line.

D R. LONG SCHEDULED surgery for the following day, after I had an MRI. The MRI showed my catheter was too long going through my brain and into my ventricle. The tip of the shunt had pushed against the wall of the ventricle, not allowing it to drain properly.

Before being taken into the operating room for the second time in four days, I asked Dr. Long to tell his residents to spare as much hair as possible. I learned after my first craniotomy at Hopkins that the residents are in charge of haircuts. While it was necessary to shave my whole head for the craniotomies, when they repaired my leaks, it seemed too extreme for the VP shunt surgery. For this surgery I had three three-to-four inch long incisions on the right side of my head. I also had a small incision at my collar bone and one in my abdomen. Dr. Long agreed, and said he would personally shave my head.

I was being prepped in the OR by the nursing staff, while the resident anesthesiologist was talking with me about anesthesia. The attending anesthesiologist was nowhere to be found, thus the resident couldn't begin sedating me. Dr. Long walked in and greeted me. It was so good to see his smile penetrating through his surgical mask. As he began shaving and prepping my head, I quickly interrupted our conversation and said, "I'm still awake. I can feel what you're doing."

He knew I was still awake and began to laugh, knowing I wasn't saying this to him, but to the resident anesthesiologist. As he left the room to scrub, he said to the resident, "I think Karen wants to be asleep by the time I come back into the room. I'm sure you can assist her with this request." She seemed nervous and made a phone call to find the doctor she was working under.

When Dr. Long returned to the OR I was still completely awake. I repeated, "I'm still awake," and added, "I don't want to know what you're doing." This seemed to amuse Dr. Long, as I said it in a joking way. Though nervous about being awake, I was most aware of my level of comfort. I had relinquished all my fears and worries, having complete confidence in Dr. Long. God was there with us, handing Dr. Long the necessary tools. I had nothing to fear but fear itself.

In the recovery room I awoke to a male nurse by my side. He was holding my hand and started talking with me as soon as he saw I was awake. I was still heavily sedated, and when I felt his hand touching mine I thought I was in heaven. I'd never awakened after surgery like this before. I felt very comforted by his presence, not having to work at relaxing at all. If I did have pain, I didn't feel it. My thoughts were temporarily preoccupied. When he wheeled me back to my room I tried to think of some way I could see him again, short of having more surgery. He talked about enjoying golf and so just as my bed was being squeezed through the doorway I said, "Well if you want to play golf sometime give me a call." He knew where to find me at least for the next couple days. Surprisingly enough, David did come visit me each night after his shift was over. I was thrilled to have some unexpected romantic excitement in my life. He called me a few times after I was discharged, but nothing ever came of our brief rendezvous.

My aunt and uncle hung in there with me the entire time I was at Hopkins. We enjoyed our time together, despite the circumstances, never without conversation and joyous laughter. On the day I was discharged, we were able to join many others in watching the big implosion of several old housing projects in Baltimore. From the parking garage we stood for only a few moments, as that was how long it took to demolish everything.

Once I was back at the Kampen's, they headed home to North Carolina. They had given so much to me, I couldn't find the words to express how thankful I was. They joined my team of angels with a split second decision to come to Maryland, not knowing how long or how intense it would be. They opened their hearts without hesitation and gave more support than I ever dreamed possible. Everything fit together, as if it were planned. We all knew it hadn't been in our plans. It fit because it was God's plan.

M ORE ANGELS WERE sent my way as my stay in Maryland again exceeded all our expectations. Mark and Karen Klug and their seven month old baby, Paul, moved from Traverse City to New Jersey the same week I left for Maryland. Mark took another job, thinking it would take him to the next level in his career. I was excited when I heard they were only two hours from Baltimore.

The weekend following this trip's second surgery, the Klugs drove to Maryland to visit for the day. It was so good to see friends from home. They were equally excited to see me, as they were already homesick. We took a drive to Annapolis and walked around the Naval Academy, had lunch, and enjoyed a very leisurely day together.

Having them so close and able to visit whenever possible brought a new level of peace and serenity to my recovery. I was in awe of how God was strategically placing my family and friends around me. There wasn't a question in my mind why this was happening, especially when I discovered how Mark and Karen felt about their move. I was certain God was using them to help me.

Mark was not happy with his job and there was a lot of uncertainty for the future of his company. He and Karen were not happy living in New Jersey. During the time I was with them I predicted they wouldn't be in the New Jersey area very long. They'd probably move elsewhere once I was back on my feet. It was as though their assignment was to care for me, and then they'd move on.

THE REPAIR OF my shunt didn't help relieve my headache at all. This prompted Dr. Long and Dr. Hanley to refer me to Dr. Pappagalo. He was the doctor I saw the previous spring for pain control. But I had no idea what he looked like, as I had no memory of my appointment with him. I never returned for the DHE treatment he suggested. Once I was de-toxed from the Phenobarbital, I wanted a break from any medical intervention.

I followed Dr. Long's advice and saw Dr. Pappagalo again. He still had a desire to try the DHE intravenous treatment. I was still apprehensive, given my fear of changing medications and what medications could do to me. Dr. Pappagalo reassured me I wouldn't have any problems with the DHE. It didn't have any side effects, and I'd be monitored very closely.

Before making a decision, I needed to talk with someone else about this. Dr. Long had just left for China, so I talked with Dr. Hanley. I liked Dr. Hanley from the very beginning. He was always very easy to talk with, and he was a good listener. When I was in the EMU and having difficulty with Dr. Krauss, I asked to see Dr. Hanley, knowing he would be understanding of my struggles. He was sensitive of other people's feelings, and acknowledged Dr. Krauss's inability to talk with and be sensitive to patients. I knew I could always count on Dr. Hanley to help me.

I discussed my concerns about doing the DHE treatment in respect to what happened the previous spring. I told him I was disappointed in the way my overdose of Phenobarbital was handled, among other things. He listened intently, remembering very clearly what happened. He reassured me the DHE would not cause any problems and that he would follow my case very closely, so that nothing would happen. Dr. Hanley wanted me to try the treatment. He also wanted to repeat the CSF pressure study for a few days. He wanted to find the cause of my problem, too high or too low CSF pressure. After our discussion, I agreed to do the treatment and monitoring.

I was admitted to NICU on Labor Day. The pressure study started all over again. Dr. Hanley found that there were dramatic positional changes in my CSF pressure. This was undoubtedly contributing to my pain. My ventricles were very small and noncompliant. They were no longer capable of adapting to pressure changes, thus even the slightest change affected my head. He relayed his findings to Dr. Long.

After three days of monitoring, Dr. Pappagalo took over and began his treatment. I became excited, when by the third day of treatment my headache ceased. This was the first time in over six years I was free of pain. I remained cautiously optimistic, however, wanting to believe it was permanent, but thinking it might be too good to be true.

The DHE was a three-day treatment that somehow interrupted the pain messages to my brain. It was completely harmless. It had no side effects, was not sedating, in fact I didn't feel any different, except for a slowly diminishing headache. After three days, I was put on maintenance medications. This was the part I didn't care for. Dr. Pappagalo named three drugs which he prescribed for me. I recognized one of the three, Calan. It was a medication that decreased blood pressure.

I asked him to describe how these drugs were going to keep me from having head pain again. I appreciated the time he took to explain the physiological effects and interactions of each drug. He was very patient with my questions. I asked about the side effects. This also required a very detailed explanation. There were many side effects, making me extremely uncertain whether I wanted to continue. He kept reassuring me the chances of the side effects manifesting themselves in me were minimal. This didn't lessen my fear. He said he'd start with the first combination, and then alter it if needed. I agreed, with a great deal of apprehension.

My first day off DHE, my headache returned, even with the mainte-nance medications. I immediately developed the one side effect we were afraid would be an issue for me. Even in a low dose the Calan decreased my already low blood pressure to an extremely low level. Plan B had to be initiated. Dr. Pappagalo came up with another cocktail of medications, monitored me for another two days, and then sent me back to the Kampen's.

My time at the Kampen's was getting longer and longer, just like in December of 1994. I felt very uncomfortable with this, even though the Kampens were very understanding. It wasn't fair to impose on their lives in this way. While I enjoyed being a part of their family, my presence created a great deal of stress for them. When I was discharged after under-going the DHE treatment, two follow-up appointments were made. I had to see Dr. Long the next week and then talk with Dr. Pappagalo on the telephone the following week.

Meanwhile, I was supposed to take the medications prescribed by Dr. Pappagalo and let him know if there were any changes, for better or worse. When I went to the pharmacy to fill my prescriptions, the pharmacist, who came to know me quite well, asked me if I knew what these medications were. I told her about the treatment I received and the purpose of com-bining these medications. She seemed quite surprised, and then stated, "This one medication is usually given to women after they have just had a baby to stop the bleeding." This caught me by surprise.

"What in the world is he doing to me?" I thought.

She continued, "Did Dr. Pappagalo tell you that when you take this medication you must have frequent kidney and liver tests, because it can cause severe damage to both organs?"

"No, he didn't say anything about that. Thanks for telling me. I think I'll wait to fill them, until I can talk to him about this."

I made up my mind right there. I wasn't going to continue taking this cocktail of medications. The only one I'd continue was Oxycodone. It was similar to Tylox, which I took a couple of years for my pain. It was a class two narcotic and was effective in dulling my pain. It didn't take it away, but at least it made me more comfortable. It was in liquid form, which made it a faster-acting medication. This was the only medication I was comfortable taking for pain. I knew I wouldn't have any side effects or complications from taking Oxycodone along with the 150mg per day of Phenobarbital for seizure control.

I called Dr. Pappagalo's office and talked with his nurse. I asked her to have Dr. Pappagalo call me to discuss these medications. He never called, so I continued with the recommendations of Dr. Long. Dr. Long wanted to go back into my head and put an anti-siphon device on my VP shunt. He scheduled this for two weeks later.

E VERYTHING SEEMED TO be repeating itself, multiple surgeries and doctors' appointments, lots of idle time in-between, and the ever present factor of the unknown. I didn't like how it felt, nor did anyone else, especially Carol. Carol was one who went beyond understanding a loved one's feelings. She took them upon herself and felt them. She felt the pain, worry, sorrow, fear, and heartache, just as much as the one who experienced them. It was the same for joys and excitement. She shared one's victories. This required a great deal of energy and stamina, even with her own family, let alone someone outside of her family.

I observed how Carol reacted when her daughter was struggling with hydrocephalus and what was thought to be the effects of her tumor. I watched as Carol turned her entire life over to helping Kathleen. It drained her, both physically and emotionally. It tore her apart to see her daughter's condition deteriorate. She not only carried the emotions of a mother, she also carried the emotions of Kathleen. Carol's faith was strong, but she still couldn't let go of feeling responsible.

Carol's love for me created the same heart-wrenching feelings. From the very first day I met Carol, she treated me like a daughter. I was drawn to her like a magnet. Her unconditional love was powerful. She road the medical roller coaster right beside me. Everything I felt, she felt. She felt a sense of responsibility for me, just like a mother. When my condition deteriorated, it wrenched at her heart of gold. Watching me go through multiple surgeries and an endless battle to curtail my headache ripped her to shreds.

When I needed someone to talk with, to listen, to understand, and to comfort me, she was always there. Being so far away from my own family and friends, I relied heavily on her to help me through the pain. Unfortunately, I wasn't aware of what it was doing to her inside. Revealing my pain made it even more difficult for Carol. She knew how much I was struggling emotionally, and she felt helpless.

I'm sure all of this was floating in fear. Fear of losing her daughter, fear of losing me, it was fear she had no control over. Carol experienced riding the roller coaster with Kathleen and me, feeling every up, down, twist, turn, and flip upside-down. At first, Kathleen and I had seat belts on to hold us in place. When our seat belts tore loose from stress, Carol grabbed hold of each of us. Neither of us had the ability to help ourselves. Carol became our care giver, and presumably, our only means to survive. It was an immense responsibility. To Carol it wasn't a choice, it was love.

Everything Carol felt as a parent and as a friend, I know my own parents felt. Carol wore her feelings on her sleeve most times, while my parents kept theirs concealed. I know they were being ripped to shreds, just the same. With so many unknowns, I felt helpless. I reached out to Carol, wanting to protect my parents from the whirlwind of emotions. When I realized the impact it was having on Carol, I began to protect her also.

During my time with the Kampens, Carol's father had to have emergency heart bypass surgery. Carol and her family weren't just riding a medical roller coaster, they were on a runaway coaster that wouldn't stop. All the stress Carol was carrying got turned up ten notches.

I knew Carol was starting to feel dragged under when one night I said, "Carol, please let me know what you and Ken want me to do about staying here. This is obviously going on much longer than any of us realized, again."

To which she replied, "Yes, this is going on longer than we expected. If you have surgery after your next appointment, it could be another month before you go home."

I took a deep breath. While I invited Carol to say what she felt, I wasn't prepared for it. Of course, when she said this, my imagination ran wild, trying to think of anything I might have done to offend them. I tried to figure out more ways in which I could repay them, or how I was imposing on their life-style. I needed to talk more about it with Carol, soon, before my imagination took over. She was very stressed after having been at the hospital all day with her father. I knew it wasn't the best time to talk. There was a harshness to her words that wasn't typical of Carol. I knew I'd find a better time to talk the next day, and I was hoping she'd bring it up. She did.

She started by saying, "Karen, I don't want you to think this is because of anything you have done. I love you dearly, and it is because I love you so much, I cannot do this anymore." She went on to say how much it had affected her, seeing me in such pain. She was worn down, couldn't sleep, and worried sick over me.

I was feeling every emotion under the sun. I was overwhelmed that she felt so close to me, while also feeling abandoned and hurt because she loved me so much. The predominant feeling, however, was one of love for her. Here was a friend I had known only one year, and she loved me so much that it caused her pain to see me hurt. This was a remarkable demonstration of love.

Carol was extremely scared this was going to affect our relationship. The night before, she and Ken left in the car so they could talk, and so Carol could cry. She had once been terrified of losing me physically, now she was twice as terrified because she feared losing me emotionally. There was a tremendous amount of pain in the Kampen home for a long, long time. It's a wonder any of us survived emotionally. We survived because our Heavenly Father's presence was surely felt. There was twice as much love as pain. There was more faith and hope than doubt.

What I heard Carol say to me was, "Karen, I love you so much, and I trust you just the same. I feel I can be totally honest with you. I love you as though you are my own daughter. I am having a difficult time handling the pain that goes along with being so close to you."

Carol took a huge risk by being honest with me, but it was the highest compliment she could display. She had to have a great deal of trust in me to tell me how she felt. She had to trust that I loved her and I'd never want anything to hurt her in any way, nor scar our friendship.

With the help of God I proved worthy of this trust. From the very beginning of her first words to me, I saw it only as an act of love. I cared only for the welfare of Carol and her family. She didn't deserve to feel such pain and heartache. By the time she told me of her pain, I had already decreased the amount of information I was sharing with her. I had already started to protect her, sensing she was getting close to the edge.

I reassured Carol that nothing could ever come between our friendship. As Michael W. Smith writes, "A friend's a friend forever, if the Lord's the Lord of them, and a friend will not say never, if the welcome will not end." I appreciated her honesty. Carol needed to turn the responsibility over to someone else, preferably my own mother.

The whole Kampen family had gone above and beyond to accommodate my needs and to care for me. Never once did I take this for granted, but I had become very comfortable being with them. They gave me a great sense of security in a very uncertain world.

With my eighth craniotomy scheduled in two weeks, there was even more pressure building. Carol suggested I ask my mother to fly out and be with me. She offered to let her stay in their home. I talked with Mom, and for the first time I said, "Mom, I need you. Can you please come to Baltimore to be with me." I didn't think my father would be able to travel the distance. I suggested she fly out and stay with the Kampens. After discussing it, my parents decided they would drive to Baltimore to be with me.

I was overjoyed to hear they were coming. It had been very difficult to go through the most recent surgeries without them. Then, after only a few conversations, we were at odds with one another again. The tension that had remained between us throughout my recovery put up a huge barrier between us. They decided not to come. I was devastated.

I couldn't stop crying long enough to even talk with my sister. What was I going to do? Where was I going to go? Everyone was giving up on me. Was this the end of my hope to relieve my pain? If everyone else was giving up, did that mean I had to, also? I still had ten days until surgery. I couldn't stay at the Kampen's, knowing how much it was hurting Carol, not to mention Ken and Kathleen.

I had experienced this before, on a smaller scale. Friends were very supportive, following my progress tenaciously, but were eventually met with interference in their own lives. It was entirely impossible for any friend to maintain the steadfast pace that I had to endure in my own recovery. While their love and prayers didn't falter, the amount of time they could devote to my support, understandably diminished. I was fortunate to have many different shifts of friends who kept passing the baton to others. It was hard enough for me to keep up the pace, and I had more than a personal interest in it. I could never have expected others to stick with me to the same degree.

When Carol told me of her need to back away, I was not without emotion. Initially, I hid it, but she saw it firsthand later. I felt lonely, as though I were holding on by myself. I never realized how painful loneliness is. Everyone else was giving up, not necessarily by choice, but because of lack of endurance. I couldn't allow myself to do the same. I had to hang on, even if it was by a thread.

I called the House of Ruth near Hopkins, which houses patients and families of patients at a low cost. There was a huge waiting list. I called and made reservations at a hotel in Baltimore, knowing I couldn't afford it, but I couldn't afford not to move there and risk losing one of my most valuable friendships. I wasn't going to allow anything to jeopardize my friendship with the Kampens.

When Carol found out my bags were packed and that I planned to have the Klugs drop me off in Baltimore, when they came to see me on the weekend, she wouldn't let me go. She felt the pain of me leaving, as well as the pain of me staying. She suggested I call my aunt and uncle to see if they could be with me, again, for this surgery. She wondered if the Klugs might be able to take me to their house for the week after surgery to recover. This worked out perfectly. My aunt and uncle gladly returned to be with me for surgery and until I was discharged.

O N THE DAY of my eighth craniotomy, the three of us took the elevator to the seventh floor to Same Day Surgery. A messenger got on the elevator with a cart loaded with patient files, also heading to the seventh floor. Not being able to distinguish whether it was one file or fifty, I made the comment, "Now they have to use a cart to transport my medical records." We all had a good laugh, realizing I probably wasn't too far from guessing the size of my patient file at this point.

We knew the routine all too well. Dr. Long was pleased with the surgery. He really hoped this device would be the answer to my headache. Time would tell. When I was returned to my room, I was still groggy, but alert enough to laugh at the story my nurse had to tell. She was surprised when she peered into my bathroom and saw a toilet. Of course, this prompted inquiries as to why there might not be a toilet in the bathroom. She said, "The toilet fell off the wall when the last patient sat on it." We were greatly amused, picturing how it must have felt to have been the patient.

Aunt Jean and Uncle Howard returned me to the Kampen's after I was discharged. We said our good-byes and thank-yous and they were on their way home once again. The following day, Mark and Karen picked me up and took me to their home in New Jersey for a week. It was a wonderful opportunity to spend time with them. People have wondered why the Klugs moved to New Jersey and were there only a very short time. It was long enough to help me. My prediction came true. They moved from New Jersey to Cincinnati shortly after I returned to Michigan.

I was at the Kampen's one more week, before finally returning home to Michigan. In a follow-up visit with Dr. Long he gave me the go ahead to return home. I had not felt a decrease in my headache, but it was time to let things settle down before proceeding further. He did everything short of installing the experimental VP shunt. This shunt was designed to allow the physician to regulate CSF pressure externally, rather than having to do a surgical procedure each time to change a valve. It would be ideal for me, because it also allows the physician to fine-tune CSF pressure with very small increments. We proved the high pressure valve was too high and the low pressure valve was too low. I needed something in-between and there wasn't anything.

During my last week in Maryland I filled out an application to become a volunteer at the 1996 Olympic Games in Atlanta, Georgia. I had an Olympic dream since a very young age. I had surpassed the time in which I could accomplish that dream as an athlete, but I still had the chance to fulfill it in a different capacity. I didn't know how much of a chance I had of being selected, but it was worth a try. This, along with the book I was writing, were two very positive things in my life. They were both goals I had in front of me, and they were far from competitive. I felt as though I was heading in a very positive direction.

A few days before my departure, we encountered one more medical adventure. Carol needed to have foot surgery. It was time for us to take care of her. While her need for surgery wasn't a positive circumstance, I welcomed the opportunity to finally give back a minute portion of what she had given me.

American Airlines was getting used to wheeling me through Chicago airport by now. I'm surprised some of their employees didn't start calling me by name. It was so good to be home again and to see the water as we approached Traverse City. There wasn't much left of the autumn, as the leaves on the trees had already fallen.

I was exhausted and weak, but it didn't matter—I was home. I could feel my life heading in a more positive direction, despite having to bear the constant pain in my head. I had no idea what was in store for the future, but I had learned that a gift is very special when unexpected, unknown, and unrecognized. Yesterdays are lessons, today is a day to enjoy, and tomorrow is a gift.

Part V

THE RAINBOW

Twenty-Five

Winning Gold

*I used to wait for rainbows,
now I go looking for them.*

KAREN WELLS

*We expect God to speak through peace,
but sometimes He speaks through pain.*

MAX LUCADO

A NEW LIFE HAD been waiting for me for many years, twenty-seven to be exact. I just never knew how to get there. I chose my own path, one that was of selfish ambition as opposed to glorifying my Lord and Savior. Then one day, as quick as lightning can strike, pain became my teacher. The world became my classroom, and there were many lessons to be learned. God spoke through pain of many forms, physical, emotional, and spiritual. In order to move forward along His path, I needed to leave some things behind. I needed to let go of all that dominated and manipulated my life, accepting and living only according to God's plan. Trusting His ways as if they were my own was essential in the process of letting go of control and grabbing hold of hope.

I used to wait for rainbows to appear in the sky, now I go looking for them. It takes both the sun and rain to make a rainbow. So, I can search for hope within the most hopeless storm, knowing the "Son" will always shine.

I thought my competitive, athletic background was an asset, when part of it truly had become a liability. My instinctual desire to be the best, controlled my life. I never took time to celebrate my victories, there were always more to achieve. My intensity was accelerated, never slowing or idling to see that which surrounded me. When I slowed my pace, I began to see the beauty of life, the love of others, and the love of our Lord.

An old cliché of athletics, which many have disputed for years is: No pain, no gain. This was one facet of my athletic background that helped me through life. When I look back at the times I grew the most, it was when I was experiencing pain. The emotional pain of losing my grandfather took me to a new level of awareness. The pain of a complete life-style change from my head injury has exceeded all other avenues for personal growth. Even the physical pain of enduring a constant headache has brought me to a new level of consciousness.

I learned pain was not the end of my journey. While holding onto hope, I was carried through pain, and learned from it. Pain was there for a reason, if only to stir me into awareness of a need to change. It got my attention.

M Y CONNECTION WITH Jesus was one of admiration from a distance. I knew Him well, but never took the time to embrace Him. My love for Him originated in my mind, more than my heart. My unbridled soul was restricting God's work in my life. It was a "do it myself" and "my own way" attitude. I used Him in my fast-paced world as a Band-Aid, turning to Him only when I had a problem.

Fortunately, as I was catapulted over my handlebars, on my way to a life-changing injury, God caught me in His arms. He carried me through the tough times and the not so tough times, even when I thought He had abandoned me. When I was waiting for a quick fix and wondering if He wasn't going to answer my prayers, He was hard at work developing patience, endurance, and a sense of moment-to-moment trust in Him. It became obvious that I had been in a hurry; but He wasn't.

Initially, I had my own plan and thought it possible to manipulate God into cooperating with my desires. This was related to my imbedded desire to have control. Once I accepted I had no control, and only God did, there came an awareness that all things happen for a reason. I was on the wrong path and I had a great deal to learn, including how to let go of control. There was a constant need to resist the temptation, to take back what I had given to God, until my faith grew stronger. I could have gone through the tough times kicking and screaming, instead I chose quiet confidence in God to restore new life. Confidence in the midst of turmoil was a peace beyond my understanding. This faith lifted a huge blanket off my back, uncovering my true self, revealing the depth of the Holy Spirit within me.

Nothing was going to separate me from the love of my Savior. This was not because of anything I could do, but solely from God's eternal love. God's love is always there, we need only open our hearts to it. The apostle Paul writes in his letter to the Romans, "Who shall separate us from the love of Christ? Shall trouble or hardship or persecution or famine or nakedness or danger or sword?" And to this he answers:

No, in all these things we are more than conquerors through Him who loved us. For I am convinced that neither death nor life, neither angels nor demons, neither the present nor the future, nor any powers, neither height nor depth, nor anything else in all creation, will be able to separate us from the love of God that is in Christ Jesus our Lord. Romans 8:35-39 NIV

My Heavenly Father's love remained constant within me, but my relationship with Him changed. His love moved from my head to my heart. As I learned to trust, even in the face of the impossible, the gift of hope was received. The vibrant colors of hope preceded and followed every challenge, every pain, and every disappointment. The times when I was completely out of my comfort zone were the times when I experienced the most growth.

A S I TRAVEL further along my journey, I'm confident I will be amidst many more storms. I'll hear the rumbles, feel the rain, and see more rainbows. Right now, I'm content with wherever God wants me to be. There is so much more peace in His place than in mine.

My cognitive deficits have, for the most part, been overcome, except for an occasional transposed letter or word, or an unbanked memory. Every now and then I'll say hello when attempting to say good-bye, or wichsand instead of sandwich. I know that I recognize my mistakes more than others, but it is a subtle reminder that there is still work to be done. I continue retraining areas of my brain that were damaged by using computer software designed for this purpose.

I experience visual changes quite frequently. Double vision and blurry vision are unpredictable and less frequent, whereas my difficulty in changing focus from one thing to another remains constant. It takes a conscious effort to bring a new object into focus, whereas before my craniotomies, this was automatic. Little things like this demand a great deal of energy, especially when feeling the cumulative effects over the course of a day. My balance remains marginal, and I've learned to accept being a bit of a klutz.

Life remains fascinating, as I continue finding treasures in unsuspecting places. I haven't found my sneakers in the refrigerator lately, but my dinners, which need to be baked, have been found in the dishwasher and pantry a few times. I'm getting used to Kool-aid finding its way onto my cereal, but of course it doesn't matter since I cannot taste.

My sense of smell and taste are permanently gone. The loss of taste doesn't worry me as much as my loss of smell. My inability to smell has presented some dangers. I've come to enjoy food more for its texture, than for flavor. I'm thankful I wasn't a gourmet chef or a food connoisseur, thus my loss has had a minimal effect on my life. Of all the senses that were vulnerable to lose, I feel very fortunate to have lost only smell and taste.

While all the swelling in my face has disappeared, I have permanently lost feeling in my upper lip, upper teeth, and a small area of my face around my mouth. It's a strange feeling, but one I've grown accustomed to. Frequently it will cause a problem with my speech, but I'm undoubtedly aware of it more than anyone. It seems to effect me more when I am tired and not concentrating on the movement of my lips when speaking.

There are few remaining visible signs of my injury. Like most closed head injuries, the damage is not easily recognized. My only scars are on my head, abdomen, and in my heart. The scars from my incisions on my head are covered by my hair, but the scars on my abdomen are apparent. The scars in my heart will remain but a memory. All of these scars are noticed more by me than by others, yet they do not bother me. The dent in my forehead is the only other sign of my injury that remains, a remnant of multiple craniotomies. It is the lower edge of the pie shaped piece of skull, which was removed during my first five craniotomies. It is only a fitting reminder, when I look in the mirror, of the impact, or dent, this injury has had on my life.

I continue to live with the pain of a headache. It's with me twenty-four hours every day, just as surely as the sun rises and sets. I cannot escape it. Its intensity varies, allowing me days when I can function adequately, knowing that some days I will be hiding under my pillow. My pain medication helps regulate it somewhat, but will not take it completely away. I have learned to accept this pain as a part of my life, but still hold onto hope of someday being pain-free.

It is uncertain as to whether a new shunt will help relieve this pain. Dr. Long is cautiously optimistic. The only assurance we have is that my case will continue to rank at an unusual and exceptionally difficult level. Dr. Long does believe, however, that if he can fine-tune my CSF pressure to correspond with the permanent damage to my ventricles, my headache may diminish. Once the new shunt is approved, he will replace my old shunt. As long as there is a chance it can help me, I'm willing to give it a try. At this point, it is my best hope for relief.

In the great scheme of things, all of my losses have been minor. All of my prayers, and the countless prayers of family and friends have been answered in the most favorable way.

I now take life one day at a time, realizing the tremendous stress imparted by living in the future. I have difficulty seeing the beauty of today if my sights are on tomorrow. I've learned to love, laugh, and sing more, and to worry less. I carry a much lighter load from day to day, carrying no regrets or expectations into tomorrow.

My seizure disorder is controlled with anti-convulsants and causes very little disruption in my life. I still have fear of the possibility for seizures, but it is a healthy fear. It keeps a check on my decisions to control my fatigue, which often precipitate my seizures. My fear was reduced, however, after a seizure occurred in the presence of my one year old golden retriever. The story of his birth into my life began four months after my last craniotomy.

There was still something missing in my life. An emptiness was left from interrupted grieving for the loss of Akita. I thought about getting another dog. Since my medical roller coaster had slowed, I felt it might be a good time, but I wasn't sure. I should have known better. I just needed to listen to God. My prayers were answered and my uncertainty disappeared when I was given an eight week golden retriever puppy. There was no question in my mind it was the right time. He chose me.

I named him Shado. We instantly became inseparable. Shado is a very special companion, and comes about as close as a canine can come to being human. He graduated from puppy kindergarten and basic obedience as valedictorian. We spend our days at home together, or else he rides with me as my copilot when I run errands. Our bond is indivisible. Shado has learned more about me than I ever thought possible.

The most miraculous story of our connectedness happened shortly after his first birthday. I was outside, pushing the freshly fallen inch of snow off the sidewalk. Shado was wandering around the yard, as he normally does. Suddenly, I noticed him standing at the door of the house, as if he wanted to go inside. He never wants to go in, especially when there's snow on the ground. He came over to me and got in my way of pushing snow, then ran back to the door. I thought he must want a drink or something, so we went inside. He didn't drink any water. He continued to pester me, as I walked around inside the house, more than his usual attention-seeking acts. I decided to sit down on the floor with him and play, since he wouldn't leave me alone. Within five minutes I had a grand mal seizure. I'm certain he sensed the seizure was going to happen, and wanted to make sure I was safe. Had I not heeded his warning, I probably would have been outside, in fifteen degree temperatures. When I regained consciousness, Shado was lying right by my side, with his head on my chest. I had a slight scratch on my arm, the mark of three claws, which had pawed at me, undoubtedly in attempts to wake me.

I wondered what he might do when I had a seizure, but thought it unlikely he'd be able to sense it coming and help me without having been trained.

Shado makes me laugh. He snuggles like a puppy, showing his love and devotion. He watches, listens to, and analyzes my every move. Waiting, wondering, and following me, he appears to be ready to help. Shado's a wonderful companion, alert and attentive, protecting me, helping me to feel more secure.

T HE RAGING RIVER has calmed, the roller coaster has slowed. My parents and I, once independently battling to survive, are now floating together in a pool of peace, absorbing the magnificent beauty surrounding us. My injury has enhanced my relationship with my parents and taken it to deeper levels of love and understanding.

I credit my parents for my voyage of survival, for formulating the voice of my human spirit. They planted the seed, watered, fed, and nurtured me, introducing me to my Lord and Savior. They did all they could to make sure my roots grew deep and strong, wanting to be certain nothing could uproot my life. They taught me survival techniques, the power of prayer. They generated a commitment of completion within me, the desire never to give up. Standards were set high, recognizing it was best to shoot for the moon, even if it meant ending up in the stars. They supported and encouraged me every step of the way, ready to pick me up when I'd fall, and cheer when I'd succeed. They cultivated a desire to learn within me, that outweighs any threat of loss through adversity.

Thanks to my parents, my roots kept growing beneath the surface, without the vine revealing how deep or how strong. My parents prayed for guidance, so they might set their children on the right path to achieve their fullest, God-given potential. And just as Jesus said to Simon Peter, they heard, "Feed my lambs." (John 21:15 NIV) Their faith was unwavering, trusting that God would guide them and protect me, even when my life appeared hopeless.

After my head injury, the essence of all that was planted began to blossom. I started to learn and grow to a higher level of awareness, a greater stage of well-being. Had it not been for my parents, I'm certain there wouldn't have been new growth. My roots would not have held their ground, given the strength of the relentless storm.

We now talk of the storm and the feeling of being tossed about in the raging river. We are able to share with one another our perspective and what was felt at various points of bewilderment. With some tragedies such as this, a family is brought closer right from the beginning, whereas ours was fragmented. We'll never know God's reasoning, but I'm confident He had good reason to orchestrate our lives in this way. Who knows, it may have been a mixture of His plan and each of us fighting to play out our own plan.

At the time I was terrified. There were too many unknowns, including where my relationship with my parents would go. While I knew I would never lose their love as parents, I was scared to death I would lose their love as friends. Given the force of the rapids and the constant thrashing, they had good reason to step out of the river, freeing them of the pain. Instead, they chose to stay in it with me, right through to the end. Not only did they feel their own pain, they felt every bit of my pain, too.

As the waters began to calm, we emerged in each other's arms. Our prayers were indeed answered. God's presence within us kept our heads above water and guided our way. We were baptized with hope and faith. New life was restored. This truly had been a *Blessed Tragedy*.

I RECEIVED A letter in the Spring of 1996, telling me I was selected to become a volunteer at the 1996 Summer Olympic Games in Atlanta. I was thrilled. Not only was my life more stable medically, but a lifetime dream was about to come true. As the weeks passed, I received more and more information about my assignment. I was selected for security at the venue where both men's and women's basketball games would be held.

Many positive things were happening in my life. It was hard to believe that only one year ago I couldn't stand up without assistance or tend to my personal needs. This is one of many reference points I use to keep every-thing in its proper perspective. I had come a long way; but the exciting part was that there would be more roads to travel and more lessons to learn.

Having this outlook helps me anytime the question, "When will this end?" pops in my head. There are no finish lines. I'll continue to learn and grow for the rest of my life, no matter what challenge crosses my path.

Some are envious of my current life-style. What they see on the out-side is that I haven't worked in almost three years. I've been able to do some things that I'd never have time to do if I were working, like read and

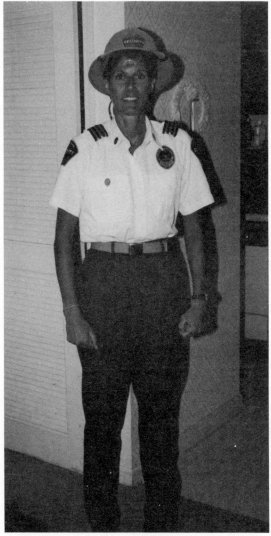

A dream fulfilled.

write a book. Then I ask them if they'd trade their life for mine, given they'd have to go through all the pain and suffering I have endured and also continue to endure my constant headache. Their answer is always, "No, not when you put it that way." It's easy to forget what I've been through, when you see me walking and talking. Brain damage is not always visible, nor are my losses.

Last summer, I was sorting through files and pitching nonessentials. I came across a file that held a call letter for a teaching position at a Lutheran high school. I received this letter while in graduate school, six years before my accident. When I saw the letter I couldn't help but think, "Maybe if I would have taken that job I wouldn't have a head injury." Then it occurred to me, "But that wasn't part of God's plan. Look at all the good things that wouldn't have happened if I didn't have a head injury." Right now God wants me just where I am. I can honestly say I wouldn't desire to have my life any other way.

T HE ARENA WAS full of over 35,000 people, clapping, whistling, and cheering, enjoying the sweet taste of victory. All became silent or sang as the United States National Anthem was played. I was among them, standing proud. This was the culmination of all that I had ever hoped and dreamed. I had just finished my volunteer position for the 1996 Summer Olympic Games in Atlanta and the United States Women's Basketball Team had just won the gold medal. My position as volunteer, not athlete, paralleled my new life: a noncompetitive, "giving-of-self" lifestyle. Whereas it was once my dream to compete in the Olympics as an athlete, it seemed only fitting that I fulfilled my dream in a noncompetitive way, given the radical changes in my life since my head injury.

It was also fitting that I was standing with my parents and sister, people who had helped me fulfill this dream. I stood, attempting to sing, but too choked up to utter a word, tears rolling down my cheeks, picturing myself standing on the podium.

I remembered how, sixteen years ago, during my competitive years, I came close to fulfilling my Olympic dream as an athlete. I thought of how seven years ago that dream still lived, only to be completely shattered, as quickly as a bolt of lightning. One year ago, I would never have been able to participate, even as a volunteer. Now, here I was, standing, hearing the words "Oh say can you see...," as our flag was raised.

My life had changed dramatically. My competitive Olympic dream had long since died, yet a dream just the same survived. This dream was fulfilled because of Jesus Christ. There was always hope, even in the midst of the most hopeless storm. I gave my self. I gave my time. I gave 100 percent. I played through pain. I denied, and I accepted. I resisted, and I let go. I laughed, and I cried. I shared faith, hope, peace, and love with everyone who crossed my path. I kept my sights set on my goal. I endured the challenge. I lived. I survived. I won the gold.

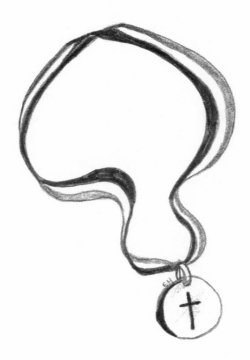

Bibliography

Chambers, Oswald. *My Utmost For His Highest*, Grand Rapids: Discovery House Publishers, 1992.

God's Little Instruction Book, Tulsa: Honor Books, Inc., 1993.

Hample, Stuart and Marshall, Eric. *Children's Letters to God*, New York: Workman Publishing, 1991.

Johnson, Barbara. *Mama, Get the Hammer! There's a Fly on Papa's Head!*, Dallas: Word Publishing, 1994.

_____. *Pack Up Your Gloomies in a Great Big Box, Then Sit on the Lid and Laugh!*, Dallas: Word Publishing, 1993.

_____. *Splashes of Joy in the Cesspools of Life*, Dallas: Word Publishing, 1992.

Lucado, Max. *And The Angels Were Silent*, Portland: Multnomah, 1992.

_____. *He Still Moves Stones*, Dallas: Word Publishing, 1993.

_____. *The Applause From Heaven*, Dallas: Word Publishing, 1995.

_____. *When God Whispers Your Name*, Dallas: Word Publishing, 1994.

McNally, David. *Even Eagles Need A Push*, New York: Dell Publishing, 1990.

Siegel, Bernie S. *Love, Medicine & Miracles*, New York: Harper & Row Publishers, 1986.

Swindoll, Charles. *The Grace Awakening*, Dallas: Word Publishing, 1990.

Williams, Margery. *The Velveteen Rabbit*, New York: Henry Holt and Company, 1983.

Index

Additional Information

IF YOU ARE UNABLE TO OBTAIN A COPY OF
Blessed Tragedy from your local bookstore,
you may send $23.95 plus $3.50
shipping and handling to:

KAREN WELLS
P.O. Box 6424
Traverse City, MI 49684-6424
(616) 943-9628
(616) 943-3422 fax
kdub20@aol.com e-mail

If you would like to contact the author,
Karen Wells, you may write to her
at the above address.

BLESSED TRAGEDY

Cover design by Eric Norton

Text design by Mary Jo Zazueta in ITC Galliard

Text stock is 50 lb. Royal Antique

*Printed and bound by Royal Book,
Norwich, Connecticut*

Production Editor: Alex Moore